Handbook of Metastatic Breast Cancer

Handbook of Metastatic Breast Cancer

Second Edition

Charles Swanton PhD, FRCP

*University College London Hospital and UCL Cancer Institute
and Cancer Research U.K. London Research Institute,
Translational Cancer Therapeutics Laboratory, London, U.K.*

Stephen R. D. Johnston, MA, PhD, FRCP

*The Royal Marsden NHS Foundation Trust
and The Institute of Cancer Research, London, U.K.*

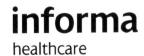

CRC Press
Taylor & Francis Group
6000 Broken Sound Parkway NW, Suite 300
Boca Raton, FL 33487-2742

First issued in paperback 2019

© 2012 by Taylor & Francis Group, LLC
CRC Press is an imprint of Taylor & Francis Group, an Informa business

No claim to original U.S. Government works

ISBN-13: 978-1-84184-811-2 (hbk)
ISBN-13: 978-0-367-38218-6 (pbk)

Library of Congress Cataloging-in-Publication Data

Handbook of metastatic breast cancer / edited by Charles Swanton, Stephen R.D. Johnston. -- 2nd ed.
      p. ; cm.
   Includes bibliographical references and index.
   Summary: "There used to be limited therapeutic options for women who developed metastatic breast cancer. However, recent development with novel systemic drugs and palliative surgical techniques, together with advances in diagnostic imaging, have given new hope for these patients and made the treatment of these patients considerably more challenging. One convenient source bringing together the various relevant aspects is long overdue. This handbook covers treatment for both the cancer and the complications that can arise from treatment itself"--Provided by publisher.
   ISBN 978-1-84184-811-2 (hardback : alk. paper)
   I. Swanton, Charles. II. Johnston, Stephen R. D.
   [DNLM: 1. Breast Neoplasms--pathology. 2. Breast Neoplasms--therapy. 3. Neoplasm Metastasis. WP 870]
   LC-classifi cation not assigned
   616.99′449--dc23

2011029662

Visit the Taylor & Francis Web site at
http://www.taylorandfrancis.com

and the CRC Press Web site at
http://www.crcpress.com

Contents

Contributors

Andy Adam Department of Radiology, Guy's, King's and St. Thomas' School of Medicine, London, U.K.

Asim Afaq Department of Diagnostic Radiology, The Royal Marsden NHS Foundation Trust, London and Sutton, U.K.

Gerhardt Attard Drug Development Unit, The Institute of Cancer Research and The Royal Marsden NHS Foundation Trust, Sutton, U.K.

Hatem A. Azim, Jr. Breast Cancer Translational Research Laboratory JC Heuson (BCTL), Institut Jules Bordet–Université Libre de Bruxelles, Brussels, Belgium

Sarah Barton Breast Unit, Royal Marsden Hospital, London, U.K.

David A. Cameron University of Edinburgh, Cancer Services, NHS Lothian, Edinburgh, Scotland

Adrian T. H. Casey Royal National Orthopaedic Hospital, Stanmore and National Hospital for Neurology and Neurosurgery, London, U.K.

Anthony Chalmers Beatson Institute for Cancer Research and Beatson West of Scotland Cancer Centre, Glasgow, Scotland

Javier Cortés Breast Cancer Unit, Oncology Department, Vall d'Hebron University Hospital, Barcelona, Spain

Stuart C. Evans The Chelsea and Westminster Hospital, London, U.K.

Roberta Ferraldeschi Signal Transduction and Molecular Pharmacology Team, Division of Cancer Therapeutics, The Institute of Cancer Research, Sutton, U.K.

Debora Fumagalli Breast Cancer Translational Research Laboratory JC Heuson (BCTL), Institut Jules Bordet–Université Libre de Bruxelles, Brussels, Belgium

Syed M. R. Kabir Royal National Orthopaedic Hospital, London, U.K.

Stephen R. D. Johnston The Royal Marsden NHS Foundation Trust and The Institute of Cancer Research, London, U.K.

George Ladas Department of Thoracic Surgery, Royal Brompton Hospital, and Imperial College School of Medicine, London, U.K.

Diane Mackie Secondary Breast Cancer, The Royal Marsden NHS Foundation Trust, London, U.K.

David MacVicar Department of Diagnostic Radiology, The Royal Marsden NHS Foundation Trust, London and Sutton, U.K.

David Miles Mount Vernon Cancer Centre, London, U.K.

Maurizio Scaltriti Massachusetts General Hospital Cancer Center, Boston, Massachusetts, U.S.A.

Bhupinder Sharma Department of Diagnostic Radiology, The Royal Marsden NHS Foundation Trust, London and Sutton, U.K.

Richard Simcock Sussex Cancer Centre, Brighton and Sussex University Hospitals NHS Trust, Brighton, U.K.

Christos Sotiriou Breast Cancer Translational Research Laboratory JC Heuson (BCTL), Institut Jules Bordet–Université Libre de Bruxelles, Brussels, Belgium

Anna-Marie Stevens Department of Palliative Medicine, The Royal Marsden NHS Foundation Trust, London, U.K.

Kuldeep K. Stöhr Starship Hospital, Auckland, New Zealand

Charles Swanton University College London Hospital and UCL Cancer Institute; and Cancer Research U.K. London Research Institute, Translational Cancer Therapeutics Laboratory, London, U.K.

Nicholas C. Turner The Institute of Cancer Research and Royal Marsden Hospital, Breakthrough Breast Cancer Research Centre, The Institute of Cancer Research, London, U.K.

Melissa Warren Secondary Breast Cancer, The Royal Marsden NHS Foundation Trust, Sutton, U.K.

Jayne Wood Department of Palliative Medicine, The Royal Marsden NHS Foundation Trust, London, U.K.

1 Introduction

Stephen R. D. Johnston and Charles Swanton

Despite significant advances in the diagnosis and treatment of breast cancer, approximately one-third of patients still develop and subsequently die from metastatic breast disease. Globally, half a million deaths each year are attributable to metastatic breast cancer and the median survival time from the diagnosis of secondary disease is approximately 3 years. The range is very wide however, with some patients having more indolent disease that they can live with for 10–15 years, while for others with widespread metastatic disease, the prognosis may only be a matter of months from the time of diagnosis. While this may represent the extent and distribution of metastatic disease, in part it reflects the biological diversity of breast cancer, with some women having disease that exhibits extreme sensitivity to hormonal treatments, whereas others with so-called triple-negative breast cancer may display relative resistance to all systemic therapies. In recent years, the increasing recognition that different molecular subtypes of breast cancer exist has substantially changed not only the way we classify and treat the disease, but also the impact that certain novel therapeutics in the metastatic setting can have on specific types of breast cancer.

In a rapidly evolving field in modern medicine where cancer genetics, molecular profiling, and targeted therapeutics have all had a huge impact over the last 5 years, it is timely to update the first edition of this "Handbook of Metastatic Breast Cancer" that was first published in 2006. Although the principles of treating the disease remain unchanged, there have been sufficient advances in several aspects of clinical management to merit a second edition that includes the most up-to-date information and results of clinical trials, and discusses the impact of these developments on the management of patients with metastatic breast cancer. There is a new chapter that discusses the molecular taxonomy of breast cancer, focusing on the relevance of gene expression signatures and predictive and prognostic biomarkers in the treatment of metastatic breast cancer. In addition, there are three new chapters on specialist systemic treatment options, including targeting HER2+ and issues relating to trastuzumab-resistant metastatic breast cancer, management of triple-negative sporadic and BRCA germline metastatic disease, and the role of angiogenesis inhibitors in the treatment of advanced breast cancer. We have provided significant updates to the existing chapters that discuss various systemic treatments for breast cancer, including endocrine therapy, chemotherapy, targeted therapies, and bisphosphonates. In addition we have updated the information on diagnostic imaging and tumour assessment, including the role of positron emission tomography and other functional imaging modalities.

The principal aim of treatment for secondary breast cancer remains to increase the duration of symptom-free survivorship and limit treatment-related toxicity, and thereby ensure the maximum quality of life for most of the patients. It is acknowledged that metastatic breast cancer can affect many parts of the body and this requires a wide range of treatments to control local symptoms. Therefore, it is strongly recommended that these patients are now managed by a specialist, multidisciplinary secondary breast cancer team which works closely with palliative care specialists and associated medical specialities as required. These aspects of multimodality management should underpin modern day services for women with secondary breast cancer, and we have updated the chapters from allied professionals that discuss local treatment options for neurological, thoracic, orthopaedic, and hepatic complications in advanced secondary breast cancer.

The high prevalence of the disease, together with the relatively long natural history for many patients, means that in the United Kingdom approximately 100,000 women are living with a diagnosis of secondary breast cancer each year. However, for these women the true impact of living with an incurable condition and coping with an uncertain future is something that often goes unrecognised by health-care professionals. The diagnosis of metastatic breast cancer is always a devastating event for any patient who has received previous therapy for early breast cancer that was given with the hope and expectation of cure. Therefore, when secondary disease returns it is associated with the realisation that "cure" is no longer possible. The information needs of patients are now very complex, made more challenging and sometimes confusing by the vast volume of information available to patients via the Internet. This means that specialist information and support services for patients and their families are vitally important, and in many centres this is now provided by clinical nurse specialists in secondary breast cancer. The role of these support services is discussed in a new chapter.

While at present metastatic breast cancer cannot be cured, modern systemic and loco-regional treatment can be very effective in maximising the duration of a patient's quality time without disease-related symptoms, which if significant in itself will often manifest as prolonged survival. With the introduction of more effective therapies over the last two decades, there has been a substantial improvement in clinical outcomes for women with metastatic breast cancer compared to treatment therapies available 30 years ago. Indeed many patients can now expect to live with metastatic secondary breast cancer for several years. However, many challenges continue to remain in the development of novel therapies proving that a given intervention on its own impacts on overall survival; this is because with so many effective therapies to offer patients with advanced disease, randomised trials against no therapy or "best supportive care" are impossible and indeed unethical to conduct in this disease. Furthermore, because breast cancer in general is relatively sensitive to the various drug- and radiation-based therapies that are available, with multiple lines of treatment often being used during the course of a patient's illness, subsequent therapies given in sequence will undoubtedly have a major impact on patient outcome. This makes the likelihood of a novel therapy in the first-line setting having a significant impact on overall survival almost impossible to demonstrate. Because of this, "progression-free survival" has become in some instances a recognised primary endpoint that is used to demonstrate to regulatory authorities the clinical utility of any given novel therapeutic. For most patients and their health-care professionals, an effective therapy that controls disease without toxicities, from which life expectancy may be prolonged, remains the most important objective in the management of the disease.

As outcomes for women with secondary breast cancer continue to improve, there are now genuine grounds for optimism, despite the sense of uncertainty and loss of control that many women inevitably feel once diagnosed. During the past two decades there have been significant advances in the diagnosis and treatment of early breast cancer, reflected by the significant improvement in mortality from the disease observed both in the United States and Europe since the early 1990s (1). The United Kingdom has witnessed perhaps the largest single improvement in survival rates form breast cancer, with a 40% reduction in mortality since 1990 (2). Reasons for this progress are multifactorial and have been attributed to the possible impact of screening and detection of earlier-stage disease, better multidisciplinary management of breast cancer by dedicated specialists, together with a more widespread use of systemic adjuvant therapies including combination chemotherapy and hormonal treatment. Furthermore, the introduction of novel targeted therapies, in particular biological therapies such as trastuzumab for HER2-positive disease, has altered the natural history of advanced breast cancer, with an unprecedented impact on survival from such treatments. As such, it is likely that many patients will now live considerably longer with their secondary breast cancer under control, although cure in this setting still remains an elusive goal.

We hope that the updated second edition of this handbook will be a useful source of information for all health-care professionals involved in the management of patients with metastatic breast cancer. Sharing knowledge helps improve practice, which ultimately benefits women afflicted by this disease.

REFERENCES

1. Peto R, Boreham J, Clarke M, et al. UK and USA breast cancer deaths down 25% in years at year 2000 in ages 20–69 years. Lancet 2000; 355: 1822–3.
2. Beral V, Peto R. UK cancer survival statistics. BMJ 2010; 341.

The prognostic and predictive value of gene expression signatures in breast cancer

Hatem A. Azim, Jr., Debora Fumagalli, and Christos Sotiriou

INTRODUCTION

Gene-expression profiling with the use of DNA microarray allows measurement of thousands of messenger RNA transcripts in a single experiment. Results of such studies have confirmed that breast cancer (BC) is not a single disease, but rather a group of molecularly distinct subtypes (1). In this regard, four main molecular classes of BC have been identified which are as follows (2–5): luminal-A cancer, which is mostly low proliferative oestrogen receptor (ER) positive; luminal-B, which is mostly high proliferative ER positive; basal-like cancer, which is negative for ER, progesterone receptor (PR) and human epidermal growth factor receptor 2 (HER2) and finally HER2-positive cancer which is characterised by the amplification of the HER2 gene.

Gene-expression profiling has also been used to develop genomic tests with the aim to provide prognostic tools which are better than classical clinicopathological parameters. In addition, such tests could serve as predictive tools to systemic therapies.

Two main approaches have been adopted to develop such signatures. The "first-generation signatures," were developed focusing on epithelial cancer cells. These include MammaPrint®: Agendia, Oncotype Dx®: Genomic Health, MapQuant Dx®: Ipsogen, and Theros®: Biotheranostics (6–10). These signatures were found to be useful for determining the risk of relapse in ER-positive BC, yet much less informative for the ER-negative and HER2-positive subgroups which are assigned to the high-risk category in almost all cases (11). More recently, another group of signatures were developed, referred to as "second-generation signatures," in which other factors are taken into consideration in addition to genomics information derived from epithelial cancer cells. After conducting a comprehensive gene expression profiling of each cell type, Allinen et al. have shown that at the transcriptome level, changes occur in epithelial as well as in myoepithelial and stromal cells that are already evident at the carcinoma *in situ* stage (12,13). The appreciation of this fact has resulted in the development of second-generation signatures derived from stromal cells (14,15), the immune system (16,17), and cancer-related pathways (16,18).

In this chapter, we discuss the prognostic and predictive value of first- and second-generation gene expression signatures emphasising their potential role in improving prognostication and selection of therapy for patients with early BC.

PROGNOSTIC VALUE OF GENE EXPRESSION SIGNATURES
First-Generation Signatures

In 2002, the Dutch group published two landmark publications addressing the prognostic value of the MammaPrint, an assay that measures the expression of 70 genes and accordingly categorises patients into good and poor risk groups (6,19). In the earlier study, the assay could accurately predict the prognosis of 78 untreated women with node-negative disease and tumour size <5 cm (6). This was followed by a validation study on a series of 295 patients including those with node-positive disease (19). In the latter study, the initial results were confirmed and the assay was found to assign patients more accurately to the low-risk category compared with other clinical prognostic tools like the St. Gallen criteria and the National Institutes of Health consensus criteria (20,21). A second validation study was later published on a larger number of patients and the 70-gene signatures outperformed the clinicopathological risk assessment by the Adjuvant! Online (AOL) program (22). In this study, 87 of the 302 (29%) patients had discordant results. Of these, 68% had tumours that were rated as clinically high risk according to the clinicopathological criteria but low risk according to the gene signature; while 32% were rated as clinically low risk but high risk according to the gene signatures. Indeed, in these cases, the genomic test was more accurate in predicting prognosis. In the former group (low genomic risk, high clinical risk), the 10-year overall survival rate was 89% while in the latter group (high genomic risk, low clinical risk), it was 69%.

The genomic grade index ((GGI), MapQuant Dx) is another signature that was developed by Sotiriou et al. to explore whether gene-expression profiling could be used to grade tumours more accurately than the conventional histological grade, particularly those tumours with intermediate grade (GII) (8). In a study involving 570 patients, GGI was able to discern among GII tumours two risk groups with a significant difference in relapse-free-survival rates (high vs. low risk; HR: 2.83; 95% CI 2.13–3.77; p < 0.001). In a multivariate model that included all known clinico-pathological parameters, GGI demonstrated strong prognostic information (HR: 1.38; 95% CI 1.43–2.78; p < 0.001) while histological grade was non-informative. In this analysis, tumour size, and lymph node status were also significantly associated with prognosis.

Oncotype Dx is another assay that measures the expression of ER and HER2, as well as that of ER-regulated transcripts and several proliferation genes. Using this assay, a recurrence score (RS) is calculated based on the expression of 16 cancer-related genes and 5 reference genes and accordingly a risk group is determined (low, intermediate, or high). Paik et al. have carried out a large retrospective analysis to examine the prognostic value of RS in predicting distant recurrence in patients with node-negative, tamoxifen-treated BC patients who were enrolled in the National Surgical Adjuvant Breast and Bowel Project clinical trial B-14 (9). The 10-year distant recurrence rates were 7%, 14%, and 30% for low-, intermediate-, and high-risk groups respectively. In a multivariate model, the recurrence score provided significant prognostic power independent of age and tumour size (p < 0.001) and was predictive for overall survival (p < 0.001). In a later study, Dowsett and colleagues examined the prognostic performance of the RS in predicting relapse at a median period of 9 years in patients enrolled in the Arimidex, Tamoxifen, Alone or in Combination (ATAC) trial (23). In this study, RS was significantly associated with time to distant relapse in multivariate analysis both for node-negative (HR: 5.25; 95% CI 2.84–9.73; p < 0.001) and node-positive disease (HR: 3.47; 95% CI 1.64–7.38; p = 0.002). Of note, tumour size was also significantly associated with time to distant relapse in the multivariate analysis in patients with node-negative (HR: 2.78; 95% CI 1.70–4.57; p < 0.001) and node-positive (HR: 2.04; 95% CI 1.20–3.48; p = 0.006) disease. There was no treatment interaction observed in this study, suggesting that the assay had similar prognostic power in patients treated with anastrozole and tamoxifen. Furthermore, the RS also showed a significant prognostic value beyond that provided by AOL (p < 0.001). In another study by the South West Oncology group, RS was found to be prognostic in patients with node-positive BC treated with tamoxifen (HR: 2.64; 95% CI 1.33–5.27; p = 0.006) (24). Importantly, the RS was only significant in predicting early relapses (i.e., during the first 5 years) (p = 0.029), with no addition prediction beyond 5 years (p = 0.58), although the cumulative benefit remained significant at 10 years. This observation was consistent for distant relapse, BC-specific survival, and overall survival.

Interestingly, a meta-analysis of publically available gene expression and clinical data from almost 3000 breast tumours showed similar prognostic performance of these signatures despite the limited overlap of genes (25). Of note, testing with more than one signature did not appear to improve the prognostic performance. Importantly, tumour size, and lymph node status remained independently prognostic, which highlights the importance of considering the known clinical prognostic parameters even in the era of gene expression signatures. While no one can question the prognostic performance of such signatures, one could argue on the real added value in terms of prediction of overall survival when these signatures are added to the known clinicopathological prognostic tools like AOL, Nottingham Prognostic Index and others. In the ATAC trial, it was clear that the RS added significantly to the prognostic prediction of AOL ($\Delta x^2 = 21.9$, $p < 0.001$), yet the high costs and advanced technology needed to perform such signatures remain a major hurdle. To address this point, Dutch investigators examined the cost effectiveness of the use of MammaPrint compared to the clinically available tools; namely the St. Gallen consensus and AOL (26). For this analysis, they developed a model to compare long-term consequences of the use of the three prognostic tools in patients with node-negative BC. The three strategies were found to be on average equally effective; with the St. Gallen strategy being more costly, followed by the MammaPrint, then the AOL strategy. However, the MammaPrint yielded more quality-adjusted life years (12.44) than the AOL and St. Gallen strategies (12.20 and 11.24). Currently, two large phase III trials, microarray in node-negative and 1 to 3 positive lymph node disease may avoid chemotherapy (MINDACT) and a cancer research trial assigning individualized options for treatment (Rx) (TAILORx), are ongoing to validate the use of such signatures in daily BC management (27,28). They would also address other important technical and analytical issues such as those related to shipping, reproducibility, and standardisation of these new molecular tools.

Hence, a critical look at the prognostic performance of first-generation signatures suggests that they improve the prognostic prediction of patients with early BC, especially those with ER-positive/HER2-negative disease. However, clinical predictors, particularly tumour size and lymph node status, should still be considered in determining patients' prognosis. Another point that deserves emphasis is that although these predictors perform well in identifying early relapses, they fail to predict late relapses (24). This suggests that different molecular mechanisms are likely to be involved during the development of early and late distant metastases (29).

Second-Generation Signatures

As mentioned earlier, first-generation signatures were developed focusing on epithelial cancer cells but it is arguable that our understanding of the complexity of BC could improve by also considering the role of tumour-surrounding stroma and host-related factors like the immune system. Second-generation signatures were developed aimed at overcoming the drawbacks highlighted earlier with first-generation signatures. These include the ability to predict the prognosis of basal-like and HER2 molecular subtypes and to accurately predict late relapse.

Finak and colleagues isolated tumour stroma and matched normal stroma from breast tumours and derived a 26-gene signature called the stroma-derived prognostic predictor (SDPP) (14). In this study, the prognostic power of SDPP was tested in a multivariate Cox regression model with all clinicopathological prognostic factors across four datasets. The SDPP was highly prognostic independently of ER, HER2, lymph node status, grade, age, and systemic therapy. Interestingly and unlike the first-generation signatures, it was able to predict outcomes in the HER2-positive molecular subtype. The HR for the poor-outcome group identified by the SDPP in the HER2-positive cohorts was, on average, 2.6 times greater than for the whole populations, indicating increased utility of the predictor in this cohort. Furthermore, the SDPP predicted outcome with greater accuracy (75.6%) than MammaPrint (61.0%) and was 5.96 times more likely to identify a true poor-outcome group of patients in the HER2- positive cohort (positive diagnostic likelihood ratio of 6.86 for SDPP vs. 1.15 for MammaPrint).

A Cambridge University team provided some very interesting work in the interrogation of the immune system with the aim to identify a group of ER-negative tumours that had a good prognosis (16). In this study, they identified an immune-response-related 7-gene module and showed that downregulation of this module conferred a greater risk of distant relapse (HR 2.02; 95% CI 1.2–3.4; p = 0.009) in the ER-negative population, which was independent of lymph node status and lympho-cytic infiltration. These results were further validated in two independent datasets. These results emphasise the point that ER-negative disease is heterogeneous in terms of expression of complement and genes involved in immune response pathways that help to identify patient subgroups with distinct prognosis. Another group from Germany further confirmed the role of immune signatures in identifying a subgroup among ER-negative tumours with favorable prognosis (17). Furthermore, Yau and co-workers recently reported a 14-gene signature that was able to predict prognosis of patients with triple-negative (basal-like) BC (30). This signature showed positive correlation with three immune-related signatures (STAT1, IFN, and IR), and further analysis identified 8 out of 14 genes as being functionally linked to immune/inflammatory chemokine regulation.

In an attempt to better understand the performance of the different signatures across the different BC subtypes, a meta-analysis conducted by Desmedt and co-workers has shown that stroma and immune signatures are the most relevant in determining clinical outcome in patients with HER2-positive tumours, while for ER-negative/HER2- negative (i.e., basal-like) tumours, only the immune response module is associated with prognosis (11).

Hence, second-generation signatures appear to improve the prognostic power beyond that achieved by first-generation signatures. It must be acknowledged that studies conducted using the second-generation signatures are fewer and require fur-ther validation. However, these signatures hold promise in improving prognostica-tion particularly in HER2 and basal molecular subtypes in which first-generation signatures failed to provide prognostic information.

THE PREDICTIVE VALUE OF GENE EXPRESSION SIGNATURES

Identification of biomarkers to predict response to a particular drug remains an impor-tant challenge for oncologists, since commonly used therapeutic agents are ineffective in many patients, and the side effects are frequent and considerable. At present, only two validated predictive biomarkers are used in the clinic: ER and HER2. Despite hav-ing an optimal negative predictive value, their positive predictive value is rather lim-ited, and they do not provide information regarding regimen selection in the adjuvant setting. Moreover, their determination shows a substantial variation both within and between laboratories, and thus has a relatively poor reproducibility (31).

In the last years, different investigators attempted to define gene expression signatures that are able to predict response to chemo, endocrine, and targeted ther-apy. Of note, most of these signatures were developed in the neoadjuvant and adju-vant setting, but their findings could be potentially applicable to patients with advanced disease as well.

Predicting Response to Chemotherapy

Several chemotherapy regimens are used in the primary treatment of BC. Interest-ingly, the retrospective application of the different gene signatures previously dis-cussed showed that they are able to assign patients to diverse risk categories that benefit differentially from chemotherapy (32–36).

Paik and colleagues reported a significant interaction between a higher RS and greater benefit to adjuvant cyclophosphamide, methotrexate, and 5-florouracil (CMF) regimen (test for interaction: p = 0.038) (32), suggesting that Oncotype DX could potentially be used to predict response to chemotherapy. Another report similarly showed that GGI is associated with sensitivity to neoadjuvant paclitaxel plus fluorouracil, adriamycin, and cyclophosphamide (T/FAC) chemotherapy in both ER-negative and ER-positive patients (35). However, it has been pointed out that the predictive component of these first-generation signatures relies on their ability to measure proliferation, a biological feature known to be associated with chemosensitivity in BC. This may limit the predictive features of these signatures to the detection of "generic" chemosensitivity rather than to the chemotherapy-regimen-specific sensitivity.

In this regard, Hess and colleagues evaluated gene expression profiling as a potential tool to predict the pathological complete response (pCR) to sequential anthracycline–paclitaxel preoperative chemotherapy (37). Diverse predictors of pCR were developed from 82 patients and their accuracy was validated on 51 independent patients with stage I–III BC treated with (T/FAC) chemotherapy. Among several identified predictors that performed equally well, a 30-probe set Diagonal Linear Discriminant Analysis (DLDA-30) classifier was selected for independent validation. It showed a significantly higher sensitivity (92% vs. 61%) than a clinical predictor including age, grade, and ER status. In a recent publication by the same group (38), the performance of DLDA-30 was evaluated in a prospective, randomised neoadjuvant clinical trial comparing T/FAC and FAC, both given for six cycles. While the assay was predictive of response to T/FAC with an apparent regimen specificity, its performance was similar to that of the clinical prediction model tested in their first study. This suggests that DLDA-30, as other genomic predictors developed with a similar strategy, interrogates mostly gene expression information associated with clinical phenotype (mainly ER, HER2, and proliferation), advocating the need for a different approach to develop clinically useful genomic predictive tools.

A "Second Generation" of Predictive Signatures

In the past decade, our group led a prospective neoadjuvant clinical trial in which ER-negative BCs were treated with anthracycline monotherapy with the objective to evaluate the predictive value of topoisomerase IIα and to develop a gene expression signature to identify patients who do not benefit from anthracyclines (39). An "anthracycline-based score (A-Score)" was developed that combined three different signatures associated with the efficacy of anthracyclines: a topoisomerase IIα signature, a stroma signature, and an immune-response signature. The "A-Score" turned out to have a high negative predictive value both in the overall population and in the two subgroups of HER2-positive and HER2-negative patients.

Similar to prognostic signatures, the development of a "second-generation" of predictive signatures that are generated in targeted populations and that explore the role of tumour microenvironment (15) or pathway activation (40) is possibly a better way to move forward in defining clinically useful predictive tools.

Predictors of Response to Endocrine Therapy

Several randomised trials have assessed the value of endocrine therapy in early and advanced stage ER-positive BC (41). As one can expect, numerous investigators have tried to develop gene expression signatures that are able to predict sensitivity or resistance to both tamoxifen and aromatase inhibitors (AIs) (42–44). In a recent study, Symmans and colleagues defined a genomic index for sensitivity to endocrine therapy (SET index) from genes co-expressed with the oestrogen receptor gene (ESR1) (44). They hypothesised that the measurement of gene expression related to ER within a BC sample represents intrinsic tumour sensitivity to adjuvant endocrine therapy. The association of SET index and ESR1 levels with distant relapse risk was evaluated in 437 microarray profiles of newly diagnosed ER-positive BC. Several cohorts were included, including a group which received 5 years of adjuvant tamoxifen and another group which received neoadjuvant chemotherapy followed by tamoxifen and/or AI. This is in addition to two cohorts which received no adjuvant systemic therapy. The SET index (165 genes) was found to be significantly associated with the risk of distant relapse and death in both tamoxifen-treated and chemo-endocrine–treated cohorts independently from pathological response to chemotherapy. Yet, it was not prognostic in the two untreated cohorts. No distant relapse or death was observed after tamoxifen treatment if node-negative and high SET index or after chemo-endocrine therapy if intermediate or high SET index.

ALTERNATIVE STRATEGIES TO DEFINE MULTIGENE PREDICTORS
Development of *In Vitro* Signature Analysis
An alternative "associative" strategy that has been used to generate predictive multi-gene assays derives from *in vitro* signature analysis. In this approach, gene expression data and *in vitro* drug response information from cell line panels are used to generate drug-specific associative pharmacogenomic response predictors that can be applied to human data (45). However, several investigators failed to reproduce in humans the discriminating power of purely cell line derived drug-specific predictors (46–48). This highlights the difficulties of associative analyses that do not interrogate gene function, deriving from cell line models, to capture patient-related differences in drug metabolism and the influence of tumour microenvironment in response to treatment.

RNA Interference Technology
Recently, the use of the RNA interference (RNAi) technology has allowed the identification of genes influencing resistance and sensitivity to diverse cytotoxic drugs used in clinical practice (49–51). Starting from a small number of overexpressed and amplified genes from chromosome 8q22 significantly associated with early disease recurrence despite anthracycline-based adjuvant chemotherapy and using RNAi knockdown, Li and colleagues were able to identify two genes (YWHAZ and LAPTM4B) which sensitized tumour cells to anthracyclines when either was depleted (50). The overexpression of either of them was on the contrary associated with drug resistance. Of note, these functional genomic data could be combined with other molecular data, such as gene expression signatures, and increase their strength (52).

Finally, a kinome RNAi screen recently identified a ceramide and a mitotic module that influenced response to paclitaxel across multiple cell lines, including an ER-negative BC cell line. This module of six genes, called "functional meta-gene," was tested in two retrospective cohorts of ER-negative patients treated with T/FAC neoadjuvant chemotherapy. The functional metagene was shown to predict pCR to paclitaxel-specific regimens but not regimens that did not contain a paclitaxel backbone (49).

UNRESOLVED ISSUES AND FUTURE PERSPECTIVES
It is worthy of note that advances in molecular technologies in the last years allowed the identification of different molecular events, such as DNA mutation and chromosomal rearrangements, which could influence the response to cancer treatment (53,54). Lately, several investigators have focused on the influence of epigenetic modifications on BC behaviour and came up with epigenetic signatures that could potentially be combined with gene expression signatures and improve their performance (55).

Despite the promises, none of the signatures generated so far have been approved for use in the clinical setting. The confidence in the results obtained remains limited given the small sample sizes and multiple comparisons (56). In addition, most of the available studies have been carried out in unselected BC populations. If different molecular classes have different sensitivity to chemotherapy, using data from "all comers" will likely yield predictors that primarily discriminate between molecular classes and have less strength to predict response within a class. Hence, properly powered studies with innovative design in a clearly defined patient population will likely provide more robust conclusions on the predictive validity of such signatures in the clinic. The adoption of an integrative approach that takes into consideration the complex interplay of factors involved in response to therapy, which might include functional RNA interference approaches, could contribute immensely to the development of a new class of predictive signatures with clinical impact.

REFERENCES

1. Sotiriou C, Pusztai L. Gene-expression signatures in breast cancer. N Engl J Med 2009; 360: 790–800.
2. Perou CM, Sorlie T, Eisen MB, et al. Molecular portraits of human breast tumours. Nature 2000; 406: 747–52.
3. Sorlie T, Perou CM, Tibshirani R, et al. Gene expression patterns of breast carcinomas distinguish tumor subclasses with clinical implications. Proc Natl Acad Sci USA 2001; 98: 10869–74.
4. Sorlie T, Tibshirani R, Parker J, et al. Repeated observation of breast tumor subtypes in independent gene expression data sets. Proc Natl Acad Sci USA 2003; 100: 8418–23.
5. Sotiriou C, Neo SY, McShane LM, et al. Breast cancer classification and prognosis based on gene expression profiles from a population-based study. Proc Natl Acad Sci USA 2003; 100: 10393–8.
6. van't Veer LJ, Dai H, van de Vijver MJ, et al. Gene expression profiling predicts clinical outcome of breast cancer. Nature 2002; 415: 530–6.
7. Wang Y, Klijn JG, Zhang Y, et al. Gene-expression profiles to predict distant metastasis of lymph-node-negative primary breast cancer. Lancet 2005; 365: 671–9.
8. Sotiriou C, Wirapati P, Loi S, et al. Gene expression profiling in breast cancer: understanding the molecular basis of histologic grade to improve prognosis. J Natl Cancer Inst 2006; 98: 262–72.
9. Paik S, Shak S, Tang G, et al. A multigene assay to predict recurrence of tamoxifen-treated, node-negative breast cancer. N Engl J Med 2004; 351: 2817–26.
10. Ma XJ, Wang Z, Ryan PD, et al. A two-gene expression ratio predicts clinical outcome in breast cancer patients treated with tamoxifen. Cancer Cell 2004; 5: 607–16.
11. Desmedt C, Haibe-Kains B, Wirapati P, et al. Biological processes associated with breast cancer clinical outcome depend on the molecular subtypes. Clin Cancer Res 2008; 14: 5158–65.
12. Cleator SJ, Powles TJ, Dexter T, et al. The effect of the stromal component of breast tumours on prediction of clinical outcome using gene expression microarray analysis. Breast Cancer Res 2006; 8: R32.
13. Allinen M, Beroukhim R, Cai L, et al. Molecular characterization of the tumor microenvironment in breast cancer. Cancer Cell 2004; 6: 17–32.
14. Finak G, Bertos N, Pepin F, et al. Stromal gene expression predicts clinical outcome in breast cancer. Nat Med 2008; 14: 518–27.
15. Farmer P, Bonnefoi H, Anderle P, et al. A stroma-related gene signature predicts resistance to neoadjuvant chemotherapy in breast cancer. Nat Med 2009; 15: 68–74.
16. Teschendorff AE, Miremadi A, Pinder SE, et al. An immune response gene expression module identifies a good prognosis subtype in estrogen receptor negative breast cancer. Genome Biol 2007; 8: R157.
17. Rody A, Holtrich U, Pusztai L, et al. T-cell metagene predicts a favorable prognosis in estrogen receptor-negative and HER2-positive breast cancers. Breast Cancer Res 2009; 11: R15.
18. Loi S, Haibe-Kains B, Majjaj S, et al. PIK3CA mutations associated with gene signature of low mTORC1 signaling and better outcomes in estrogen receptor-positive breast cancer. Proc Natl Acad Sci USA 2010; 107: 10208–13.

19. van de Vijver MJ, He YD, van't Veer LJ, et al. A gene-expression signature as a predictor of survival in breast cancer. N Engl J Med 2002; 347: 1999–2009.
20. Goldhirsch A, Ingle JN, Gelber RD, et al. Thresholds for therapies: highlights of the St Gallen International Expert Consensus on the primary therapy of early breast cancer 2009. Ann Oncol 2009; 20: 1319–29.
21. Eifel P, Axelson JA, Costa J, et al. National Institutes of Health Consensus Development Conference Statement: adjuvant therapy for breast cancer, November 1–3, 2000. J Natl Cancer Inst 2001; 93: 979–89.
22. Buyse M, Loi S, van't Veer L, et al. Validation and clinical utility of a 70-gene prognostic signature for women with node-negative breast cancer. J Natl Cancer Inst 2006; 98: 1183–92.
23. Dowsett M, Cuzick J, Wale C, et al. Prediction of risk of distant recurrence using the 21-gene recurrence score in node-negative and node-positive postmenopausal patients with breast cancer treated with anastrozole or tamoxifen: a TransATAC study. J Clin Oncol 2010; 28: 1829–34.
24. Albain KS, Barlow WE, Shak S, et al. Prognostic and predictive value of the 21-gene recurrence score assay in postmenopausal women with node-positive, oestrogen-receptor-positive breast cancer on chemotherapy: a retrospective analysis of a randomised trial. Lancet Oncol 2010; 11: 55–65.
25. Wirapati P, Sotiriou C, Kunkel S, et al. Meta-analysis of gene expression profiles in breast cancer: toward a unified understanding of breast cancer subtyping and prognosis signatures. Breast Cancer Res 2008; 10: R65.
26. Retel VP, Joore MA, Knauer M, et al. Cost-effectiveness of the 70-gene signature versus St. Gallen guidelines and Adjuvant Online for early breast cancer. Eur J Cancer 2010; 46: 1382–91.
27. Cardoso F, Van't Veer L, Rutgers E, et al. Clinical application of the 70-gene profile: the MINDACT trial. J Clin Oncol 2008; 26: 729–35.
28. Sparano JA, Paik S. Development of the 21-gene assay and its application in clinical practice and clinical trials. J Clin Oncol 2008; 26: 721–8.
29. Fumagalli D, Sotiriou C. Treatment of pT1N0 breast cancer: multigene predictors to assess risk of relapse. Ann Oncol 2010; 21(Suppl 7): vii103–6.
30. Yau C, Esserman L, Moore DH, et al. A multigene predictor of metastatic outcome in early stage hormone receptor-negative and triple-negative breast cancer. Breast Cancer Res 2010; 12: R85.
31. Gown AM. Current issues in ER and HER2 testing by IHC in breast cancer. Mod Pathol 2008; 21(Suppl 2): S8–15.
32. Paik S, Tang G, Shak S, et al. Gene expression and benefit of chemotherapy in women with node-negative, estrogen receptor-positive breast cancer. J Clin Oncol 2006; 24: 3726–34.
33. Gianni L, Zambetti M, Clark K, et al. Gene expression profiles in paraffin-embedded core biopsy tissue predict response to chemotherapy in women with locally advanced breast cancer. J Clin Oncol 2005; 23: 7265–77.
34. Knauer M, Mook S, Rutgers EJ, et al. The predictive value of the 70-gene signature for adjuvant chemotherapy in early breast cancer. Breast Cancer Res Treat 2010; 120: 655–61.
35. Liedtke C, Hatzis C, Symmans WF, et al. Genomic grade index is associated with response to chemotherapy in patients with breast cancer. J Clin Oncol 2009; 27: 3185–91.
36. Straver ME, Glas AM, Hannemann J, et al. The 70-gene signature as a response predictor for neoadjuvant chemotherapy in breast cancer. Breast Cancer Res Treat 2010; 119: 551–8.
37. Hess KR, Anderson K, Symmans WF, et al. Pharmacogenomic predictor of sensitivity to preoperative chemotherapy with paclitaxel and fluorouracil, doxorubicin, and cyclophosphamide in breast cancer. J Clin Oncol 2006; 24: 4236–44.
38. Tabchy A, Valero V, Vidaurre T, et al. Evaluation of a 30-gene paclitaxel, fluorouracil, doxorubicin, and cyclophosphamide chemotherapy response predictor in a multicenter randomized trial in breast cancer. Clin Cancer Res 2010; 16: 5351–61.
39. Desmedt C, Di Leo A, De Azambuja E. Multi-factorial approach to predicting resistance to anthracyclines. In press, 2011.
40. Bild AH, Yao G, Chang JT, et al. Oncogenic pathway signatures in human cancers as a guide to targeted therapies. Nature 2006; 439: 353–7.
41. Early Breast Cancer Trialists' Collaborative Group (EBCTCG) Effects of chemotherapy and hormonal therapy for early breast cancer on recurrence and 15-year survival: an overview of the randomised trials. Lancet 2005; 365: 1687–717.

42. Mello-Grand M, Singh V, Ghimenti C, et al. Gene expression profiling and prediction of response to hormonal neoadjuvant treatment with anastrozole in surgically resectable breast cancer. Breast Cancer Res Treat 2010; 121: 399–411.
43. Miller WR, Larionov A, Renshaw L, et al. Gene expression profiles differentiating between breast cancers clinically responsive or resistant to letrozole. J Clin Oncol 2009; 27: 1382–7.
44. Symmans WF, Hatzis C, Sotiriou C, et al. Genomic index of sensitivity to endocrine therapy for breast cancer. J Clin Oncol 2010; 28: 4111–19.
45. Potti A, Dressman HK, Bild A, et al. Genomic signatures to guide the use of chemotherapeutics. Nat Med 2006; 12: 1294–300.
46. Coombes KR, Wang J, Baggerly KA. Microarrays: retracing steps. Nat Med 2007; 13: 1276–7; author reply 1277–8.
47. Lee JK, Coutant C, Kim YC, et al. Prospective comparison of clinical and genomic multivariate predictors of response to neoadjuvant chemotherapy in breast cancer. Clin Cancer Res 2010; 16: 711–18.
48. Liedtke C, Wang J, Tordai A, et al. Clinical evaluation of chemotherapy response predictors developed from breast cancer cell lines. Breast Cancer Res Treat 2010; 121: 301–9.
49. Juul N, Szallasi Z, Eklund AC, et al. Assessment of an RNA interference screen-derived mitotic and ceramide pathway metagene as a predictor of response to neoadjuvant paclitaxel for primary triple-negative breast cancer: a retrospective analysis of five clinical trials. Lancet Oncol 2010; 11: 358–65.
50. Li Y, Zou L, Li Q, et al. Amplification of LAPTM4B and YWHAZ contributes to chemotherapy resistance and recurrence of breast cancer. Nat Med 2010; 16: 214–18.
51. Swanton C, Marani M, Pardo O, et al. Regulators of mitotic arrest and ceramide metabolism are determinants of sensitivity to paclitaxel and other chemotherapeutic drugs. Cancer Cell 2007; 11: 498–512.
52. Swanton C, Szallasi Z, Brenton JD, et al. Functional genomic analysis of drug sensitivity pathways to guide adjuvant strategies in breast cancer. Breast Cancer Res 2008; 10: 214.
53. Martin SA, Hewish M, Lord CJ, et al. Genomic instability and the selection of treatments for cancer. J Pathol 2010; 220: 281–9.
54. Swanton C, Nicke B, Schuett M, et al. Chromosomal instability determines taxane response. Proc Natl Acad Sci USA 2009; 106: 8671–6.
55. Parrella P. Epigenetic signatures in breast cancer: clinical perspective. Breast Care (Basel) 2010; 5: 66–73.
56. Michiels S, Koscielny S, Hill C. Prediction of cancer outcome with microarrays: a multiple random validation strategy. Lancet 2005; 365: 488–92.

3 | Endocrine therapy for advanced disease

Stephen R. D. Johnston

INTRODUCTION

In the United Kingdom, breast cancer affects up to 1 in 8 women during their lifetime; with an annual incidence that has now reached more than 41,000, the death rate is approximately 12,000 per year (1). Approximately 5–10% of newly diagnosed breast cancer patients have locally advanced/metastatic disease at the outset, and 20–70% of patients (depending on their tumour biology, initial stage of disease and subsequent therapy) will develop recurrent/metastatic disease in the future. It is estimated that in the United Kingdom over 100,000 women are living with advanced/metastatic breast cancer (MBC) at any one time. Once the metastatic disease is diagnosed it cannot be cured, and the overall median survival from the time metastatic disease is confirmed is between 2 and 3 years.

The optimal management of patients with metastatic disease remains a challenge, with systemic drug treatments such as chemotherapy, endocrine therapy, biological targeted therapy, and supportive therapies being the mainstay of care. The decision as to which is the most appropriate treatment option is based on a number of patient- and disease-related factors. Approximately two-thirds of human breast carcinomas express oestrogen receptors (ERs) and thus may be dependent on oestrogen for their growth, and for patients in whom their breast cancer (either primary tumour or biopsy of accessible metastatic disease) is positive for ER and/or progesterone receptor (PgR) endocrine therapy is an important treatment option with minimal toxicity. For patients with ER-/PgR-positive breast cancer and an estimated low risk of rapid progression of their advanced disease (i.e., soft tissue and/or bone metastasis as their dominant site, absence of life threatening visceral involvement, disease-free interval greater than 2 years, and limited sites of metastatic involvement), endocrine therapies can be very effective in the treatment of their advanced/metastatic disease (Table 1). For example, locally advanced ER-positive disease within the breast of elderly women is often slow growing and extremely hormone sensitive. Excellent clinical responses can be achieved with simple well-tolerated endocrine therapy such as tamoxifen, albeit maximal response and tumour shrinkage may take between 6 and 9 months to occur (Fig. 1A, B). However, sites of visceral metastases such as the liver may also respond well to endocrine therapy provided an appropriate selection of patients is undertaken. For example, post-menopausal patients with strongly ER/PgR-positive disease with a long treatment-free interval of many years after completion of adjuvant tamoxifen, may then develop metastatic disease within the liver but with a limited number of tumours and preserved organ function (i.e., normal liver function tests), lack of any symptoms from their advanced disease, and a good overall performance status. Such patients can have an excellent clinical response to endocrine therapy alone with, for example, aromatase inhibitors (AIs), which may last for 18–24 months before their disease progresses and patients require chemotherapy (Fig. 1C, D). Therefore, appropriate selection of patients that are suitable for initial endocrine therapy is therefore crucially important in order to maximise the benefits from such treatments.

In this chapter the evidence for the current endocrine therapy options that are available for advanced disease are reviewed in more detail, together with the emerging strategies that might be used in future to further enhance their effectiveness.

TABLE 1   Clinical Parameters Utilised in Decision Making Regarding Systemic Therapy Options in Advanced Breast Cancer

Patient Factors
   Age
   Menopausal status
   Performance status
   Severity and nature of symptoms
   Presence/absence of visceral disease
   Prior adjuvant systemic therapies
   Organ function (i.e., liver/renal functions)
Disease-Related Factors
   Tumour biology (ER/PgR status; HER2 status)
   Duration of treatment-free period (i.e., sensitive vs. resistant disease)
   Dominant site of disease (i.e., bone/soft tissue vs. visceral metastasis)
   Number of sites of metastasis
   Tumour burden

Abbreviations: ER, oestrogen receptor; PgR, progesterone receptor; HER2, human epidermal growth factor receptor 2.

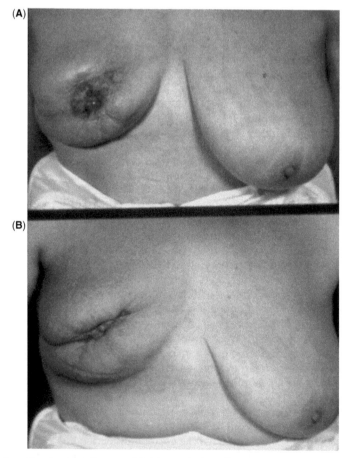

FIGURE 1   Locally advanced disease of the breast before (**A**) and 6 months after (**B**) therapy with tamoxifen, showing a substantial tumour shrinkage. Metastatic disease within the liver with three isolated tumours developing many years after prior adjuvant tamoxifen. (*Continued*)

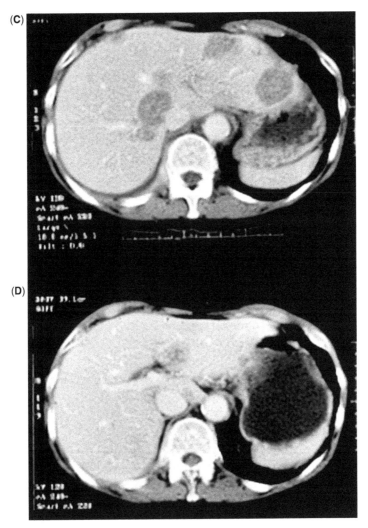

FIGURE 1 (*Continued*) Before (**C**) and after (**D**) 6 months, therapy with an aromatase inhibitor.

ENDOCRINE THERAPY OPTIONS FOR MBC

Historically, tamoxifen has been the approved "gold standard" endocrine therapy for the treatment of MBC, both of pre- and postmenopausal women. Tamoxifen is a non-steroidal ER antagonist which inhibits breast cancer growth by the competitive antagonism of oestrogen at the receptor site (Fig. 2). However, its actions are complex due to partial oestrogenic agonist effects which in some tissues (i.e., bone) can be beneficial (2), but in others may be harmful increasing the risk of thromboembolism and uterine cancer (3). Although this being an effective treatment for advanced breast cancer, the partial agonist effects may account for the development of tamoxifen resistance after prolonged treatment. Furthermore, the majority of women with ER-positive breast cancer who then develop metastatic disease have already been treated with tamoxifen in the adjuvant setting. In the past, tamoxifen therapy was used again if tamoxifen had been stopped several years previously, but now alternative endocrine approaches that deprive tumours of circulating oestrogens are utilised in preference.

Within the last 5 years third-generation potent oral AIs have become a standard treatment option for postmenopausal patients with ER-positive advanced/metastatic breast cancer. Oral AIs such as anastrozole (Arimidex™), letrozole (Femara™), and exemestane (Aromasin™) all reduce serum oestrogen levels in postmenopausal women by preventing the conversion of adrenal androgens into oestrogens (Fig. 2). Oestrogens are normally synthesised in the ovary in premenopausal women, but following the menopause, mean plasma oestradiol (E2) levels fall from about 400–600 pmol/L to around 25–50 pmol/L. These residual oestrogens come solely from peripheral aromatase conversion, particularly in subcutaneous fat, and plasma E2 levels correlate with body mass index in postmenopausal women (4). As discussed below, in postmenopausal women with advanced breast cancer several clinical trials have demonstrated that AIs are more effective and better tolerated than tamoxifen as first-line management of MBC. Since the late 1990s AIs have become the new "gold standard" for first-line endocrine treatment in postmenopausal women with advanced breast cancer.

For premenopausal women with ER-positive advanced breast cancer, oestrogen deprivation through ovarian ablation has been the main endocrine approach when tamoxifen has been used previously in the adjuvant setting. This can be achieved either by surgical oophorectomy, radiation of the ovaries, or medical ablation with luteinising hormone-releasing hormone (LHRH) agonists such as goserelin (Zoladex™) (Fig. 2). Such an approach can be effective in premenopausal women with endocrine-sensitive advanced disease, and at the time of further progression the addition of AIs to LHRH agonists has been a successful additional second-line option.

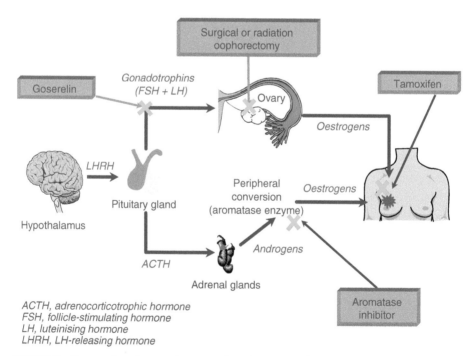

ACTH, adrenocorticotrophic hormone
FSH, follicle-stimulating hormone
LH, luteinising hormone
LHRH, LH-releasing hormone

FIGURE 2 Source of oestrogens in pre- and postmenopausal women, together with endocrine therapy options to either antagonise oestrogens (tamoxifen), or induce oestrogen deprivation via aromatase inhibition (postmenopausal) or ovarian ablation (premenopausal) via surgical, radiation, or medical means.

As discussed below, for women initially presenting with endocrine-sensitive advanced disease who have not received prior tamoxifen, tamoxifen combined with LHRH agonists appears to be a more effective strategy than tamoxifen alone.

Recently oestrogen suppressive therapies with either AIs or LHRH agonists have started to move into the adjuvant setting for post- and premenopausal women, respectively. This has led to new questions about the optimal sequence of endocrine therapies for subsequent use in advanced disease. The ER downregulator fulvestrant (Faslodex™) is a novel treatment option for women with progressive disease following prior tamoxifen therapy, and current trials are investigating whether fulvestrant is a suitable treatment option for postmenopausal women following progression with an AI. Research in endocrine therapy has been focusing on understanding the mechanisms of acquired resistance and the molecular pathways which allow ER-positive cells to escape from endocrine therapy. As discussed at the end of this chapter, several new strategies that combine endocrine therapies with various signal transduction inhibitors are now being investigated in ongoing clinical trials in advanced breast cancer. The ultimate goal will be to overcome and/or prevent the development of endocrine resistance in ER-positive breast cancer, and thus further enhance the benefits of existing endocrine therapy.

CLINICAL EFFICACY OF AIS IN ADVANCED BREAST CANCER
Pharmacology
Anastrozole and letrozole are third-generation non-steroidal AIs that have similar pharmacokinetics with half-lives of approximately 48 hours allowing a once-daily schedule (5,6). Exemestane is a steroidal aromatase inactivator with a longer half-life of 27 hours (7) (Fig. 3). All three compounds are orally active, reducing serum oestrogen levels in postmenopausal women by preventing conversion of adrenal androgens (androstenedione and testosterone) into oestradiol (E1) and oestrone (E2) via the cytochrome P450 enzyme aromatase. Based on the clinical trials outlined below, all

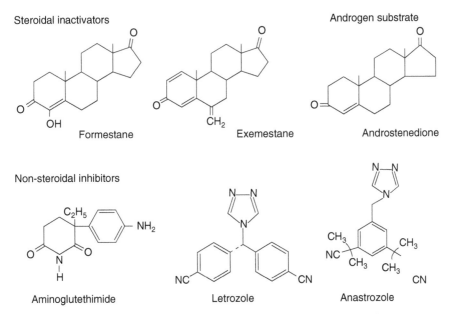

FIGURE 3 Structures of steroidal and non-steroidal aromatase inhibitors.

three AIs are licensed and approved as endocrine treatment for postmenopausal women with ER-positive advanced breast cancer.

Second-Line Therapy Post Tamoxifen

Between 1995 and 2000 the three third-generation AIs established themselves clinically when a series of randomised controlled trials (RCTs) in over 2000 women demonstrated clinical superiority over megestrol acetate (MA) as second-line therapy after tamoxifen (8–13) (Table 2). An analysis of two randomised phase III trials of 764 patients treated with either anastrozole or MA as second-line therapy after tamoxifen failure demonstrated an equivalent efficacy in terms of objective response rates (10.3% and 7.9%, respectively) and disease stabilisation for 6 months (25.1% and 26.1 %, respectively), although showed a better tolerability for anastrozole (8). A subsequent analysis following a median of 31 months follow-up showed a significant improvement in overall survival for anastrozole (hazard ratio (HR) 0.78, $p = 0.02$) (9). For letrozole, improvements were seen in objective tumour response rate (HR 1.82, $p = 0.04$) and time to treatment failure compared with MA, although no impact on survival was detected (10). In the trial with exemestane duration of objective response, time to disease progression, and overall survival were all significantly better than with MA (11). A subsequent second trial of letrozole (12), together with a study or the AI vorozole (no longer in development) (13) showed less substantial improvements over MA.

This was in contrast with previous trials with the second-generation inhibitors, fadrozole and formestane, which had all failed to show any such advantage (14,15).

TABLE 2　Comparative Second-Line Trials of Third-Generation Aromatase Inhibitors vs. Megestrol Acetate

Author	Comparators	n	Response (%)	Clinical benefit (%)[a]	Median time to progression (months)	Median overall survival (months)
Buzdar et al. (8,9)	Anastrozole 1 mg	263	13	42		27[b]
	Megestrol acetate	253	12	40		23[b]
Dombernowsky et al. (10)	Letrozole 2.5 mg	174	24[b]	35	5.6	25
	Megestrol acetate	189	16[b]	32	5.5	22
Buzdar et al. (12)	Letrozole 2.5 mg	199	32	53	3.0	29
	Megestrol acetate	201	30	47	3.0	26
Kaufmann et al. (11)	Exemestane 25 mg	336	15	37	4.7[b]	Not reached[b]
	Megestrol acetate	403	12	35	3.8[b]	28[b]
Goss et al. (13)	Vorozole 2.5 g	225	11		2.7	26
	Megestrol acetate	227	8		3.6	29

[a]Defined as the total percentage of patients responding or achieving stable disease for at least 6 months.
[b]Significant difference.

The improvements in clinical endpoints for the third-generation AIs, together with their consistent superior tolerability profile over MA (i.e., reduced weight gain and thromboembolic events), defined the AIs by the late 1990s as the standard endocrine treatment for advanced postmenopausal breast cancer following tamoxifen failure (16). In practice, however, developments in first-line endocrine therapy rapidly diminished the clinical relevance of these findings.

First-Line Therapy vs. Tamoxifen
Subsequent trials in advanced breast cancer questioned whether AIs could challenge tamoxifen as the first-line endocrine agent of choice. Previously, no first- or second-generation AI had proved superior to tamoxifen (17–19). In addition to comparing tolerability, the potential of these studies with the new third-generation AIs was to see whether the nearly complete oestrogen blockade provided by these drugs could deliver greater control of hormone-sensitive breast cancer than tamoxifen, thus circumventing the problem of acquired resistance due to the partial agonist effects of tamoxifen (20).

The first published data came from two parallel multi-centre double-blind RCTs in which anastrozole was compared with tamoxifen as first-line therapy in ER-positive breast cancer (Table 3). The first study in 353 women showed that anastrozole significantly prolonged the time to disease progression from 5.6 to 11.1 months (p = 0.005) (21). While there was no significant difference in objective tumour response rate (21% anastrozole vs. 17% tamoxifen), the clinical benefit rate (defined as the proportion of patients who responded or had stable disease for at least 6 months) was significantly better for anastrozole (59% vs. 46%). By contrast, in the larger trial with 668 patients no difference was found between the treatments in terms of median time to progression [(TTP) 8.2 vs. 8.3 months], response rate (33% both arms), or clinical benefit rate (56% both arms) (22). The explanation for the different results may have involved a higher proportion of patients with unknown ER status in the second trial, and a subsequent combined analysis of women with just ER-positive disease from both trials confirmed a significant improvement in disease-free survival in favour of anastrozole (23). Short-term side effects such as hot flashes, vaginal dryness, and headaches were infrequent and similar in both trials in comparison with tamoxifen.

The largest single trial was conducted with letrozole in comparison with tamoxifen in over 900 women with advanced breast cancer (24). Patients treated with

TABLE 3 Comparative First-Line Trials of Aromatase Inhibitors vs. Tamoxifen

Author	Comparators	n	Response %	Clinical benefit %[a]	Median time to progression (months)
Nabholtz et al. (21)	Anastrozole	171	21	59[b]	11.1[b]
	Tamoxifen	182	17	46	5.6
Bonneterre et al. (22,23)	Anastrozole	340	33	56	8.2
	Tamoxifen	328	33	56	8.3
Mouridsen et al. (24,25)	Letrozole	453	30[b]	49[b]	9.4[b]
	Tamoxifen	454	20[b]	38	6.0
Paridaens et al. (26)	Exemestane	182	46[b]	66[b]	9.9[b]
	Tamoxifen	189	31	49	5.8

[a]Defined as the total percentage of patients responding or achieving stable disease for at least 6 months.
[b]Significant difference vs. tamoxifen.

letrozole had a significantly higher objective tumour response rate (30% vs. 20%, p < 0.001), clinical benefit rate (49% vs. 38%, p < 0.001), and prolonged time to disease progression (TTP) (median TTP of 9.4 months vs. 6.0 months, HR 0.72, p < 0.0001). Of particular note in this trial, nearly 20% patients had received tamoxifen prior in the adjuvant setting, although had ceased more than a year (median 3 years) prior to the development of metastatic disease; in this subgroup, re-treatment with tamoxifen had a low response rate of 8% compared with a 32% response rate with letrozole. The improvements in clinical efficacy for letrozole resulted in an early improvement in survival during the first 2 years, with overall 64% of patients treated with letrozole alive at 2 years compared with 58% treated with tamoxifen (p = 0.02) (25), although with a longer follow-up this difference was lost. The explanation for this may relate to the high number (>50%) of patients who prospectively crossed over to the alternate treatment at the time of progression, as significantly more patients benefited from second-line letrozole after progression on tamoxifen than from second-line tamoxifen after letrozole. Again, there were no significant differences in toxicity between the two treatments.

Finally, a large European study in 383 patients has compared the efficacy and tolerability of the steroidal aromatase inactivator exemestane with tamoxifen as first-line therapy (26). After a median follow-up of 29 months, there was an improvement in progression-free survival from 5.8 months for tamoxifen to 9.9 months for exemestane (HR 0.84, p = 0.028 by Wilcoxon sensitivity test). There was a significantly higher objective response rate (ORR) with exemestane than tamoxifen (46% vs. 31%, ORR 1.85, p = 0.005). Likewise the clinical benefit rate was significantly higher (66% vs. 49%). Both treatments were well tolerated, with more grade 1 myalgia in the exemestane treated group, and more grade 2 edema, grade 1 hot flashes, vaginal bleeding, and sweating in the tamoxifen group.

Thus, the available data from the four RCTs of the inhibitors in advanced disease suggest consistent improved efficacy over tamoxifen, and as such all are approved as first-line endocrine therapy for post-menopausal women with ER-positive advanced breast cancer, especially where prior adjuvant endocrine therapy was with tamoxifen. Since 2001, the third-generation AIs have become the standard of care as first-line endocrine therapy in this setting.

Tolerability in Advanced Disease

All the third-generation AIs are in general very well tolerated with a remarkably low incidence of serious short-term side effects, reflecting the extreme specificity of their action. The commonest include hot flashes, vaginal dryness, musculoskeletal stiffness/pain and headache, but are usually mild. Comparative trials in general show these to be very similar in nature and frequency to those of tamoxifen, and less troublesome than with the progestins. A better indication of the drug-specific side effects, particularly the long-term effects of AIs on bone and cognition over many years, has come from large-scale adjuvant trials. Furthermore, unlike the advanced breast cancer studies these adjuvant trials are not confounded by tumour-related symptoms and have reported that patients treated with AIs had a significantly lower incidence of hot flashes, vaginal bleeding, vaginal discharge, weight gain, and venous thromboembolism than with tamoxifen. However, musculoskeletal symptoms and fractures were more common than with tamoxifen.

Comparisons Between Different Third-Generation AIs in Advanced Disease

Letrozole achieved greater aromatase inhibition than anastrozole in a cross-over pharmacodynamic trial (27), and the clinical data for its superiority over tamoxifen in advanced disease are more solid. Preliminary data from a comparative trial of these two inhibitors in advanced breast cancer after tamoxifen are confusing, with letrozole achieving significantly more regressions overall than anastrozole, but not in the key subgroup with known ER-positive tumours (28). Overall current clinical evidence suggests that there are unlikely to be major direct clinical differences among the different AIs in advanced disease. There are no comparative data for exemestane with anastrozole or letrozole, although as discussed below further responses have been reported for this drug and the second-generation inhibitor formestane in patients relapsing after anastrozole, letrozole, or the other non-steroidal inhibitors suggesting a partial non-cross resistance (29,30).

POSTMENOPAUSAL SECOND-LINE TREATMENT OPTIONS POST AIS

It has become important to develop effective endocrine therapies that will work following non-steroidal AIs, and to date clinical options have included treatment with tamoxifen (especially if this had not been used prior to the AI), use of the steroidal aromatase inactivator exemestane based on phase II data suggesting non-cross resistance), or the ER downregulator fulvestrant based on its novel endocrine mechanism of action. Likewise, other endocrine approaches including progestins, corticosteroids, oestrogens, and inhibitors of androgen biosyntheses are being evaluated. Evidence for each of these seven approaches of further endocrine therapies in advanced disease is reviewed below.

Tamoxifen Following Prior Non-Steroidal AIs

There are few prospective data to show the true efficacy of tamoxifen in those who had progressed on a non-steroidal AI (i.e., anastrozole or letrozole). The largest available data come from the letrozole versus tamoxifen study where over 50% of the patients prospectively crossed over to an alternative treatment at the time of progression (25). Median overall survival from the date of cross-over was 19 months for patients who crossed to second-line tamoxifen, compared with 31 months for patients who crossed to second-line letrozole. The only other data come from retrospective questionnaire data from the combined analysis of the two international phase III anastrozole versus tamoxifen TARGET trials (21,22). This analysis suggested that of the 119 patients who went on to receive tamoxifen following progression on anastrozole, 58 (49%) derived clinical benefit and 12 (10%) had an objective response (31). A subsequent double-blind crossover study by the Swiss centres in the TARGET trial (SAKK 21/95 sub-trial) further investigated the clinical impact of the sequence anastrozole followed by tamoxifen, and reported that 8 of the 16 (50%) derived clinical benefit from tamoxifen (32). Thus, tamoxifen may have some efficacy as second-line therapy after AI therapy. However, data are sparse to confidently determine the optimal sequence. Furthermore, preclinical studies (discussed below) suggest that tamoxifen may be an agonist in cells resistance to long-term oestrogen deprivation (LTED), and more effective endocrine/signalling strategies may exist for use following failure of first-line AI therapy.

While the clinical data with the third-generation AIs suggest they are more effective if given as first-line therapy for advanced breast cancer; they are more expensive and in some health-care systems will only gain greater acceptance if they can also demonstrate cost effectiveness. Life table analyses have been used to compare the costs and benefits of treating post-menopausal women with advanced breast cancer with the first-line AI letrozole with the option of second-line tamoxifen, compared with first-line use with tamoxifen with the option of second-line letrozole. The results of a U.K.-based analysis showed that the mean cost of providing first- and second-line hormonal therapy was £4765 if letrozole was first-line therapy, compared with £3418 if tamoxifen was provided first (a difference of £1347) (33). However, patients who received letrozole as first-line therapy gained an additional 0.228 life years, or 0.158 quality-adjusted life years (QALYs). In public-health care terms, these values were highly cost effective compared with many other generally accepted medical treatments.

Exemestane Following Prior Non-Steroidal AI

Steroidal AIs such as exemestane have an androgen structure and compete with the aromatase substrate androstenedione. They inactivate aromatase by irreversibly binding to its catalytic site, and additional aromatase must be produced before oestrogen biosynthesis can resume. This is in contrast with non-steroidal AIs that reversibly interact with the cytochrome P450 moiety of aromatase, and the interference with oestrogen biosynthesis is dependent on the continued presence of the non-steroidal agent (34). Preliminary data suggest that there may be a lack of cross resistance between steroidal AIs and non-steroidal AIs, and that steroidal AIs may be an option in non-steroidal AI-resistant disease (35–38).

In a phase II, open-label, multinational trial, 24% of patients overall achieved clinical benefit with exemestane following either aminoglutethimide (n = 136) or non-steroidal AI treatment (n = 105) (37). The objective response and clinical benefit rates were 8% and 27% respectively, for patients who received prior aminoglutethimide. The corresponding rates were 5% and 20% respectively, for those who had previously received non-steroidal AIs. A separate retrospective analysis of 96 patients receiving exemestane, 89 of whom had received prior non-steroidal AIs, reported that 37 (39%) patients experienced clinical benefit with exemestane (38).

Fulvestrant Following Prior Endocrine Therapy

Fulvestrant (Faslodex) is a novel type of ER antagonist that unlike tamoxifen, has no known agonist effects (39,40). Fulvestrant binds to the ER, but due to its steroidal structure and long side-chain, induces a different conformational shape with the receptor to that achieved by the non-steroidal anti-oestrogen tamoxifen. Because of this, fulvestrant prevents ER dimerisation and leads to the rapid degradation of the fulvestrant–ER complex, producing the loss of cellular ER. Thus fulvestrant, unlike

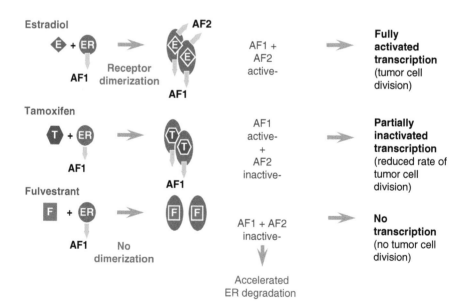

FIGURE 4 Mechanism of action of oestradiol, tamoxifen, and fulvestrant on oestrogen receptor dimerisation and transcription of oestrogen-regulated genes.

tamoxifen, inhibits ER binding with DNA and produces abrogation of oestrogen-sensitive gene transcription (41) (Fig. 4). It has been shown that due to its unique mechanism of action, fulvestrant delays the emergence of acquired resistance compared with tamoxifen in an MCF-7 hormone-sensitive xenograft model (42). The lack of agonist effects means that fulvestrant did not support the growth of tumours that became resistant to, and subsequently stimulated by, tamoxifen.

Fulvestrant entered clinical trials after preclinical studies suggested it was active in tamoxifen-resistant cancer (43). An initial phase II study analysing the pharmacokinetic, pharmacological, and anti-tumour effects of fulvestrant demonstrated that fulvestrant was not cross-resistant with tamoxifen in the clinical setting and was well tolerated (44). Subsequent two large phase III trials (45,46) compared fulvestrant with anastrozole in postmenopausal women with locally advanced or metastatic breast carcinoma who had progressed after prior endocrine therapy, and these trials were prospectively designed to allow a combined analysis of data (47). At a median follow-up of 15.1 months, fulvestrant was at least as effective as anastrozole in terms of median TTP (5.5 months vs. 4.1 months, respectively) and objective response (19% vs. 17%, respectively) (47). A subsequent survival analysis after a median follow-up of 27 months has shown there was no significant difference in the median time to death between fulvestrant and anastrozole (27.4 months vs. 27.7 months, respectively) (48). Thus fulvestrant is therefore unique among ER antagonists as it is effective in tamoxifen-resistant disease.

Evidence for clinical efficacy of fulvestrant after prior non-steroidal AI therapy came from several phase II studies which showed that fulvestrant produced clinical benefit in 20–52% patients who had received, and had progressed on, prior treatment with tamoxifen and a non-steroidal AI (49–53) (Table 4). On the basis of these findings, several phase III clinical trials of fulvestrant investigated the role of fulvestrant

TABLE 4 Clinical Benefit Rates with Fulvestrant Following Disease Progression on Prior Endocrine Therapy, Including Aromatase Inhibitors (AIs)

Study	Treatment	Prior treatment	No. of patients	Clinical benefit[a] (%)
Perey et al. 2004 (49)	Fulvestrant (3rd line)	Includes tamoxifen and AIs	67	28
Ingle et al. 2004 (50)	Fulvestrant (2nd and 3rd line)	Includes AIs	77	32
Petruzelka & Zimovjanova 2003 (51)	Fulvestrant (2nd to 5th line)	Includes non-steroidal AIs, adjuvant tamoxifen, goserelin formestane	44	52
Franco et al., 2003 (52)	Fulvestrant (mean prior endocrine therapies = 3.4)	Includes non-steroidal AIs, tamoxifen, toremifene, megestrol acetate, exemestane, androgens, high-dose oestrogens	42	20
Steger et al. 2005 (53)	Fulvestrant (2nd to 5th line)	Includes non-steroidal AIs, tamoxifen, exemestane, goserelin, formestane	88	44

[a]Clinical benefit includes patients who had a complete response, partial response, or stable disease for >24 weeks.

in breast cancer therapy either following prior non-steroidal AI treatment, or in combination with AIs (to maintain low estradiol levels) as first-line therapy. The comparator for several of these studies is the steroidal aromatase inactivator, exemestane, which in phase II studies has shown some efficacy following progression on non-steroidal AIs. The Evaluation of Faslodex vs Exemestane Clinical Trial (EFECT) assessed the efficacy of fulvestrant vs. exemestane in patients who had progressed on treatment with non-steroidal AIs, and found no significant difference in clinical effectiveness between either approaches, with a clinical benefit rate of 32.2 % and 31.5% respectively (54). Both treatments were well tolerated with no significant differences observed in adverse events or quality of life. In the Fulvestrant and Anastrozole in Combination Trial (FACT) trial, the combination of fulvestrant plus anastrozole did not improve the TTP compared with anastrozole alone in the first-line setting (55). However, the results of two completed trials (SoFEA and SWOG-226) are awaited, which have further evaluated the potential benefit of combined fulvestrant and AIs in advanced disease, including in the second-line setting.

Finally, recent studies have suggested that the most effective dose for fulvestrant in advanced disease may be 500 mg intramuscular given monthly after a loading dose schedule. The FIRST study established that the 500-mg dosing regimen of fulvestrant when used in the first-line setting resulted in a similar clinical benefit rate (72% vs. 67%), yet a significantly longer TTP compared with anastrozole (HR 0.63, p = 0.049) (56). The CONFIRM study subsequently established that fulvestrant 500 mg had a superior TTP compared with the previously approved 250 mg dose (median 6.5 vs. 5.5 months, p = 0.006) (57), leading to the recent approval by the U.S. Food and Drug Administration of this 500-mg monthly dosing regimen for fulvestrant.

Progestogens

Synthetic progestogens/androgens, such as medroxyprogesterone (MPA) (usually 500–1500 mg/day p.o.) and MA (100–200 mg/day p.o.), have been used in the treatment of advanced breast cancer although their main benefit is the relief of metastatic bone pain. Their mechanism of action is unclear but may be a combination of adrenal and/or gonadal suppression, "anti-oestrogenic" effects on oestradiol dehydrogenase and the oestrogen receptor and direct effects through the progesterone receptor. In doses sufficient to be effective, they cause steroidogenic side effects such as weight gain and cardiovascular and thromboembolic complications in most patients. The results of trials evaluating the new generation of AIs have now clearly shown them to be more effective and less toxic than MA or MPA and these agents have now largely been replaced as second-line therapy for treatment of advanced breast cancer.

Androgens and Corticosteroids

Androgens are used rarely for the treatment of advanced breast cancer due to side effects but the mechanism of action probably overlaps that of progestogens. Corticosteroids have been used although less than 10% of patients with advanced breast cancer respond. However, corticosteroids particularly at higher doses are often effective at controlling symptoms, particularly those associated with inflammation, local oedema, and pain. Dexamethasone at 8 mg twice a day for short periods is very effective in controlling the symptoms of neurological metastases, especially for raised intracranial pressure and cord compression during radiotherapy treatment.

Oestrogens

High-dose oestrogen therapy was used in the treatment of advanced breast cancer until the introduction of tamoxifen in the 1970s, which was shown to be both effective and better tolerated. A recent phase II trial has explored the use of high-dose oestrogen therapy in highly refractory advanced breast cancer (58), using diethylstilbestrol 15 mg/day or oestradiol 30 mg/day. The clinical benefit rate was 40% with a median duration of response of 9 months. Another trial compared low dose oestradiol 6 mg/day with high dose 30 mg/day (59) in women with AI resistant advanced breast cancer. The lower dose was found to be equally as effective as the higher dose with a clinical benefit rate of 29% but with fewer side effects.

Abiraterone
Abiraterone acetate, an inhibitor of cytochrome P 17 is a key enzyme in androgen and oestrogen biosynthesis. Abiraterone has previously shown activity in castration-resistant prostate cancer which is thought to remain driven by ligand dependent androgen receptor (AR) signalling (60). Around 60–70% of breast cancers are thought to be AR positive; however, the role of the androgen receptor in breast cancer is yet to be understood completely. A phase I study of abiraterone in breast cancer patients is currently underway.

ENDOCRINE THERAPY FOR PREMENOPAUSAL WITH ADVANCED BREAST CANCER
For women with ER-positive MBC who are still premenopausal when they develop advanced disease, the available endocrine therapy options include ovarian abla-tion [via surgery, radiotherapy, or luteinising hormone-releasing hormone ana-logues (LHRHa)], tamoxifen, or a combination of ovarian ablation with tamoxifen or with an AI (Fig. 2). While oophorectomy and ovarian irradiation induce perma-nent ovarian ablation, the most widely used method involves using an LHRHa to induce a potentially reversible medical ovarian ablation. Goserelin (Zoladex) is the most widely used LHRHa in ER-positive advanced disease, and is administered as a 3.6 mg subcutaneous monthly depot injection. The most common side effects are those of oestrogen suppression including hot flushes and less frequently reduced libido, vaginal dryness, and headache, and a local injection is well tolerated. A pooled analysis of several phase II studies that included 228 pre- and peri-meno-pausal women with advanced breast cancer showed that 36% had an objective response to goserelin, with an additional 50% showing stabilisation of their disease (61). The median duration of response was 10 months, with an overall sur-vival of 26 months. These results were comparable to previously published data with either tamoxifen or surgical oophorectomy in this group of premenopausal patients with advanced disease (62).

Combined therapy of goserelin plus tamoxifen has been compared with goser-lin alone as first-line endocrine therapy in 318 pre- and peri-menopausal women with advanced breast cancer (63). In this study objective response rates were statistically similar (38% for goserelin plus tamoxifen, 31% for goserelin), but there was a signifi-cant improvement in median time to disease progression (6.5 months vs. 5.3 months). Overall survival was similar (32 months vs. 29 months), and there was no difference in tolerability for the combination. In another trial 161 premenopausal patients with advanced breast cancer were randomly assigned to treatment with the LHRHa buserelin, tamoxifen, or both (64). Combined treatment with buserelin and tamoxifen was superior to treatment with buserelin or tamoxifen alone by ORR (48% vs. 34% and 28%, respectively), median progression-free survival (9.7 months vs. 6.3 months and 5.6 months respectively, p = 0.03), and overall survival (3.7 years vs. 2.5 years and 2.9 years respectively, p = 0.01). Subsequently, there was a meta-analysis of four ran-domised trials of LHRHa + tamoxifen vs. LHRHa alone, and significant benefits were found for the combination in terms of improved ORR (39% vs. 30%, p = 0.03), median progression-free survival (8.7 months vs. 5.4 months, HR 1.31, p < 0.001), and most importantly overall survival (34.8 months vs. 30.0 months, p = 0.02) (65). As such, standard practice is now to recommend LHRHa plus tamoxifen as first-line endocrine therapy in hormone-sensitive advanced breast cancer (66).

Several unanswered questions remain in the endocrine therapy of premeno-pausal patients. In particular, it is unclear whether complete oestrogen suppression using LHRHa and an aromatase inhibitor will be superior to using LHRHa plus tamoxifen as first-line endocrine therapy for advanced disease. Given the superiority of AI over tamoxifen in postmenopausal women, it is not unreasonable to suppose that LHRHa plus AI could further enhance endocrine responsiveness over LHRHa plus tamoxifen; however, there are no randomised data yet to answer this, and there are concerns that the hormonal toxicities of maximal oestrogen blockade might out-weigh the benefits. Likewise it is unclear whether sequential oestrogen suppression might not be a better long-term strategy compared with maximal oestrogen suppres-sion up-front. In the past, further clinical benefit has been reported for premeno-pausal women with advanced breast cancer initially treated with goserelin, and then at progression given an AI combined with goserelin (67). New randomised trials will be required to see whether a sequential approach of LHRHa alone or LHRHa plus tamoxifen followed by switch at progression to LHRHA plus AI would produce over-all greater disease control and improved survival than using LHRHa plus AI upfront. Unfortunately, the relatively small number of suitable patients for such trials makes them difficult to undertake, and answers to these clinical questions are unlikely to occur quickly.

OVERCOMING ENDOCRINE RESISTANCE

Despite adjuvant chemotherapy and endocrine therapy a proportion of patients with ER-positive breast cancer will still relapse and ultimately die of the disease. Further developments depend on finding methods to prevent and overcome resistance to endocrine therapy. Endocrine resistance may occur both initially (*de novo*) or subse-quently (acquired) in ER-positive breast cancer. Laboratory studies using ER-positive breast cancer cells exposed to LTED (i.e. analogous to AI use) or tamoxifen therapy have demonstrated that various growth factor pathways and oncogenes involved in the signal transduction cascade become activated and utilised by breast cancer cells to bypass normal endocrine responsiveness (68–70). Exposure to LTED and subse-quent development of acquired resistance, may be accompanied by adaptive increases in ER gene expression and intercellular signalling resulting in hypersensitivity to low oestradiol levels (71–74)

There is evidence for increased cross-talk between various growth factor recep-tor signalling pathways and ER at the time of relapse on LTED, with ER becoming activated and supersensitised by a number of different intracellular kinases, includ-ing mitogen-activated protein kinases (MAPKs), epidermal growth factor receptor (EGFR)/human epidermal growth factor receptor (HER1) and HER2/HER3 signal-ling, and the insulin-like growth factor (IGFR)/Akt pathway (Fig.5) (74–77). As such, these various signaling pathways, including activated ER itself have become the tar-gets for pharmacological intervention (78). Approaches used have included maximal blockade of ER signalling as with fulvestrant, combining endocrine therapy with agents targeted against the HER family of growth factor receptors and combinations with drugs that target downstream signalling pathways. A variety of agents have been developed including monoclonal antibodies and tyrosine kinase inhibitors (TKIs) which target key proteins along signal transduction cascades with the aim of blocking tumour cell access to pathways that facilitate resistance to hormone therapy. Clinically, trials utilising these approaches in advanced breast cancer have yielded mixed results thus far (Table 5) (79–85).

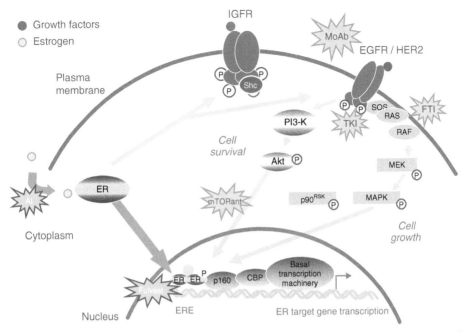

FIGURE 5 A schematic diagram of molecular pathways for endocrine resistance involving "cross-talk" between ER and growth factor receptor signalling, with an enhanced activation of ER/co-activator phosphorylation & gene transcription via the PI3-kinase/Akt cell survival pathway and Ras/Raf/mitogen-activated protein kinase (MAPK) cell growth pathway. Site of action for signal transduction inhibitors (e.g., MoAB, monoclonal antibodies to growth factor receptors; TKI, tyrosine kinase inhibitors; FTIs, farnesyl transferase inhibitors; mTORant, mammalian target of rapamycin antagonists) that are being studied in combination with endocrine agents (AIs or fulvestrant) in an attempt to produce maximal endocrine blockade.

Based on preclinical evidence that endocrine resistance can be delayed by the use of EGFR/HER1 inhibition in vitro (86) a number of studies have explored the use of the small-molecule TKI of EGFR/HER1, gefitinib (79,80). However, the benefits were relatively modest (Table 5) with no improvements in objective response rates. These studies did not pre-select patients with EGFR/HER1 overexpression and it is possible that with a relatively biologically heterogeneous trial population the true benefits may be underestimated.

Enhanced expression of the HER2 and subsequent downstream MAPK activation has been found in breast cancer cells that become resistant to endocrine therapy. A randomised phase II trial (TAnDEM) compared the monoclonal antibody against HER2 trastuzumab plus anastrazole versus anastrazole alone in ER-positive HER2-positive advanced breast cancer, and found improved progression-free survival (PFS) from 2.4 to 4.8 months in favour of the combination arm (81). Similarly, dual targeting of EGFR and HER2 with the orally active small-molecule TKI, lapatanib, has been assessed in combination with endocrine therapy in the first-line treatment of ER-positive MBC in a trial in over 1200 patients. The results of the large phase III trial EGF30008 demonstrated a significantly improved PFS in patients with ER-positive HER2-positive tumours from 3 months in the letrozole alone arm to 8.2 months with the combination (p = 0.019), with an associated improvement in clinical benefit rates from 29% to 48% (82). Interestingly, although no improvement in PFS was observed for the combination arm in the ER-positive HER2-negative population, overall there did appear to be a trend for improvement with the combination arm in HER2-negative

TABLE 5 Results from Randomised Trials of Combinations of Endocrine Therapies and Targeted Agents in Metastatic Breast Cancer

Author (ref)	N=	Population	Intervention	Progression-free survival in months		Clinical benefit Rate (%)	
				Endocrine alone	Combination	Endocrine alone	Combination
Osborne et al. (79)	290	ER/PgR+	Tamoxifen +/- gefitinib	8.8	10.9	45.5	50.5
Cristofanili et al. (80)	94	ER/PgR+	Anastrazole +/- gefitinib	8.2	14.5	34	49
Kaufman et al. (81)	208	HER2+ER/PgR+	Anastrazole +/- trastuzumab	2.4	4.8	27.9	42.7
Johnston et al. (82)	952	ER/PgR+HER2-	Letrozole +/- lapatanib	<6-m tam[a] 3.1	8.3	32	44
				>6-m tam[b] 15	3		
Baselga et al. (83)	219	ER/PgR+HER2+	Letrozole +/- temsirolimus	11.6	14.7	64	62
	92	ER/PgR+			8.2	29	48
					13.2	45	40
Chow et al. (84)	992	ER/PgR+	Letrozole +/- temsirolimus	9.2	9.2	43	40
Bachelot et al. (85)	111	ER+	Tamoxifen +/- everolimus	4.5	8.6	42	61

[a]Less than 6 months since prior adjuvant tamoxifen.
[b]Greater than 6 months since prior adjuvant tamoxifen.

patients who were classified as endocrine resistant (i.e., they had relapsed during adjuvant tamoxifen, or within less than 6 months since completion of adjuvant tamoxifen). This suggests that resistance to prior endocrine therapy may be an important determinant of who is most likely to benefit from combined targeted and endocrine therapy combinations.

Downstream from the cell surface growth factor receptors, pathways such as the phosphoinositide-3 kinase (PI3K)/Akt/mammalian target of rapamycin (mTOR) have also been targeted as a therapeutic means to overcome endocrine resistance. The mTOR inhibitor temsirolimus has been combined with letrozole in the advanced setting (Table 4), but despite initial promising results from a small phase II study (83) this approach failed to demonstrate any significant benefit for the combination in the larger definitive phase III study (84). This may, in part, be due to a failure to identify patients in whom tumours depend on PI3K/mTOR activation, or due to the activation of compensatory feedback loops in the Akt pathway that exist following mTOR blockade. Despite these negative data, a more recent phase II study of the mTOR antagonist everolimus given in combination with tamoxifen in 111 patients with advanced ER-positive metastatic disease who had received prior AI therapy suggested substantially greater efficacy than tamoxifen alone (TAMRAD) (85). Time to disease progression was significantly prolonged from a median of 4.5 to 8.6 months (HR 0.53, p = 0.0026), with clinical benefit rate improving from 41% to 62% (p = 0.045). A subsequent analysis suggested that the majority of this benefit was seen in those patients with acquired secondary resistance, rather than those with primary de-novo resistance. This was further confirmed in the BOLERO-II trial (87), which assessed the benefit of adding everolimus to exemestane following prior therapy with a non-steroidal aromatase inhibitor, in particular when most patients (>80%) had demonstrated responsiveness to their previous aromatase inhibitor in the metastatic setting prior to subsequent progression with acquired resistance. The results showed a highly significant 2.6-fold prolongation in median PFS (10.6 months versus 4.1 months), resulting in a 64% risk reduction of progression or death (HR 0.36), suggesting that this could be a very effective new therapeutic endocrine strategy in advanced disease.

Further progress in this field will depend on understanding the various mechanisms behind the development of endocrine resistance, and the compensatory pathways that emerge in individual patients at any one particular time. Numerous studies are underway with various novel therapies combined with endocrine therapy, including insulin-like growth factor receptor antibodies or TKIs, PI3K/Akt inhibitors, cyclin-dependent kinase inhibitors, angiogenesis inhibitors, fibroblast growth factor receptor inhibitors, src inhibitors, and histone deacetylase (HDAC) inhibitors. The identification of the key pathways and relevant biomarkers predictive of response to these various signalling therapies in endocrine resistant ER-positive breast cancer is crucial to the success of these trials, and it is encouraging that many of these studies are now selecting patients for these trials based on the expression of the relevant marker in tumour tissue. This approach should allow a better selection of patients for treatment with specific combinations of targeted and endocrine therapies, and maximise the chance of success to this novel strategy to improve on the benefit of endocrine therapy in advanced disease.

CONCLUSION: NEW OPPORTUNITIES FOR ENDOCRINE THERAPY IN ADVANCED DISEASE

Endocrine therapy is an important part of the systemic treatment for women with hormone-sensitive advanced/MBC. Appropriate selection of patients for this approach is crucial, and it is well recognised that substantial clinical benefit in both pre- and postmenopausal women can be achieved by use of such therapies ahead of the need for chemotherapy. AIs have had a major impact on the treatment of breast cancer over the last decade, and shown substantial improvements over the previous standard of care tamoxifen. As these treatments now move into the adjuvant scenario, there is an urgent need to establish which endocrine strategies are still effective following disease progression on oestrogen deprivation approaches. Progress in this area critically depends on understanding mechanisms of resistance to AIs, and may involve utilising novel approaches such as fulvestrant or various signal transduction inhibitors to combat resistance pathways and block cross-talk. Many studies in advanced disease have started recently, and over the next few years we should learn whether such an approach will produce significant further gains in clinical benefit from endocrine therapy.

REFERENCES

1. Quinn MJ, Babb P, Brock A, et al. Cancer Trends in England and Wales 1950-1999. London: Studies on Medical Populations Subjects No. 66. The Stationery Office, 2001.
2. Powles TJ, Hickish T, Kanis JA, Tidy A, Ashley S. Effect of tamoxifen on bone mineral density measured by dual-energy x-ray absorptiometry in healthy premenopausal and postmenopausal women. J Clin Oncol 1996; 14: 78–84.
3. Fisher B, Constantino JP, Wickerham DL, et al. Tamoxifen for prevenation of breast cancer: report of the National Surgical Adjuvant Breast and Bowel Project P-1 Study. J Natl Cancer Inst 1998; 90: 1371–88.
4. Longcope C, Baker R, Johnston CC Jr. Androgen and estrogen metabolism: relationship to obesity. Metabolism 1986; 35: 235–7.
5. Lamb HM, Adkins JC. Letrozole. A review of its use in postmenopausal women with advanced breast cancer. Drugs 1998; 56: 1125–40.
6. Wiseman LR, Adkins JC. Anastrozole. A review of its use in the management of postmenopausal women with advanced breast cancer. Drugs Aging 1998; 13: 321–32.
7. Lonning PE. Pharmacological profiles of exemestane and formestane, steroidal aromatase inhibitors used for treatment of postmenopausal breast cancer. Breast Cancer Res Treat 1998; 49(Suppl 1):S45–52; discussion S73–7.
8. Buzdar A, Jonat W, Howell A, et al. Anastrozole, a potent and selective aromatase inhibitor, versus megestrol acetate in postmenopausal women with advanced breast cancer: results of overview analysis of two phase III trials. Arimidex Study Group. J Clin Oncol 1996; 14: 2000–11.
9. Buzdar AU, Jonat W, Howell A, et al. Anastrozole versus megestrol acetate in the treatment of postmenopausal women with advanced breast carcinoma. Cancer 1998; 83: 1142–52.
10. Dombernowsky P, Smith I, Falkson G, et al. Letrozole, a new oral aromatase inhibitor for advanced breast cancer: double-blind randomized trial showing a dose effect and improved efficacy and tolerability compared with megestrol acetate. J Clin Oncol 1998; 16: 453–61.
11. Kaufmann M, Bajetta E, Dirix LY, et al. Exemestane is superior to megestrol acetate after tamoxifen failure in postmenopausal women with advanced breast cancer: results of a phase III randomized double-blind trial. The Exemestane Study Group. J Clin Oncol 2000; 18: 1399–411.
12. Buzdar A, Douma N, Davidson N, et al. Phase III, multicenter, double-blind, randomized study of letrozole, an aromatase inhibitor, for advanced breast cancer versus megestrol acetate. J Clin Oncol 2001; 19: 3357–66.
13. Goss PE, Winer EP, Tannock IF, Schwartz LH. Randomized phase III trial comparing the new potent and selective third-generation aromatase inhibitor vorozole with megestrol acetate in postmenopausal advanced breast cancer patients. J Clin Oncol 1999; 17: 52–63.
14. Thurlimann B, Castiglione M, Hsu-Schmitz SF, et al. Formestane versus megestrol acetate in postmenopausal breast cancer patients after failure of tamoxifen: a phase III prospective randomised cross over trial of second-line hormonal treatment (SAKK 20/90). Swiss Group for Clinical Cancer Research (SAKK). Eur J Cancer 1997; 33: 1017–24.

15. Buzdar AU, Smith R, Vogel C, et al. Fadrozole HCl (CGS-16949A) versus megestrol acetate treatment of postmenopausal patients with metastatic breast carcinoma: results of two randomized double blind controlled multi-institutional trials. Cancer 1996; 77: 2503–13.
16. Hamilton A, Piccart M. The third-generation non-steroidal aromatase inhibitors: a review of their clinical benefits in the second-line hormonal treatment of advanced breast cancer. Ann Oncol 1999; 10: 377–84.
17. Smith IE, Harris AL, Morgan M, et al. Tamoxifen versus aminoglutethimide in advanced breast carcinoma: a randomised cross-over trial. Br Med J 1981; 283: 1432–4.
18. Falkson CI, Falkson HC. A randomised study of CGS 16949A (fadrozole) versus tamoxifen in previously untreated postmenopausal patients with metastatic breast cancer. Ann Oncol 1996; 7: 465–9.
19. Thurlimann B, Beretta K, Bacchi M, et al. First-line fadrozole HCl (CGS 16949A) versus tamoxifen in postmenopausal women with advanced breast cancer. Prospective randomised trial of the Swiss Group for Clinical Cancer Research SAKK 20/88. Ann Oncol 1996; 7: 471–9.
20. Johnston SRD. Acquired tamoxifen resistance in human breast cancer - potential mechanisms and clinical implications. Anti Cancer Drugs 1997; 8: 911–30.
21. Nabholtz JM, Buzdar A, Pollak M, et al. Anastrozole is superior to tamoxifen as first-line therapy for advanced breast carcinoma in postmenopausal women: results of a North American multicenter randomized trial. J Clin Oncol 2000; 18: 3758–67.
22. Bonneterre J, Thurlimann B, Robertson JFR, et al. Anastrozole versus tamoxifen as first-line therapy for advanced breast cancer in 668 postmenopausal women: results of the Tamoxifen or Arimidex Randomized Group Efficacy and Tolerability Study. J Clin Oncol 2000; 18: 3748–57
23. Bonneterre J, Buzdar A, Nabholtz JM, et al. Anastrozole is superior to tamoxifen as first-line therapy in hormone-receptor positive advanced breast carcinoma. Cancer 2001; 92: 2247–58.
24. Mouridsen H, Gershanovich M, Sun Y, et al. Superior efficacy of letrozole versus tamoxifen as first-line therapy for postmenopausal women with advanced breast cancer: results of a phase III study of the International Letrozole Breast Cancer Group. J Clin Oncol 2001; 19: 2596–606.
25. Mouridsen H, Gershanovich M, Sun Y, et al. Phase III study of letrozole versus tamoxifen as first—line therapy of advanced breast cancer in postmenopausal women: analysis of survival and update of efficacy from the International Letrozole Breast Cancer Group. J Clin Oncol 2003; 21: 2101–9.
26. Paridaens R, Therasse P, Dirix L, et al. First-line treatment for metastatic breast cancer with exemestane or tamoxifen in post-menopausal patients; a randomized phase III trial of the EORTC Breast Group. Proc Am Soc Clin Oncol 2004; 23: Abstract 515.
27. Geisler J, Haynes B, Anker G, Dowsett M, Lonning PE. Influence of letrozole and anastrozole on total body aromatization and plasma estrogen levels in postmenopausal breast cancer patients evaluated in a randomized, cross-over study. J Clin Oncol 2002; 20: 751–7.
28. Rose C, Vtoraya O, Pluzanska A, et al. An open randomised trial of second-line endocrine therapy in advanced breast cancer: comparison of the aromatase inhibitors letrozole and anastrozole. Eur J Cancer 2003; 39: 2318–27.
29. Carlini P, Frassoldati A, De Marco S, et al. Formestane, a steroidal aromatase inhibitor after failure of non-steroidal aromatase inhibitors (anastrozole and letrozole): is a clinical benefit still achievable? Ann Oncol 2001; 12: 1539–43.
30. Lonning PE, Bajetta E, Murray R, et al. Activity of exemestane in metastatic breast cancer after failure of nonsteroidal aromatase inhibitors: a phase II trial. J Clin Oncol 2000; 18: 2234–44.
31. Thurlimann B, Robertson JRF, Nabholtz JM, Buzdar A, Bonneterre J. Efficacy of tamoxifen following anastrozole compared with anastrozole following tamoxifen as first-line treatment for advanced breast cancer in post-menopausal women. Eur J Cancer 2003; 39: 2310–17.
32. Thurlimann B, Hess D, Koberle D, et al. Anastrozole versus tamoxifen as first-line therapy in post-menopausal women with advanced breast cancer; results of the double-blind cross-over SAKK trial 21/95 – a sub study of the TARGET (Tamoxifen or Arimidex Randomised Group Efficacy and Tolerability) trial. Breast Cancer Res Treat 2004; 85: 247–54.

33. Karnon JR, Johnston SRD, Jones T, Glendenning A. A trial based economic evaluation of first-line letrozole followed by second-line tamoxifen versus first-line tamoxifen followed by second-line letrozole for post-menopausal advanced breast cancer. Ann Oncol 2003; 14: 1629–33.
34. Campos SM. Aromatase inhibitors for breast cancer in postmenopausal women. Oncologist 2004; 9: 126–36.
35. Bertelli G, Garrone O, Merlano M. Sequential use of aromatase inactivators and inhibitors in advanced breast cancer. Proc Am Soc Clin Oncol 2002; 21: 60a Abstract 238.
36. Carlini P, Michelotti A, Giannarelli D, et al. Exemestane (EXE) is an effective 3rd line hormonal therapy for postmenopausal metastatic breast cancer (MBC) patients (pts) pretreated with 3rd generation non steroidal aromatase inhibitors (nSAI). Ann Oncol 2002; 13(Suppl 5): 48.
37. Lønning PE, Bajetta E, Murray R, et al. Activity of exemestane in metastatic breast cancer after failure of nonsteroidal aromatase inhibitors: a phase II trial. J Clin Oncol 2000; 18: 2234–44.
38. Fernie NL, Zekri JM, Leonard RCF, Coleman RE, Cameron DA. Exemestane in metastatic breast cancer: effective therapy after 3rd generation aromatase inhibitor failure. Breast Cancer Res Treat 2003; 82(Suppl 1): S104 Abstract 435.
39. Robertson JF, Nicholson RI, Bundred NJ, et al. Comparison of the short-term biological effects of 7alpha-[9-(4,4,5,5,5-pentafluoropentylsulfinyl)-nonyl]estra-1,3,5, (10)-triene-3, 17beta-diol (Faslodex) versus tamoxifen in postmenopausal women with primary breast cancer. Cancer Res 2001; 61: 6739–46.
40. Wakeling AE, Dukes M, Bowler J. A potent specific pure antiestrogen with clinical potential. Cancer Res 1991; 51: 3867–73.
41. Dauvois S, White R, Parker MG. The antiestrogen ICI 182780 disrupts estrogen receptor nucleocytoplasmic shuttling. J Cell Sci 1993; 106: 1377–88.
42. Osborne CK, Coronado-Heinsohn EB, et al. Comparison of the effects of a pure steroidal anti-estrogen with those of tamoxifen in a model of human breast cancer. J Natl Cancer Inst 1995; 87: 746–50.
43. Hu XF, Veroni M, De Luise M, et al. Circumvention of tamoxifen resistance by the pure anti-estrogen ICI 182,780. Int J Cancer 1993; 55: 873–6.
44. Howell A, DeFriend DJ, Robertson JF, et al. Pharmacokinetics, pharmacological and anti-tumour effects of the specific anti-oestrogen ICI 182780 in women with advanced breast cancer. Br J Cancer 1996; 74: 300–8.
45. Howell A, Robertson JFR, Quaresma Albano J, et al. Fulvestrant, formerly ICI 182,780, is as effective as anastrozole in postmenopausal women with advanced breast cancer progressing after prior endocrine treatment. J Clin Oncol 2002; 20: 3396–403.
46. Osborne CK, Pippen J, Jones SE, et al. Double-blind, randomized trial comparing the efficacy and tolerability of fulvestrant versus anastrozole in postmenopausal women with advanced breast cancer progressing on prior endocrine therapy: results of a North American trial. J Clin Oncol 2002; 20: 3386–95.
47. Robertson JF, Osborne CK, Howell A, et al. Fulvestrant versus anastrozole for the treatment of advanced breast carcinoma in postmenopausal women - a prospective combined analysis of two multicenter trials. Cancer 2003; 98: 229–38.
48. Pippen J, Osborne CK, Howell A, Robertson JFR. Fulvestrant (Faslodex) versus anastrozole (Arimidex) for the treatment of advanced breast cancer: a prospective combined survival analysis of two multicenter trials. Breast Cancer Res Treat 2003; 82(Suppl 1): S101 Abstract 426.
49. Perey L, Paridaens R, Nole F, et al. Fulvestrant (Faslodex) as hormonal treatment in postmenopausal patients with advanced breast cancer progressing after treatment with tamoxifen and aromatase inhibitors – update of a phase II SAKK trial. Breast Cancer Res Treat 2004; 88(Suppl 1): S236 (A6048).
50. Ingle JN, Rowland KM, Suman VJ, et al. Evaluation of fulvestrant in women with advanced breast cancer and progression on prior aromatase inhibitor therapy: a phase II trial of the North Central Cancer Treatment Group. Breast Cancer Res Treat 2004; 88(Suppl 1): S38 Abstract 409.
51. Petruzelka L, Zimovjanova M. Fulvestrant in postmenopausal women with metastatic breast cancer progressing on prior endocrine therapy – results from an expanded access programme. Eur J Cancer 2004; (Suppl 2): 132 Abstract 264.

52. Franco S, Perez A, Tan-Chiu E, Frankel C, Vogel CL. Fulvestrant demonstrates clinical benefit in heavily pre-treated postmenopausal women with advanced breast cancer: a single-center experience. Breast Cancer Res Treat 2003; (Suppl 1): S105 Abstract 439.
53. Steger GG, Bartsch R, Wenzel C, et al. Fulvestrant in pre-treated patients with advanced breast cancer; a single-centre experience. Eur J Cancer 2005; 41: 2655–61.
54. Chia S, Gradishar W, Mauriac L, et al. Double-blind, randomized placebo controlled trial of fulvestrant compared with exemestane after prior nonsteroidal aromatase inhibitor therapy in postmenopausal women with hormone receptor-positive, advanced breast cancer: results from EFECT. J Clin Oncol 2008; 26: 1664–70.
55. Bergh J, Jonsson PE, Lidbrink E, et al. First results from FACT; an open label, randomized phase II study investigating loading dose of fulvestrant combined with anstrozole versus anastrozole at first relapse in hormone receptor positive breast cancer. San Antonio Breast Cancer Symposium, 2009.
56. Roberston J, Llombart-Cussac A, Rolski J, et al. Activity of 500mg fulvestrant versus anastrozole 1mg as first-line treatment for advanced breast cancer; results from FIRST study. J Clin Oncol 2009; 27: 4530–5.
57. DiLeo A, Jerusalem G, Petruzelka L, et al. Results of the CONFIRM phase III traisl comparing fulvestrant 250mg with fulvestrant 500mg in postmenopausal women with estrogen receptor positive advanced breast cancer. J Clin Oncol 2010; 28: 4594–600.
58. Mahtani RL, SA, Vogel CL, ed. High dose oestrogen as a salvage therapy for highly refractory metastatic breast cancer "back to the future". San Antonio Breast Cancer Symposium, 2008.
59. Ellis MJ, DF, Kommareddy A, et al. A randomised phase 2 trial of low dose (6mg daily) versus high dose (30mg daily) estradiol for patients with estrogen receptor positive aromatase inhibitor resistant advanced breast cancer. San Antonio Breast Cancer Symposium, 2008.
60. Attard G, Reid AH, Yap TA, et al. Phase I clinical trial of a selective inhibitor of CYP17, abiraterone acetate, confirms that castration-resistant prostate cancer commonly remains hormone driven. J Clin Oncol 2008; 26: 4563–71.
61. Blamey R, Jonat W, Kaufmann M, Bianco AR, Namer M. Goserelin depot in the treatment of premenopausal advanced breast cancer. Eur J Cancer 1992; 28A: 810–14.
62. Buchanan RB, Blamey R, Durrant KR, et al. A randomized comparison of tamoxifen with surgical oophorectomy in premenopausal patients with advanced breast cancer. J Clin Oncol 1986; 4: 1326–30.
63. Jonat W, Kaufmann M, Blamey R, et al. A randomised study to compare the effect of the luteinising hormone releasing hormone (LHRH) analogue goserelin with or without tamoxifen in pre- and perimenopausal patients with advanced breast cancer. Eur J Cancer 1995; 31A: 137–42.
64. Klijn JGM, Beex L, Mauriac L, et al. Combined treatment with buserelin and tamoxifen in premenopausal metastatic breast cancer: a randomized study. J Natl Cancer Inst 2000; 92: 903–11.
65. Klijn JGM, Blamey RW, Boccardo F, et al. Combined tamoxifen and Luteinizing Hormone-Releasing Hormone (LHRH) agonist versus LHRH agonist alone in premenopausal advanced breast cancer: a meta-analysis of four randomized trials. J Clin Oncol 2001; 19: 343–53.
66. Blamey R. Guidelines on endocrine therapy of breast cancer EUSOMA. Eur J Cancer 1992; 38: 615–34.
67. Stein RC, Dowsett M, Hedley A, Coombes RC. The clinical and endocrine effects of 4-hydroxyandrostenedione alone and in combination with goserelin in pre-menopausal women with advanced breast cancer. Br J Cancer 1990; 62: 679–83.
68. Johnston SR, Dowsett M. Aromatase inhibitors for breast cancer: lessons from the laboratory. Nat Rev Cancer 2003; 3: 821–31.
69. Nicholson RI, McClelland RA, Robertson JF, Gee JM. Involvement of steroid hormone and growth factor cross-talk in endocrine response in breast cancer. Endocr Relat Cancer 1999; 6: 373–87.
70. Shou J, Massarweh S, Osborne CK, et al. Mechanisms of tamoxifen resistance: increased estrogen receptor-HER2/neu cross-talk in ER/HER2-positive breast cancer. J Natl Cancer Inst 2004; 96: 926–35.

71. Chan CM, Martin LA, Johnston SR, Ali S, Dowsett M. Molecular changes associated with the acquisition of oestrogen hypersensitivity in MCF-7 breast cancer cells on long-term oestrogen deprivation. J Steroid Biochem Mol Biol 2002; 81: 333–41.

72. Martin LA, Farmer I, Johnston SR, et al. Enhanced estrogen receptor (ER) alpha, ERBB2, and MAPK signal transduction pathways operate during the adaptation of MCF-7 cells to long term estrogen deprivation. J Biol Chem 2003; 278: 30458–68.

73. Jeng MH, Shupnik MA, Bender TP, et al. Estrogen receptor expression and function in long-term estrogen-deprived human breast cancer cells. Endocrinology 1998; 139: 4164–74.

74. Shim WS, Conaway M, Masamura S, et al. Estradiol hypersensitivity and mitogen-activated protein kinase expression in long-term estrogen deprived human breast cancer cells in vivo. Endocrinology 2000; 141: 396–405.

75. Jeng MH, Yue W, Eischeid A, Wang JP, Santen RJ. Role of MAP kinase in the enhanced cell proliferation of long term estrogen deprived human breast cancer cells. Breast Cancer Res Treat 2000; 62: 167–75.

76. Stephen RL, Shaw LE, Larsen C, Corcoran D, Darbre PD. Insulin-like growth factor receptor levels are regulated by cell density and by long term estrogen deprivation in MCF7 human breast cancer cells. J Biol Chem 2001; 276: 40080–6.

77. Campbell RA, Bhat-Nakshatri P, Patel NM, et al. Phosphatidylinositol 3-kinase/AKT-mediated activation of estrogen receptor alpha: a new model for anti-estrogen resistance. J Biol Chem 2001; 276: 9817–24.

78. Johnston SR, Martin LA, Leary A, Head J, Dowsett M. Clinical strategies for rationale combinations of aromatase inhibitors with novel therapies for breast cancer. J Steroid Biochem Mol Biol 2007; 106: 180–6.

79. Osborne CK, Neven P, Dirix LY, et al. Gefitinib or placebo in combination with tamoxifen in patients with hormone receptor-positive metastatic breast cancer: a randomized phase II study. Clin. Cancer Res. 2011; 17: 1147–59.

80. Cristofanilli M, Valero V, Mangalik A, et al. Phase II, randomized trial to compare anastrozole combined with gefitinib or placebo in postmenopausal women with hormone receptor-positive metastatic breast cancer. Clin. Cancer Res. 2010; 16: 1904–14.

81. Kaufman B, Mackey JR, Clemens MR, et al. Trastuzumab plus anastrozole versus anastrozole alone for the treatment of postmenopausal women with human epidermal growth factor receptor 2-positive, hormone receptor-positive metastatic breast cancer: results from the randomized phase III TAnDEM study. J Clin. Oncol. 2009; 27: 5529–37.

82. Johnston SRD, Pippen J, Lichinitser M, et al. Lapatinib combined with letrozole versus letrozole and placebo as first-line therapy for postmenopausal hormone receptorpositive metastatic breast cancer. J Clin. Oncol. 2009; 27: 5538–46.

83. Baslega J, Roche H, Fumoleau P, et al. Treatment of postmenopausal women with locally advanced or metastatic breast cancer with letrozole alone or in combinations with temsirolimus; a randomized 3-arm, phase 2 study. Breast Cancer Res. Treat. 2005; 94 (Suppl 1): A1068.

84. Chow L, Sun Y, Jassem J, et al. Phase 3 study of temsirolimus with letrozole or letrozole alone in postmenopausal women with locally advanced or metastatic breast cancer. Breast Cancer Res. Treat. 2006; 100 (Suppl 28): A6091.

85. Bachelot T, Bourgier C, Cropet C, et al. TAMRAD: a GINECO randomized phase II trial of everolimus in combination with tamoxifen versus tamoxifen alone in patients with hormone receptor–positive, HER2-negative metastatic breast cancer with prior exposure to aromatase inhibitors. San Antonio Breast Cancer Symposium 2010, Abstr S1–6.

86. Gee JM, Harper ME, Hutcheson IR, et al. The antiepidermal growth factor receptor agent gefitinib (ZD1839/Iressa) improves antihormone response and prevents development of resistance in breast cancer in vitro. Endocrinology 2003; 11: 5105–17.

87. Baselga J, Campone M, Sahmoud T, et al. Everolimus in combination with exemestane for postmenopausal women with advanced breast cancer who are refractory to letrozole or anastrozole: results of the BOLERO-2 phase III trial. ECCO/ESMO Congress 2011; LBA 9.

4 Targeting HER2$^+$ and trastuzumab-resistant metastatic breast cancer

Javier Cortés and Maurizio Scaltriti

TARGETING THE HER FAMILY RECEPTORS IN BREAST CANCER: A BRIEF INTRODUCTION

Breast cancer (BC) is the most common cancer type occurring in women world-wide. During the last 25 years, the technological progress that has characterised both genetic and molecular biology has led to a greater understanding of the events underlying the normal tissue development as well as malignant transformation. This level of knowledge has enabled the identification of molecular players responsible for cell growth, survival, motility, and transformation that may serve as therapeutic targets. The human epidermal growth factor family receptors (HER) have been proposed as a rationale target for cancer therapy. This family of receptors comprises four receptors: HER1, HER2, HER3, and HER4. All four receptors share an extracellular ligand-binding domain, a trans-membrane section, and an intracellular tyrosine-kinase domain. The binding of a ligand to the extracellular domain induces the formation of receptor homodimers or heterodimers, phosphorylation of key tyrosine residues of the kinase domain and consequent recruitment of molecular adaptors and effectors that start the downstream, signalling cascade. Key pathways activated by HER signalling include the RAS-RAF-MAP kinase and the phosphatidylinositol-3-kinase (PI3K)/AKT/mammalian target of rapamycin (mTOR) pathways (1) involved in the control of several cellular processes such as apoptosis, migration, growth, adhesion, and differentiation (reviewed in (1–3)). Deregulated HER signalling is associated with malignant transformation. HER signalling can be altered via a number of mechanisms (3) including ligand overexpression, overexpression of the normal or constitutively mutated HER receptor, and defective HER receptor internalisation degradation (3). HER2 is the preferred dimerisation partner for the other HER family receptors (4).

Overexpression/amplification of HER2 occurs in approximately 20–25% of patients with BC and is associated with more aggressive disease and a decreased survival (5,6). Moreover, HER2 homodimers are constitutively active and thus able to initiate downstream signalling pathways (7). These findings stimulated interest in HER2 as a target for therapy in BC. There are two main therapeutic strategies that can be employed to target HER2-positive cells. Extracellular targeting can be achieved using monoclonal antibodies (MAbs). There are two humanised MAbs designed to be used against HER2: trastuzumab and pertuzumab, with different mechanisms of action that will be explained later in the chapter. Intracellular targeting can be achieved using small-molecule adenosine triphosphate competitors that inhibit the phosphorylation of the HER2 intracellular kinase domain. There are several types of HER tyrosine-kinase inhibitors (TKIs) (2). Some are highly specific, blocking only one receptor (erlotinib, gefitinib inhibiting HER1), and others more promiscuous that can inhibit both HER1 and HER2 because of the high degree of homology between the two kinase domains (lapatinib). Targeting HER receptors with either strategy has the knock-on effect of inhibiting HER-dependent downstream pathways (2). This has a large number of effects, including cell cycle arrest, induction of apoptosis, inhibition of tumour cell invasion, and metastasis and augmentation of the anti-tumour effects of chemotherapy/radiation therapy.

TARGETING HER2+ AND TRASTUZUMAB-RESISTANT MBC
Trastuzumab and Lapatinib in MBC Treatment

The clinical responses observed in phase II studies of trastuzumab, the high anti-tumour activity of doxorubicin and paclitaxel in BC, and the enhanced anti-tumour activity of paclitaxel and doxorubicin by trastuzumab against human breast carcinoma xenografts, led to the design of a phase III multicentre clinical trial of chemotherapy (doxorubicin based or paclitaxel based) plus trastuzumab, versus chemotherapy alone, in patients with progressive metastatic breast cancer (MBC) that overexpressed HER2, who had not previously received chemotherapy for metastatic disease (8). Four hundred sixty-nine patients were randomly assigned to receive chemotherapy alone or chemotherapy plus trastuzumab. Chemotherapy consisted of doxorubicin $60\,mg/m^2$ (or epirubicin $75\,mg/m^2$) plus cyclophosphamide $600\,mg/m^2$ for anthracycline-naïve patients or paclitaxel $175\,mg/m^2$ in a 3-hour infusion for those who had received adjuvant anthracyclines. All chemotherapeutic agents were given every 3 weeks for 6 cycles. Treatment with chemotherapy plus trastuzumab was associated with a significantly higher response rate (50% vs. 32%, P < 0.001) compared with chemotherapy alone. Statistically significant differences in the overall response rates were also found in the subgroup treated with an anthracycline, cyclophosphamide, and trastuzumab and the subgroup treated with paclitaxel and trastuzumab, as compared with the subgroups treated with anthracycline and cyclophosphamide alone or paclitaxel alone. The median survival rate was 25.1 months in the group treated with chemotherapy plus trastuzumab and 20.3 months in the group that received chemotherapy alone (P = 0.046); similarly, trends indicating a survival benefit were seen in patients who received trastuzumab plus paclitaxel (22.1 months vs. 18.4 months) and trastuzumab plus anthracycline, cyclophosphamide (AC) (27 months vs. 21 months) subgroups, relative to those who received either paclitaxel or AC alone. After a retrospective analysis of fluorescent *in situ* hybridization (FISH) status in the pivotal phase III trastuzumab combination trial, it was revealed that immunohistohemistry (IHC) 3 positivity has high concordance (89%) with FISH positivity. Analysis of patient response based on FISH status demonstrated that in FISH-negative patients, response rates were similar for patients who received chemotherapy alone and trastuzumab plus chemotherapy (39% and 41%, respectively), whereas in FISH-positive patients, response rates were significantly increased from 27% in those patients receiving chemotherapy alone to 54% in those patients receiving trastuzumab plus chemotherapy. FISH-negative patients did not appear to benefit from the addition of trastuzumab to conventional chemotherapy in terms of overall survival. The unexpected cardiac events observed in the trastuzumab arm prompted a retrospective analysis of all cases of cardiac dysfunction by an independent cardiac review and evaluation committee. This review identified 63 patients with symptomatic or asymptomatic cardiac dysfunction: 27% of patients had received AC plus herceptin, 8% AC alone, 13% paclitaxel and trastuzumab, and 1% had received paclitaxel as a single agent. Among the five patients with persistent class III or IV cardiac dysfunction, three were in the group given an anthracycline, cyclophosphamide, and trastuzumab. However, adding trastuzumab to chemotherapy did not increase the incidence of other side effects, and no patient developed detectable levels of antibodies against trastuzumab.

In a multicentre randomised phase II trial (9), patients with previously untreated HER2 overexpressing MBC were randomised to trastuzumab (loading dose $4\,mg/kg$ and weekly dose $2\,mg/kg$ until disease progression) plus docetaxel ($100\,mg/m^2$ q 3 weeks for 6 cycles) (92 patients), or docetaxel alone (94 patients). Patients who progressed on docetaxel alone were allowed to receive trastuzumab. Almost all patients were confirmed to be HER2 overexpressors (97% in the combination group and 94% in the single-agent group). The overall response rate was significantly higher in the combination group (61% vs. 34%). The addition of trastuzumab to chemotherapy was associated with significantly improved time to progression (TTP) of the disease (11.7 months vs. 6.1 months, p = 0.0001) and overall survival ((OS) 31.2 months vs. 22.7 months, p = 0.0325) compared with chemotherapy alone. Trastuzumab added little to the toxicity profile of docetaxel with only 1% incidence of congestive heart failure. Febrile neutropenia was observed in 17% and 23% of patients who received docetaxel as single treatment or the combination, respectively.

Two clinical trials explored the combination of aromatase inhibitors with anti-HER2 therapies. In the TAnDEM (10) (Trastuzumab and Anastrozole Directed against Estrogen receptor-positive HER2-positive Mammary carcinoma) trial, Kaufman et al. assessed the role of trastuzumab in patients with HER2-positive and hormone-receptor-positive MBC treated with anastrozole. In their trial, 207 patients were randomly assigned to receive anastrozole, either alone or in combination with trastuzumab. The primary objective of the trial was progression-free survival (PFS), defined as the time between randomisation and the date of progressive disease of death. The median PFS was 4.8 months for the group that received trastuzumab and anastrozole, and 2.4 months for the anastrozole group (hazard ratio (HR) with the combination group, 0.63; p = 0.0016; 95% CI 0.47–0.85). The combination therapy group also experienced a higher clinical benefit rate (42.7% vs. 27.9%, p = 0.026). These benefits, however, did not translate into an improvement in OS (median OS was 28.5 and 23.9 months for the combination group and the anastrozole group, respectively). Incidence of grade 3 and 4 adverse events was slightly more frequent in the trastuzumab-plus-anastrozole arm. Cardiac toxicity was minimal in both groups, with only one patient developing New York Heart Association Class II congestive heart failure in the trastuzumab-based arm.

In a second study, the EGF30008 trial, Johnston et al. (11) assessed the role of lapatinib in combination with letrozole in patients with hormone receptor-positive MBC. In total, 1286 patients were included, 17% of which had in addition HER2-positive tumours. Importantly, although this trial did not exclusively recruit patients with HER2-positive tumours , the primary objective of the trial was PFS in this patient population (HER2/hormone receptor co-positive tumours). The PFS-HR with the combination group was 0.71; p = 0.019; 95% CI 0.53–0.96 (median PFS rate increased from 3.0 months for the group that received lapatinib and placebo to 8.2 months for the letrozole and lapatinib group). The response rate was also higher in the combination therapy group (28% vs. 15%, p = 0.021). Again, these benefits did not translate into an improvement in OS (median OS was 33.3 and 32.3 months for the combination group and the letrozole group, respectively). Although it was not the primary endpoint, in HER2-negative tumours the combination of lapatinib and letrozole did not seem to be superior to letrozole alone in terms of PFS (HR = 0.90; p = 0.188). Interestingly, however, in 200 patients who were considered resistant to previous endocrine therapy, a trend towards an improvement in PFS was observed in the lapatinib-plus-letrozole arm. These four studies are summarised in Table 1.

Recently, lapatinib has also been tested in a blinded, randomised phase III study (12). A total of 444 patients with untreated HER2-positive MBC were randomised to receive weekly paclitaxel with placebo or lapatinib. The data showed that patients who received lapatinib-based therapy experienced a statistically significant improvement in OS when treated with lapatinib plus paclitaxel compared to those treated with paclitaxel plus placebo, (27.8 months vs. 20.5 months, respectively; p = 0.0124) equating to a 26% reduction in the risk of death. The study also showed a statistically significant improvement in median PFS for women treated with the lapatinib plus paclitaxel regimen (9.7 months lapatinib plus paclitaxel vs. 6.5 months for paclitaxel plus placebo p ≤ 0.0001). Response rates observed in the study were 69% in

TABLE 1 Randomised Pivotal Trials in HER2-Positive Metastatic Breast Cancer Activity

Study	Regimen	No. of patients	ORR (%)	TTP of the disease (months)	OS (months)
Slamon et al. (8)	Ch + T	235	50	7.4	25.1
	Ch	234	32	4.6	20.3
Marty et al. (9)	D + T	92	61	11.7	31.2
	D	94	34	6.1	22.7
Kaufman et al. (10)	A + T	103	20	4.8	28.5
	A	104	7	2.4	23.9
Johnston et al. (11)	L + Lap	111	28	8.2	33.3
	L	108	15	3.0	32.3

Abbreviations: A, anastrozole; Ch, chemotherapy; D, docetaxel; L, letrozole; Lap, lapatinib; ORR, overall response rate; OS, overall survival; T, trastuzumab; TTP, time to progression.

the lapatinib plus paclitaxel arm compared with 50% in the paclitaxel plus placebo arm (p ≤ 0.0001).

Mechanisms of Trastuzumab Resistance
The introduction of trastuzumab into the therapeutic regimens for patients with HER2-positive BC has undoubtedly improved both response rates and clinical outcomes. However, not all HER2-positive tumours respond in the same way. A significant fraction of trastuzumab-treated patients display primary (intrinsic) resistance to the therapy. Moreover, most of the patients with advanced disease who are initially sensitive to trastuzumab-based therapy will invariably develop secondary (acquired) resistance. There are several ways to classify the numerous mechanisms of trastuzumab resistance. We have chosen to group them in two categories: (i) clinically relevant, for those that have been confirmed or there is a strong indication that can occur in BC patients and (ii) proposed mechanisms, based on laboratory/pre-clinical results but still to be validated in the clinical setting.

Activation of the PI3K/Akt/mTOR Pathway
Loss of function of phosphatase and tensin homolog (PTEN) (13,14) and the presence of activating mutations of the p110α subunit of the PI3K enzyme (15) are relatively frequent in HER2-positive BC and seem to limit the efficacy of trastuzumab-based therapy. There is a correlation between presence of aberrations of the PI3K/Akt/mTOR pathway and low clinical benefit rate from trastuzumab therapy. These findings are being tested in larger cohorts of patients and may provide the rationale for the use of PI3K inhibitors in this setting.

P95HER2
P95HER2 is a truncated form of HER2 that lacks the extracellular domain (and the binding site for trastuzumab) but conserves an intact intracellular domain with a strong kinase activity. P95HER2 is present only in HER2-positive patients and can be formed by either metalloprotease cleavage (16) or alternative initiation of translation of the HER2 mRNA (17). The presence of p95HER2 has been associated with increased node metastases and worse clinical outcome among the HER2-positive patient population (18,19). Two independent studies have recently demonstrated that expression of p95HER2 also correlates with *de novo* resistance to trastuzumab-based therapy (20,21). Seeking alternative anti-HER2 therapeutic strategies, Scaltriti and colleagues investigated the activity of lapatinib, a small molecule that inhibits both epidermal growth

factor receptor (EGFR) and HER2 phosphorylation, in p95HER2-positive tumours. Lapatinib proved to be efficacious in inhibiting tumour growth in several trastuzumab-resistant p95HER2 pre-clinical models, and lapatinib-based therapy was equally effective in p95HER2-positive and p95HER2-negative patients, distinguishing from trastuzumab-based therapy (22).

HER2 Loss of Amplification/Overexpression

Prolonged treatment with trastuzumab-based therapy may result in loss of HER2 amplification and overexpression with consequent decrease of therapy response and worse clinical outcome (23,24). Interestingly, the same phenomenon occurs also in vitro in HER2-positive cells chronically exposed to increasing concentration of trastuzumab (24). This HER2 "negativisation" suggests that a few HER2-negative cells present in the original tumours were positively selected under the pressure of trastuzumab and proliferated over the HER2-positive cells, becoming the most prevalent population of the tumour. This hypothesis, however, still needs to be validated experimentally.

IGF-IR Expression and Dimerisation

Several publications have reported that expression of IGF-IR and its dimerisation with HER2 can decrease the therapeutic effects of trastuzumab both in pre-clinical models (25,26) and in the clinical setting (27), although clinical resistance should be confirmed in a larger cohort of samples derived from patients who escaped trastuzumab-based therapy. Essentially, the formation of HER2/IGF-IR heterodimers may abrogate the anti-proliferative effects of trastuzumab in IGF-IR overexpressing HER2-positive cells.

FcγRIIIa Polymorphisms

Trastuzumab (as single agent) has only cytostatic effects in vitro in contrast to the *in vivo* setting where it can lead to tumour shrinkage in pre-clinical models (28). This phenomenon can be explained by the in vivo engagement of the immune-effector system with consequent antibody-dependent cell-mediated cytotoxicity (ADCC), considered nowadays as one of the main therapeutic mechanisms of trastuzumab (29). Immune effector cells, such as natural killers or macrophages, can recognise and bind trastuzumab via their receptors for IgGs and commit HER2-positive cells to cytolysis. Some of these receptors, namely the FcγRIIIa and the FcγRIIa, seem to be crucial for the clinical response to trastuzumab. In fact, in a recent study Musolino and colleagues discovered that patients with certain germline polymorphisms in these receptors (FcγRIIIa 158 V/V and/or FcγRIIa 131 H/H) were more likely to receive clinical benefit from trastuzumab therapy (30). Another indication of the importance of ADCC in the clinical setting derives from a small study reporting that patients who achieved either a partial or a complete response to trastuzumab were found to have a higher infiltration of leukocytes in the tumour sites and a higher capability to mediate in vitro ADCC activity (31).

Cyclin E Amplification/Overexpression

High cyclin E expression has been proposed as a marker of poor clinical outcome in BC (32). Furthermore, it has been shown that cyclin E levels decrease when HER2 is downregulated/inhibited, suggesting that HER2 regulates cyclin E expression (33). In a recent study, Scaltriti and colleagues identified cyclin E amplification/overexpression as a major gain of function in HER2-positive cells that have acquired resistance to trastuzumab (34). These cells were proved to be addicted to either cyclin E ablation or CDK2 inhibition both *in vitro* and *in vivo*. Interestingly, the authors found that cyclin E amplification/overexpression is a relatively common feature in

HER2-positive BC and correlates with shorter PFS and low clinical benefit rate from trastuzumab treatment. Analyses of larger cohorts of patients are ongoing.

Other Proposed Mechanisms of Trastuzumab Resistance
Overexpression of Receptor Tyrosine Kinases

Overexpression of EGFR and EGFR ligands was found in HER2-positive cells that acquired resistance to trastuzumab (35). With this pre-clinical model it was suggested that the combined inhibition of HER2 and EGFR could be a valid therapeutic strategy in HER2-positive BC and/or could dampen the emergence of acquired resistance to anti-HER2 agents. Unfortunately, a clinical trial designed with this plausible hypothesis in mind failed to demonstrate significant therapeutic advantages of the combination of gefitinib and trastuzumab versus trastuzumab alone in HER2-positive MBC (36).

Overexpression of HER3 and its innate capacity to activate the PI3K/Akt/mTOR axis is also reported to compensate for inhibition of other HER family members, including HER2 (37,38). The same applies for c-Met, frequently co-expressed with HER2 and upregulated by trastuzumab treatment, which decreases the sensitivity to trastuzumab through sustained activation of the PI3K/Akt/mTOR pathway (39).

Prevention of Trastuzumab-Dependent Cytostatic Effects

The role of the transforming growth factor beta (TGFβ) pathway in reducing the anti-proliferative effects of trastuzumab is still controversial. Although there are indications that TGFβ interferes with anti-HER2 therapy through activation of ADAM 17, release of HER ligands, and subsequent activation of the HER3/PI3K axis (40), other data propose that overexpression of LIP, a TGFβ inhibitor, will prevent the ability of trastuzumab to inhibit proliferation and/or induce senescence (41).

Upregulation of the cyclin-dependent kinase inhibitor p27 following trastuzumab treatment has been known for a decade (42). p27 binds to and inhibits cyclin E/cdk2 complexes. Nahta and colleagues successively found a strict correlation between p27 levels and sensitivity to trastuzumab (43). This study showed that HER2-positive cells resistant to trastuzumab had low expression of p27 and that restoring the levels of p27 significantly increased trastuzumab sensitivity. Therefore, reduced p27 expression, that may generate active cyclin E/cdk2 complexes, may provide an alternative route to trastuzumab resistance over cyclin E overexpression.

Hyperactivation of HER2

Expression of mucin 4 (MUC4) has been associated with trastuzumab resistance through two different mechanisms. MUC4, in close steric association with HER2, interferes with trastuzumab binding masking the epitope recognised by the antibody (44). Furthermore, MUC4 has been described to physically interact with the receptor, enhancing its phosphorylation/activation and potentiating HER2-dependent inhibition of apoptosis (45).

A splice variant of HER2 (HER2Δ16) was recently found to be expressed in a substantial proportion of BC patients (46). This HER2 isoform, more often found in node-positive tumours, is hyperactive, promotes cell invasion and, in pre-clinical models, leads to both trastuzumab and endocrine resistance (47).

Mechanisms of Lapatinib Resistance

The development of therapeutic resistance to lapatinib is far from being understood. The occurrence of secondary mutations of the receptor is a known mechanism of acquired pharmacological resistance to small molecule TKIs (48,49). In the case of HER2, however, the frequency of somatic mutations in BC is rare (50). This suggests that other events are based on either intrinsic (primary) or acquired (secondary) resistance to lapatinib. Compared with trastuzumab, lapatinib is an excellent silencer of the HER2 downstream signalling pathway. This feature has been described to trigger the activation/expression of anti-apoptotic proteins that, in some cases, can counteract lapatinib-induced cell death.

One example is the increased phosphorylation/activation of RelA, a subunit of NF-kB, which is known to promote the expression of numerous anti-apoptotic genes (51). In cells treated with lapatinib, total RelA protein remains unvaried but the steady-state levels of the phosphorylated (Ser529) form increase soon after 24 hours of treatment. Importantly, this phenomenon has been found to occur also in HER2-positive BC patients with inflammatory disease treated with lapatinib. The possible correlation between increased levels of phospho-RelA and lack of response to lapatinib has been postulated but needs to be confirmed in a larger cohort of patients.

Increased estrogen receptor signalling has been also reported as a consequence of lapatinib-dependent HER2 inhibition. Chronic exposure to lapatinib would result in enhanced ER signalling as a consequence of FOXO3a overexpression and activation in response to lapatinib-dependent inhibition of the PI3K/Akt/mTOR pathway (52). In other words, the efficacy of lapatinib in inhibiting HER2 downstream signalling becomes the cause of the acquired resistance. Upregulation of ER-regulated proteins, such as PR and bcl2, has been described also in tissue samples from patients treated with lapatinib. This mechanism would apply only in ER-positive HER2 amplified patients.

Chronic exposure to lapatinib and acquired resistance seems to correlate also with increased expression of Axl, a membrane-bound receptor tyrosine kinase associated with poor prognosis and increased invasiveness in BC (53). Overexpression of Axl and its dimerisation with HER3 would overcome the inhibitory effects of lapatinib in this setting. As a proof of concept, both siRNA against Axl and a kinase inhibitor of the receptor succeeded in restoring lapatinib sensitivity in cells with acquired resistance to lapatinib.

Activation of the PI3K/Akt/mTOR axis has been described to limit the activity of lapatinib, when used at low doses, in HER2-positive BC pre-clinical models (54). In the clinical setting, however, the presence of activating mutations of PI3K or low levels of PTEN seem to correlate only with trastuzumab resistance (55). This discrepancy is likely due to the relatively high concentration of lapatinib (over 1 μM) achievable in the serum of treated patients.

Treatment of MBC Beyond Trastuzumab Progression

Upon progression to an initial trastuzumab-based regimen, there was the question of whether anti-HER2 therapies should be continued in combination with other chemotherapy agents. Two randomised trials were specifically designed to answer that question. In a first trial, Geyer and colleagues (56) included women with HER2-positive, locally advanced, or metastatic BC that had progressed after treatment with regimens that included an anthracycline, a taxane, and a trastuzumab and patients were randomly assigned to receive either the combination therapy (lapatinib at a dose of 1250 mg per day continuously plus capecitabine at a dose of 2000 mg/m^2 on days 1 through 14 of a 21-day cycle) or monotherapy (capecitabine alone at a dose of 2500 mg/m^2 on days 1 through 14 of a 21-day cycle). The HR for the TTP was 0.49 (95% CI, 0.34–0.71; P < 0.001), with 49 events in the combination-therapy group and 72 events in the monotherapy group. The median TTP was 8.4 months in the combination-therapy group and 4.4 months in the monotherapy group. This improvement was achieved without an increase in serious toxic effects or symptomatic cardiac events. In the GBG 26/BIG 3-05 trial (57), women with HER2-positive, locally advanced or metastatic BC that had progressed during or after a treatment with trastuzumab with or without chemotherapy as adjuvant or first-line treatment were randomly assigned to receive either capecitabine 2500 mg/m on days 1–14, q21 (78 patients) or the same capecitabine treatment simultaneously to a continuation of trastuzumab 6 mg/kg every 3 weeks (78 patients). Median times to progression were 5.6 months in the capecitabine group and 8.2 months in the capecitabine-plus-trastuzumab group with an unadjusted HR of 0.69 (95% CI, 0.48–0.97; two-sided log-rank $P = 0.0338$) and OS rates were 20.4 months (95% CI, 17.8–24.7) in the capecitabine group and 25.5 months (95% CI, 19.0–30.7) in the capecitabine-plus-trastuzumab group ($P = 0.257$).

The rationale for the dual inhibition of the HER2 receptor with MAb and TKI treatment emerged from pre-clinical experiments and early clinical studies which finally led to the design of a clinical phase III study. The EGF104900 study compared the activity of lapatinib alone or in combination with trastuzumab in patients with HER2-positive, trastuzumab-refractory MBC. The primary objective was PFS. The combination of lapatinib with trastuzumab was superior to lapatinib alone for PFS (HR: 0.73; 95% CI, 0.57–0.93; $p = 0.008$) and OS (HR: 0.74; 95% CI, 0.57–0.97; $p = 0.026$) (58). The most frequent adverse events were diarrhea, rash, nausea, and fatigue; diarrhea was higher in the combination arm ($P = 0.03$).

Novel Agents Targeting HER2-Positive MBC

Numerous treatments for HER2-positive BC are in clinical development (Table 2) (Fig. 1). It is not the purpose of this chapter to review all of them, but it is to provide an overview about those ahead in development.

HER Dimerisation Inhibitors: Pertuzumab

Pertuzumab, also known as 2C4, is a fully humanised MAb that differs from trastuzumab in the epitope-binding regions of the light and heavy chains. As a result, pertuzumab binds to a different extracellular epitope on HER2 than trastuzumab. This agent can therefore avoid HER2 homo- or heterodimerisation formation and consequently inhibits the activation of associated downstream signalling pathways, critical

TABLE 2   Treatments in the Development for HER2-Positive Breast Cancer

HER2 dimerisation inhibitor	Pertuzumab
	Monoclonal antibody that inhibits dimerisation of HER2
HER2 ADC	Trastuzumab-DM1
	Trastuzumab-based ADC delivering DM1
mTOR inhibitors	e.g., Everolimus
	Small-molecule-inhibiting mTOR signal transduction
Other TIKs	e.g., Neratinib, afatinib
	Irreversible inhibitors of EGFR and HER2
PI3K inhibitors	e.g., BKM120
	Small molecules selectively binding PI3K
PI3K/mTOR inhibitors	e.g., BEZ235 and BGT226
	Small molecules that inhibit dual PI3K/mTOR
HSP 90 inhibitors	e.g., Tanespimycin
	Antibiotic that binds to and inhibits the cytosolic chaperone functions of HSP 90
Antiangiogenic agents	e.g., Bevacizumab, sunitinib
	Monoclonal antibodies or small molecules targeting the angiogenic signalling pathway

Abbreviations: ADC, antibody–drug conjugate; DM1, maytansine; EGFR, epidermal growth factor receptor; HSP, heat-shock protein; mTOR, mammalian target of rapamycin; PI3K, phosphoinositide 3-kinase; TKIs, tyrosine kinase inhibitors.

for tumour growth (59–62). The ability of pertuzumab to inhibit dimerisation has been confirmed in cell lines with both normal and high levels of HER2. *In vivo*, pertuzumab has demonstrated potent anti-tumour activity in a variety of animals with established BT 474 (high HER2) or MCF 7 (low HER2) BC xenograft tumours (43,59). Pertuzumab showed tumour growth inhibition (85%) similar to trastuzumab (82%) against Calu-3 cells, whereas the single-agent activity was moderate against other HER2-positive models such as KPL-4 cells, with a tumour growth inhibition of 38% and 45%, respectively. However, the combination effect of both antibodies was more than additive in several lung and breast xenograft models, resulting in strong tumour growth inhibition and cases of complete tumour remission. This data indicate that the combination has resulted in a more than additive anti-tumour activity and suggests a synergistic effect.

A phase II trial with pertuzumab and trastuzumab in combination has been performed in patients with MBC (63). Patients included in the trial were women with measurable BC disease, HER2-positive treated with up to three lines of prior chemotherapy plus trastuzumab and with disease progression during the most recent treatment with trastuzumab for MBC. Patients were treated with trastuzumab plus 420 mg fixed dose of pertuzumab following a loading dose 840 mg. There were no clinical cardiac events, and a central review revealed no case of fall in left ventricular ejection fraction of ≥10 to ≤50%. Sixteen confirmed partial responses (24%) were achieved and the clinical benefit rate was 50%. The authors concluded that the combination of the pertuzumab and trastuzumab is active and well tolerated in patients with pre-treated HER2-positive BC which has progressed during treatment with trastuzumab alone. However, pertuzumab alone produced only a modest

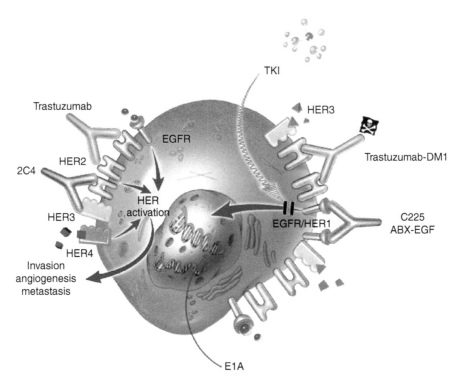

FIGURE 1   New anti-HER2 strategies against HER2-positive metastatic breast cancer. DM1, maytansine; EGFR, HER, human epidermal growth factor family receptor; TKI, tyrosine kinase inhibitor. (with permission: Nahta R, Hortobagyi G, Esteva F. The Oncologist 2003; 8: 5–17).

activity in the same patient population with only 3% of patients having a partial response. When trastuzumab was reintroduced in those patients progressing on pertuzumab, the combination showed attractive activity (64). Based on these data, a phase III trial is evaluating the efficacy of trastuzumab and docetaxel with or without pertuzumab as a first-line therapy and a second phase II trial will define the role of pertuzumab in patients being treated with capecitabine and trastuzumab in second line.

Trastuzumab-Based Antibody–Drug Conjugate: T-DM1

Trastuzumab-MCC-DM1 (T-DM1) is a first-in-class anti-HER2 antibody–drug conjugate that combines the biological activity of trastuzumab (T) with a highly potent anti-microtubule agent (DM1) and specifically targets HER2-expressing cells, conferring selectivity to the cytotoxic agent and thus increasing the therapeutic index (65). A phase I study of T-DM1 as a single agent has revealed clinical activity (ORR 44%) in patients with HER2-positive MBC who had progressed while receiving trastuzumab-based chemotherapy at the maximum tolerated dose of 3.6 mg/kg (66). Two phase II trials studied the activity and toxicity of T-DM1 in the MBC of more than 220 patients. In the first trial (67), 112 patients with HER2-positive MBC who have progressed on HER2 therapy and who have previously received trastuzumab and ≥1 line of chemotherapy in the metastatic setting received T-DM1 at a dose of 3.6 mg/kg. The overall response rate was 26%. Interestingly, in those 67 patients who were also pretreated with lapatinib, the response rate was 24%. The activity in those patients with centrally confirmed HER2-positive disease (n = 75) was 34%. In the second study (68), 39 out of 110 patients (34.5%) who had been treated with lapatinib, trastuzumab, capecitabine, anthracyclines, and taxanes and received T-DM1, achieved a partial response.

An open-label, phase II study of T-DM1 versus trastuzumab plus docetaxel in the first-line treatment of 137 HER2-positive MBC patients was presented in the European Society of Medical Oncology meeting in 2010 (69). At a median follow-up of 6 months, the ORR rates were 47.8% for the T-DM1 group versus 41.4% for trastuzumab plus docetaxel-treated patients and T-DM1 was associated with a much reduced incidence of grade ≥3 adverse events (37% vs. 75%). A phase III study of T-DM1 plus pertuzumab or T-DM1 plus placebo versus trastuzumab plus taxane in the first line of treatment is currently recruiting patients.

Irreversible Anti-HER2 TKIs

Neratinib (HKI-272), a potent, oral, irreversible pan-HER TKI (i.e., HER 1, 2, and 4) has also been tested in HER2-positiveMBC with an impressive activity reported in monotherapy in BC patients: 24% of patients with prior trastuzumab treatment and 56% in the trastuzumab-naive cohort (70). In addition, a new generation of irreversible inhibitors of EGFR and an HER2 TKI, BIBW 2992, is in early phases of clinical development (40). To better define the role of neratinib in first-line treatment, a phase III trial is being conducted comparing neratinib plus paclitaxel with the standard trastuzumab and paclitaxel regimen.

Targeting the PI3K/AKT/mTOR Pathway

As it was commented previously, there is a strong rationale to explore the combined treatment with PI3K or mTOR inhibitors with anti-HER therapies. Although there are several ongoing clinical trials, the results of combining trastuzumab and everolimus, an mTOR inhibitor, have already been presented. In a phase Ib study, Andre and colleagues (71) assessed the dose limiting toxicity of everolimus, trastuzumab, and weekly paclitaxel in patients with taxanes-pretreated and trastuzumab-resistant

HER2-positive MBC. Twenty-seven patients had measurable disease and were evaluable for efficacy. Among these patients, ORR was 44%. Overall disease was controlled for 6 months or more in 74% and median PFS was 34 weeks. In a second multicentre phase I/II trial (72), everolimus and trastuzumab were administered to trastuzumab-resistant HER2-positive MBC to determine the safety and efficacy of this combination. Forty-seven patients were evaluable for safety and efficacy. Seven (15%) patients demonstrated a partial response and nine (19%) had stable disease ≥24 weeks, equaling a clinical benefit rate of 34%.

HSP90 Inhibitors in HER2-Positive MBC

One of the last developed strategies to disturb HER2-positive tumours is the inhibition of the chaperone HSP90, essential for HER2 folding and maturation. The mechanism of action is through inhibition of HSP90 chaperone function with consequent proteasome degradation of chaperone clients. One of the most sensitive clients of HSP90 is, in fact, HER2. These drugs are in clinical trials and show promising results in combination with trastuzumab (73). After showing preliminary activity in a phase I trial, the activity of trastuzumab and tanespimycin (a water-insoluble HSP90 inhibitor) was evaluated in a phase II trial (74). Twenty-seven out of 31 patients with MBC following one prior line of trastuzumab-containing therapy were eligible for response assessment. Seven patients (26%) experienced a partial response; an additional five patients had disease regressions between 20% and 29%, and five more had sable disease for at least 4 months, giving a clinical benefit rate of 63%. Second-generation HSP90 inhibitors with higher potency, alvespimycinor or IPI-504, an agent that interconverts with tanespimycin in vivo, are currently being studied in combination with weekly trastuzumab.

Anti-Angiogenic Agents and HER2

Overexpression of HER2 is associated with the upregulation of vascular endothelial growth factor (VEGF) in BC cells (75). This is one of the most important endothelial mitogens involved in the development and differentiation of the vascular system. The correlation between micro-vessel density and engineered expression of VEGF has been observed in human breast xenografts. VEGF's role in BC progression is evident from clinical studies showing elevated serum VEGF in invasive BC. Bevacizumab, a VEGF-specific angiogenesis inhibitor, in combination with trastuzumab showed promising results in a phase II study as a first-line therapy (76). The ORR was 48% and the median TTP was 9.2 months. These data support the ongoing phase III trial that compares docetaxel and trastuzumab with or without bevacizumab.

CONCLUSION

Although trastuzumab-based therapy is the standard first-line therapy for patients with HER2-positive MBC, improved understanding of mechanisms of resistance to trastuzumab has facilitated the development of novel agents for this BC subtype. Recent data from studies of these agents indicate that the HER2 pathway remains a valid therapeutic target following progression on trastuzumab, and suggest a promising role for combined HER2 blockade with two or more agents. It is very likely that other targeted agents will have a role in the treatment of patients with HER2-positive MBC. Lapatinib, pertuzumab, neratinib, trastuzumab-DM1, bevacizumab, and everolimus are the most well-established agents in this setting, and they may emerge as a new standard of care in the forthcoming years. However, in the near future, we will have to deal with a new issue, that is, resistance to the combination of different anti-HER2 therapies.

REFERENCES

1. Atalay G, Cardoso F, Awada A, Piccart MJ. Novel therapeutic strategies targeting the epidermal growth factor receptor (EGFR) family and its downstream effectors in breast cancer. Ann Oncol 2003; 14: 1346–63.
2. Mendelsohn J, Baselga J. Status of epidermal growth factor receptor antagonists in the biology and treatment of cancer. J Clin Oncol 2003; 21: 2787–99.
3. Yarden Y, Sliwkowski M. Untangling the ErbB signalling network. Nat Rev Mol Cell Biol 2001; 2: 127–37.
4. Graus-Porta D, Beerly R, Daly JM, Hynes N. ErbB2, the prefered heterdimerization partner of all ErbB receptors, is a mediator of lateral signaling. EMBO J 1997; 16: 1647–55.
5. Slamon DJ, Clark GM, Wong SG, et al. Human breast cancer: correlation of relapse and survival with amplification of the HER-2/neu oncogene. Science 1987; 235: 177–82.
6. Slamon DJ, Godolphin W, Jones LA, et al. Studies of the HER-2/neu Proto-oncogene in human breast and ovarian cancer. Science 1989; 244: 707–12.
7. Pinkas-Kramarski R, Soussan L, Waterman H, et al. Diversification of Neu differentiation factor and epidermal growth factor signaling by combinatorial receptor interactions. EMBO J 1996; 15: 2452–67.
8. Slamon DJ, Leyland-Jones B, Shak S, et al. Use of chemotherapy plus a monoclonal antibody against HER2 for metastatic breast cancer that overexpresses HER2. N Engl J Med 2001; 344: 783–92.
9. Marty M, Cognetti F, Maraninchi D, et al. Randomized phase II trial of the efficacy and safety of trastuzumab combined with docetaxel in patients with human epidermal growth factor receptor 2-positive metastatic breast cancer administered as first-line treatment: the M77001 study group. J Clin Oncol 2005; 23: 4265–74.
10. Kaufman B, Mackey JR, Clemens MR, et al. Trastuzumab plus anastrozole versus anastrozole alone for the treatment of postmenopausal women with human epidermal growth factor receptor 2-positive, hormone receptor-positive metastatic breast cancer: results from the randomized phase III TAnDEM study. J Clin Oncol 2009; 27: 5529–37.
11. Johnston S, Pippen J, Jr, Pivot X, et al. Lapatinib combined with letrozole versus letrozole and placebo as first-line therapy for postmenopausal hormone receptor-positive metastatic breast cancer. J Clin Oncol 2009; 27: 5538–46.
12. Guan Z, Xu B, Arpornwirat W, et al. Overall survival benefit observed with Lapatinib (L) plus Paclitaxel (P) as first-line therapy in patients with HER2-overexpressing metastatic breast cancer. Proc SABCS 2010; P3-14–24.
13. Nagata Y, Lan KH, Zhou X, et al. PTEN activation contributes to tumor inhibition by trastuzumab, and loss of PTEN predicts trastuzumab resistance in patients. Cancer Cell 2004; 6: 117–27.
14. Pandolfi PP. Breast cancer—loss of PTEN predicts resistance to treatment. N Engl J Med 2004; 351: 2337–8.
15. Berns K, Horlings HM, Hennessy BT, et al. A functional genetic approach identifies the PI3K pathway as a major determinant of trastuzumab resistance in breast cancer. Cancer Cell 2007; 12: 395–402.
16. Codony-Servat J, Albanell J, Lopez-Talavera JC, Arribas J, Baselga J. Cleavage of the HER2 ectodomain is a pervanadate activable process that is inhibited by the tissue inhibitor of metalloproteases TIMP-1 in breast cancer cells. Cancer Res 1999; 59: 1196–201.
17. Anido J, Scaltriti M, Bech Serra JJ, et al. Biosynthesis of tumorigenic HER2 C-terminal fragments by alternative initiation of translation. EMBO J 2006; 25: 3234–44.
18. Molina MA, Saez R, Ramsey EE, et al. NH(2)-terminal truncated HER-2 protein but not full-length receptor is associated with nodal metastasis in human breast cancer. Clin Cancer Res 2002; 8: 347–53.
19. Saez R, Molina MA, Ramsey EE, et al. p95HER-2 predicts worse outcome in patients with HER-2-positive breast cancer. Clin Cancer Res 2006; 12: 424–31.
20. Scaltriti M, Rojo F, Ocana A, et al. Expression of p95HER2, a truncated form of the HER2 receptor, and response to anti-HER2 therapies in breast cancer. J Natl Cancer Inst 2007; 99: 628–38.
21. Sperinde J, Jin X, Banerjee J, et al. Quantitation of p95HER2 in paraffin sections by using a p95-specific antibody and correlation with outcome in a cohort of trastuzumab-treated breast cancer patients. Clin Cancer Res 2010; 16: 4226–35.

22. Scaltriti M, Chandarlapaty S, Prudkin L, et al. Clinical benefit of lapatinib-based therapy in patients with human epidermal growth factor receptor 2-positive breast tumors coexpressing the truncated p95HER2 receptor. Clin Cancer Res 2010; 16: 2688–95.
23. Hurley J, Doliny P, Reis I, et al. Docetaxel, cisplatin, and trastuzumab as primary systemic therapy for human epidermal growth factor receptor 2-positive locally advanced breast cancer. J Clin Oncol 2006; 24: 1831–8.
24. Mittendorf EA, Wu Y, Scaltriti M, et al. Loss of HER2 amplification following trastuzumab-based neoadjuvant systemic therapy and survival outcomes. Clin Cancer Res 2009; 15: 7381–8.
25. Nahta R, Yuan LX, Zhang B, Kobayashi R, Esteva FJ. Insulin-like growth factor-I receptor/human epidermal growth factor receptor 2 heterodimerization contributes to trastuzumab resistance of breast cancer cells. Cancer Res 2005; 65: 11118–28.
26. Lu Y, Zi X, Zhao Y, Mascarenhas D, Pollak M. Insulin-like growth factor-I receptor signaling and resistance to trastuzumab (Herceptin). J Natl Cancer Inst 2001; 93: 1852–7.
27. Harris LN, You F, Schnitt SJ, et al. Predictors of resistance to preoperative trastuzumab and vinorelbine for HER2-positive early breast cancer. Clin Cancer Res 2007; 13: 1198–207.
28. Scaltriti M, Verma C, Guzman M, et al. Lapatinib, a HER2 tyrosine kinase inhibitor, induces stabilization and accumulation of HER2 and potentiates trastuzumab-dependent cell cytotoxicity. Oncogene 2009; 28: 803–14.
29. Clynes RA, Towers TL, Presta LG, Ravetch JV. Inhibitory Fc receptors modulate in vivo cytoxicity against tumor targets. Nat Med 2000; 6: 443–6.
30. Musolino A, Naldi N, Bortesi B, et al. Immunoglobulin G fragment C receptor polymorphisms and clinical efficacy of trastuzumab-based therapy in patients with HER-2/neu-positive metastatic breast cancer. J Clin Oncol 2008; 26: 1789–96.
31. Gennari R, Menard S, Fagnoni F, et al. Pilot study of the mechanism of action of preoperative trastuzumab in patients with primary operable breast tumors overexpressing HER2. Clin Cancer Res 2004; 10: 5650–5.
32. Keyomarsi K, Tucker SL, Buchholz TA, et al. Cyclin E and survival in patients with breast cancer. N Engl J Med 2002; 347: 1566–75.
33. Mittendorf EA, Liu Y, Tucker SL, et al. A novel interaction between HER2/neu and cyclin E in breast cancer. Oncogene 2010; 29: 3896–907.
34. Scatriti M, Eichhorn PJ, Cortes J, et al. Cyclin E amplification/overexpression is a mechanism of trastuzumab resistance in HER2⁺ breast cancer patients. Proc Natl Acad Sci USA 2011; 108: 3761–6.
35. Ritter CA, Perez-Torres M, Rinehart C, et al. Human breast cancer cells selected for resistance to trastuzumab in vivo overexpress epidermal growth factor receptor and ErbB ligands and remain dependent on the ErbB receptor network. Clin Cancer Res 2007; 13: 4909–19.
36. Arteaga CL, O'Neill A, Moulder SL, et al. A phase I-II study of combined blockade of the ErbB receptor network with trastuzumab and gefitinib in patients with HER2 (ErbB2)-overexpressing metastatic breast cancer. Clin Cancer Res 2008; 14: 6277–83.
37. Sergina NV, Rausch M, Wang D, et al. Escape from HER-family tyrosine kinase inhibitor therapy by the kinase-inactive HER3. Nature 2007; 445: 437–41.
38. Baselga J, Swain SM. Novel anticancer targets: revisiting ERBB2 and discovering ERBB3. Nat Rev Cancer 2009; 9: 463–75.
39. Shattuck DL, Miller JK, Carraway KL 3rd, Sweeney C. Met receptor contributes to trastuzumab resistance of Her2-overexpressing breast cancer cells. Cancer Res 2008; 68: 1471–7.
40. Wang SE, Xiang B, Guix M, et al. Transforming growth factor beta engages TACE and ErbB3 to activate phosphatidylinositol-3 kinase/Akt in ErbB2-overexpressing breast cancer and desensitizes cells to trastuzumab. Mol Cell Biol 2008; 28: 5605–20.
41. Arnal-Estape A, Tarragona M, Morales M, et al. HER2 silences tumor suppression in breast cancer cells by switching expression of C/EBPss isoforms. Cancer Res 2010; 70: 9927–36.
42. Lane HA, Motoyama AB, Beuvink I, Hynes NE. Modulation of p27/Cdk2 complex formation through 4D5-mediated inhibition of HER2 receptor signaling. Ann Oncol 2001; 12(Suppl 1): S21–2.
43. Nahta R, Takahashi T, Ueno NT, Hung MC, Esteva FJ. P27(kip1) down-regulation is associated with trastuzumab resistance in breast cancer cells. Cancer Res 2004; 64: 3981–6.

44. Nagy P, Friedlander E, Tanner M, et al. Decreased accessibility and lack of activation of ErbB2 in JIMT-1, a herceptin-resistant, MUC4-expressing breast cancer cell line. Cancer Res 2005; 65: 473–82.
45. Workman HC, Sweeney C, Carraway KL 3rd. The membrane mucin Muc4 inhibits apoptosis induced by multiple insults via ErbB2-dependent and ErbB2-independent mechanisms. Cancer Res 2009; 69: 2845–52.
46. Mitra D, Brumlik MJ, Okamgba SU, et al. An oncogenic isoform of HER2 associated with locally disseminated breast cancer and trastuzumab resistance. Mol Cancer Ther 2009; 8: 2152–62.
47. Cittelly DM, Das PM, Salvo VA, et al. Oncogenic HER2{Delta}16 suppresses miR-15a/16 and deregulates BCL-2 to promote endocrine resistance of breast tumors. Carcinogenesis 2010; 31: 2049–57.
48. Gorre ME, Mohammed M, Ellwood K, et al. Clinical resistance to STI-571 cancer therapy caused by BCR-ABL gene mutation or amplification. Science 2001; 293: 876–80.
49. Pao W, Miller VA, Politi KA, et al. Acquired resistance of lung adenocarcinomas to gefitinib or erlotinib is associated with a second mutation in the EGFR kinase domain. PLoS Med 2005; 2: e73.
50. Lee JW, Soung YH, Seo SH, et al. Somatic mutations of ERBB2 kinase domain in gastric, colorectal, and breast carcinomas. Clin Cancer Res 2006; 12: 57–61.
51. Xia W, Bacus S, Husain I, et al. Resistance to ErbB2 tyrosine kinase inhibitors in breast cancer is mediated by calcium-dependent activation of RelA. Mol Cancer Ther 2010; 9: 292–9.
52. Xia W, Bacus S, Hegde P, et al. A model of acquired autoresistance to a potent ErbB2 tyrosine kinase inhibitor and a therapeutic strategy to prevent its onset in breast cancer. Proc Natl Acad Sci USA 2006; 103: 7795–800.
53. Liu L, Greger J, Shi H, et al. Novel mechanism of lapatinib resistance in HER2-positive breast tumor cells: activation of AXL. Cancer Res 2009; 69: 6871–8.
54. Eichhorn PJ, Gili M, Scaltriti M, et al. Phosphatidylinositol 3-kinase hyperactivation results in lapatinib resistance that is reversed by the mTOR/phosphatidylinositol 3-kinase inhibitor NVP-BEZ235. Cancer Res 2008; 68: 9221–30.
55. Dave B, Migliaccio I, Gutierrez MC, et al. Loss of phosphatase and tensin homolog or phosphoinositol-3 kinase activation and response to trastuzumab or lapatinib in human epidermal growth factor receptor 2-overexpressing locally advanced breast cancers. J Clin Oncol 2011; 29: 166–73.
56. Geyer CE, Forster J, Lindquist D, et al. Lapatinib plus capecitabine for HER2-positive advanced breast cancer. N Engl J Med 2006; 355: 2733–43.
57. von Minckwitz G, du Bois A, Schmidt M, et al. Trastuzumab beyond progression in human epidermal growth factor receptor 2-positive advanced breast cancer: a german breast group 26/breast international group 03-05 study. J Clin Oncol 2009; 27: 1999–2006.
58. Blackwell KL, Burstein HJ, Storniolo AM, et al. Randomized study of Lapatinib alone or in combination with trastuzumab in women with ErbB2-positive, trastuzumab-refractory metastatic breast cancer. J Clin Oncol 2010; 28: 1124–30.
59. Agus DB, Akita RW, Fox WD, et al. Targeting ligand-activated ErbB2 signaling inhibits breast and prostate tumor growth. Cancer Cell 2002; 2: 127–37.
60. Baselga J. A new anti-ErbB2 strategy in the treatment of cancer: prevention of ligand-dependent ErbB2 receptor heterodimerization. Cancer Cell 2002; 2: 93–4.
61. Cho HS, Mason K, Ramyar KX, et al. Structure of the extracellular region of HER2 alone and in complex with the Herceptin Fab. Nature 2003; 421: 756–60.
62. Sliwkowski MX. Ready to partner. Nat Struct Biol 2003; 10: 158–9.
63. Baselga J, Gelmon KA, Verma S, et al. Phase II trial of pertuzumab and trastuzumab in patients with human epidermal growth factor receptor 2-positive metastatic breast cancer that progressed during prior trastuzumab therapy. J Clin Oncol 2010; 28: 1138–44.
64. Cortes J, Baselga J, Petrella T, et al. Pertuzumab monotherapy following trastuzumab-based treatment: activity and tolerability in patients with advanced HER2- positive breast cancer. Proc Am Soc Clin Oncol 2009; A1022.
65. Lewis Phillips GD, Li G, Dugger DL, et al. Targeting HER2-positive breast cancer with trastuzumab-DM1, an antibody-cytotoxic drug conjugate. Cancer Res 2008; 68: 9280–90.

66. Krop IE, Beeram M, Modi S, et al. Phase I study of trastuzumab-DM1, an HER2 antibody-drug conjugate, given every 3 weeks to patients with HER2-positive metastatic breast cancer. J Clin Oncol 2010; 28: 2698–704.
67. Burris HA 3rd, Rugo HS, Vukelja SJ, et al. Phase II study of the antibody drug conjugate trastuzumab-DM1 for the treatment of human epidermal growth factor receptor 2 (HER2) - positive breast cancer after prior HER2-directed therapy. J Clin Oncol 2011; 29: 398–405.
68. Krop I, LoRusso P, Miller K, et al. A phase II study of trastuzumab-DM1 (T-DM1), a novel HER2 antibody–drug conjugate, in HER2⁺ metastatic breast cancer (MBC) patients previously treated with conventional chemotherapy, lapatinib and trastuzumab. Proc SABCS 2009; A710.
69. Perez E, Dirix L, Kocsis J, et al. Efficacy and safety of trastuzumab-DM1 versus trastuzumab plus docetaxel in HER2-positive metastatic breast cancer patients with no prior chemotherapy for metastatic disease: preliminary results of a randomized, multicenter, open-label phase 2 study (TDM4450G). Proc Eur Soc Med Oncol 2010; LBA3.
70. Burstein HJ, Sun Y, Dirix LY, et al. Neratinib, an irreversible ErbB receptor tyrosine kinase inhibitor, in patients with advanced ErbB2-positive breast cancer. J Clin Oncol 2010; 28: 1301–7.
71. Andre F, Campone M, O'Regan R, et al. Phase I study of everolimus plus weekly paclitaxel and trastuzumab in patients with metastatic breast cancer pretreated with trastuzumab. J Clin Oncol 2010; 28: 5110–15.
72. Morrow P, Wulf G, Booser D, et al. Phase I/II trial of everolimus (RAD001) and trastuzumab in patients with trastuzumab-resistant, HER2-overexpressing breast cancer. Proc Am Soc Clin Oncol 2010; A1014.
73. Modi S, Stopeck AT, Gordon MS, et al. Combination of trastuzumab and tanespimycin (17-AAG, KOS-953) is safe and active in trastuzumab-refractory HER-2 overexpressing breast cancer: a phase I dose-escalation study. J Clin Oncol 2007; 25: 5410–17.
74. Modi S, Sugarman S, Stopeck A, et al. Phase II trial of the Hsp90 inhibitor tanespimycin (Tan) + trastuzumab (T) in pts (patients) with HER2-positive metastatic breast cancer (MBC). Proc Am Soc Clin Oncol 2008; A1027.
75. Konecny GE, Meng YG, Untch M, et al. Association between HER-2/neu and vascular endothelial growth factor expression predicts clinical outcome in primary breast cancer patients. Clin Cancer Res 2004; 10: 1706–16.
76. Hurvitz S, Pegram P, Lin L, et al. Final results of a Phase II trial evaluating trastuzumab and bevacizumab as first line treatment of HER2-amplified advanced breast cancer. Proc SABCS 2009; A6094.

5

Targeting triple-negative sporadic and hereditary BRCA-related metastatic breast cancer

Sarah Barton and Nicholas C. Turner

INTRODUCTION

Metastatic triple-negative breast cancer (TNBC) presents a management challenge with a poor prognosis compared to other subtypes of breast cancer. In part, this reflects the inherent characteristics of TNBC, which is an aggressive, highly proliferative breast cancer with a preponderance of visceral and brain metastases. Most importantly, there is a relative lack of targeted therapy options compared to cancers that express either the oestrogen receptor (ER) or have HER2 amplification. This is compounded by high levels of heterogeneity in the cancers, which in part contributes to the frequently observed clinical pattern of response to chemotherapy being maintained for short durations prior to progression.

In this chapter we will discuss the biology of TNBC, how this impacts on the current treatment options, and clinical trials of targeted therapies. In addition, we cover the topic of hereditary breast cancer related to germline BRCA1 and BRCA2 mutations. This topic is covered in this chapter due to the overlap of hereditary BRCA1-related breast cancer and TNBC, and the use of poly (ADP-ribose) polymerase (PARP) inhibitors.

BIOLOGY OF TNBC AND ITS RELATIONSHIP WITH HEREDITARY BREAST CANCER

Triple-Negative and Basal-Like Breast Cancer

TNBCs are those that do not express oestrogen or progesterone receptors, as measured by immunohistochemistry (IHC), and lack HER2 amplification, as measured by IHC or *in situ* hybridisation (1–3). TNBCs account for 10–15% of invasive breast cancers (4–7) and are more prevalent in women at an age below 50. There is an increased prevalence in African-Americans (8), with an association with abdominal obesity (9).

The term TNBC is often used interchangeably with the term basal-like breast cancer (BLBC), but whilst these two entities have a significant overlap, they do not describe exactly the same subsets of breast cancer (Fig. 1). The term BLBC originated from micro-array gene expression profiling that led to the description of three broad subtypes of breast cancer (10,11): luminal (which has substantial overlap with ER$^+$ cancers), HER2 overexpressed, and basal like. The luminal group can be further split into luminal A and B in part reflecting low- and high-proliferation, respectively (12,13). Further refining these subtypes, the claudin low subtype has recently been defined, which is also triple-negative (14).

The BLBC subtype was labelled as such because of its resemblance to the basal–myoepithelial layer of a normal breast duct (10,15), with the expression of basal cytokeratins 5 (often referred to as CK5/6 when assayed by IHC), 14, and 17. Further studies showed that BLBCs characteristically lack ER and HER2 overexpression, and approximately 80% are triple-negative (16–18). The tumours frequently have a very high proliferative rate, with central necrosis pushing the borders of invasion, and may have a stromal lymphocytic response (Fig. 1) (19–26).

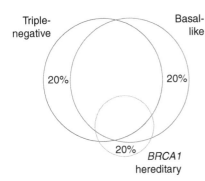

Basal-like phenotype

Ductal Carcinomas
High histological grade
Pushing borders
Central Necrosis
Lymphocytic infiltrate

Triple nagative
Basal keratin expression
TP53 mutations
High level of genomic instability

FIGURE 1   Relationship between triple-negative breast cancer and the basal-like phenotype. (**A**) The terms triple-negative, tumour lacking hormone receptor expression and without HER2 amplification, and basal-like describe similar but not overlapping subsets of breast cancer. Approximately 20% of basal-like breast cancers, as defined by expression profiling, are not triple-negative and likewise approximately 20% of triple-negative cancers are not basal like (19,112). Breast cancers occurring in women with germline BRCA1 mutations are frequently basal like (70–80%) although only 10–15% of sporadic cancers are basal like (24,36–39). (**B**) Pathological characteristics of basal-like breast cancer (16–26).

Basal-like breast cancers frequently express epidermal growth factor receptor (EGFR), c-KIT, and c-MET and this has led to clinical trials of therapies targeting these receptor kinases. The androgen receptor is also expressed in a subset of TNBCs (27). TP53 mutations are very often seen in BLBC, and the tumour suppressor PTEN may be mutated (28). Breast cancer stem cells (as signified by the CD44$^+$/CD24$^-$ phenotype) appear to be most common in BLBC (29).

Heterogeneity of TNBC and Its Influence on Management
The majority of TNBC and BLBC are invasive ductal breast cancers of no special type. However, a number of pathological special types are characteristically triple-negative including metaplastic, medullary, and adenoid cystic tumours (1,6,12), and the very rare secretory breast cancers of childhood. In general, there is no evidence to suggest that the management of TNBC should be different whether the pathological type is ductal, metaplastic, or medullary. The limited available evidence suggests that metaplastic cancers are less likely to respond to chemotherapy in the metastatic setting (30). However, adenoid cystic carcinomas do form a distinct group that should not be considered with other TNBCs. Adenoid cystic carcinomas behave in an indolent fashion, characterised by a high risk of local recurrence but with only infrequent and usually late distant metastases, with limited evidence suggesting poor chemotherapy responsiveness (31).
TNBCs are highly heterogeneous at the genetic level. There is substantial heterogeneity between different cancers, with no common oncogenic aberrations yet identified and this complicates the development of targeted therapies (32). In addition intra-tumoural heterogeneity may in part contribute to the short duration of response seen in metastatic TNBC.
A significant proportion of TNBCs (approx. 20%) do not express basal-like markers (17,33,34) (Fig. 1). At present there is no indication that the management of TNBC should differ between basal-like and non-basal-like cancers.

Hereditary BRCA1-Related Cancer and the Basal-Like Phenotype
Hereditary breast cancer caused by BRCA1 or BRCA2 mutations account for approximately 2% of breast cancers in the Western world (35). Breast cancer that arises in

carriers of BRCA1 mutations characteristically has a basal-like phenotype, with 70–80% of hereditary BRCA1-related cancers having a basal-like phenotype compared to only 10–15% of sporadic cancers (24,36–39) (Fig. 1). Consequently, a majority of BRCA1-related cancers have the same clinicopathological features as sporadic basal-like breast cancers and are frequently triple-negative (40,41) (Fig. 1).

Both *BRCA1* and *BRCA2* are tumour suppressor genes. BRCA mutation carriers have an inactivating germline mutation in one allele of a BRCA gene. In BRCA-related cancer, the wild-type, or normal, allele is also inactivated and consequently BRCA tumour suppressor function is lost. The similarity between hereditary BRCA1-related and sporadic BLBC has raised the possibility that sporadic basal-like breast cancers may also harbour an underlying defect in BRCA1, which has been termed "BRCAness" (42). Recent data have supported this by suggesting that BRCA1 is required for normal differentiation of breast stem and progenitor cells, and when BRCA1 is lost in the cancer this drives the development of a basal-like phenotype (43,44).

Although in this chapter we review the treatment of BRCA2-related cancers, it is important to emphasise that BRCA2-related cancers do not have an association with TNBC or the basal-like phenotype (37). BRCA2 mutation carriers develop predominantly ER-expressing breast tumours, and develop a spectrum of breast cancer subtypes similar to sporadic breast cancers.

BRCA1 in Sporadic TNBC

BRCA1 mutations are only very rarely found in sporadic breast cancers, but despite this there is now substantial evidence for a link between loss of BRCA1 function and sporadic TNBC. BRCA1 expression is suppressed in potentially up to half of sporadic TNBC (37,45–47). BRCA1 promoter methylation that leads to silencing of BRCA1 expression is found in 10–15% of sporadic cancers overall (48–50), but in 20–36% of TNBC (47,51). X chromosomal inactivation has been described to occur frequently in BLBC, which may indicate BRCA1 dysfunction (52).

Not all sporadic TNBC and basal-like cancers share the same features as hereditary BRCA1-related breast cancer. Hereditary BRCA1-related cancers are characterised by high levels of genomic instability and specific TP53 mutations (53). Within sporadic TNBC a group of BRCA1-like cancers can be identified that share the same pattern of genomic instability and TP53 mutations (54), and similar gene expression patterns (55,56). It is assumed that these BRCA1-like sporadic cancers are those that are likely to have a defect in BRCA1 function, but this is unproved.

It is clear that there is heterogeneity in the loss of BRCA1 in TNBC, and this may have importance in the delivery of targeted therapy as we discuss later. The pathologically defined special types of breast cancers with a basal-like phenotype, including metaplastic and medullary, have a very high frequency of BRCA1 promoter methylation (47). This may reflect that these are cancers with a "strong" basal-like phenotype.

BRCA1/2 and HR-Based DNA Repair

Both BRCA1 and BRCA2 functions are required for DNA double strand break (DSB) repair by homologous recombination (HR) (57,58). There are two principal repair pathways for DNA DSB repair. Non-homologous end joining is one pathway that is active throughout the cell cycle and essentially rejoins the two ends of the DNA DSB, deleting DNA on either side of the break in the process. HR is the second pathway and is active only during the S and G2 phases of the cell cycle. HR is the most accurate mechanism of repair, frequently restoring the original sequence at the break without error, and is the only repair pathway that can adequately repair DNA DSBs that occur at collapsed replication forks.

As the normal function of both BRCA1 and BRCA2 is required for HR, tumours arising in carriers of BRCA1/2 germline mutations have a defect in HR. This DNA repair defect leads to increased genomic instability, and it is this genomic instability that is thought to drive tumourigenesis.

HR repairs the damage of many commonly used chemotherapy drugs, and consequently HR-deficient cell lines are more sensitive to certain chemotherapy drugs *in vitro*. Alkylating agents cause DNA interstrand cross-links which lead to the arrest of DNA replication forks and double strand DNA breaks. Topoisomerase II inhibitors such as anthracyclines cause an arrest of DNA replication forks and DNA DSBs. Platinum chemotherapies form adducts with DNA and DNA DSBs, and when HR function is lost cell lines are highly sensitive to cisplatin (37,59–62). In mouse mammary tumour models of BRCA1 deficiency, 100% of tumours had a complete response to platinum given in high dose (62).

Conversely, cancer cell lines defective specifically of BRCA1 show resistance to microtubule interfering agents such as paclitaxel and vincristine *in vitro* (63). It is unclear whether this translates into a lack of sensitivity in the clinic. This effect is not seen in BRCA2-deficient tumours, and the resistance seen *in vitro* is likely explained by the additional functions that BRCA1 has in transcriptional control and cell cycle checkpoints (63).

CHARACTERISTICS OF METASTATIC TNBC

TNBCs have a poor prognosis in the adjuvant setting, characterised in particular by early recurrence compared to other subtypes of breast cancer (64,65) (Fig. 2). This occurs despite a high sensitivity to (neo)adjuvant chemotherapy (66). Although cancers that have a pathological complete response (pathCR) to neoadjuvant chemotherapy have a good prognosis, those cancers that do not achieve a pathCR have a marked poor prognosis with frequent and, in particular, early relapse (66). Distant disease-free survival at 4 years was 87% for those who had a pathCR, compared to 69% in those who did not (p = 0.03) (Fig. 2). A vast majority of relapses from TNBC and BLBC occur in the first 5 years following diagnosis (64).

A similar pattern is carried over into the metastatic setting where TNBCs have a marked poor prognosis compared to other cancer types. In one study the median survival time from recurrence to death was 9 months in TNBC, compared to 20 months for other cancers (p = 0.02 for difference) (67). These results were supported by a recently published study which showed the median survival time from the diagnosis of metastatic disease. It was just 0.5 years for BLBC and 0.9 years for TNBC, compared with 2.2 years for low proliferation ER-positive cancers (64).

The reasons for this poor prognosis in the metastatic setting are multifactorial. In part this reflects the lack of targeted therapies for TNBC and the highly proliferative nature of TNBC. In part, this reflects the pattern of metastasis seen in TNBCs, which are characterised by less frequent bone and liver metastasis and more frequent lung and brain metastasis (64,65) (Table 1). Current evidence suggests that triple-negative basal-like and non-basal-like breast cancers have a similar pattern of metastatic disease (64).

Molecular subtype is also predictive for risk of locoregional recurrence ensuing after breast-conserving surgery and mastectomy. BLBC and HER2-enriched cancer molecular subtypes are reported to have the highest rates of local and regional nodal recurrence after breast conserving surgery (10-year local relapse-free survival 86% BLBC, 79% HER2, and 92% luminal A) (68) . However, this evidence pre-dates the introduction of adjuvant trastuzumab. With contemporary trastuzumab containing adjuvant systemic therapy the outcome of the HER2-enriched group is now likely to have improved, leaving BLBC as the cancer subtype with the highest risk of local relapse.

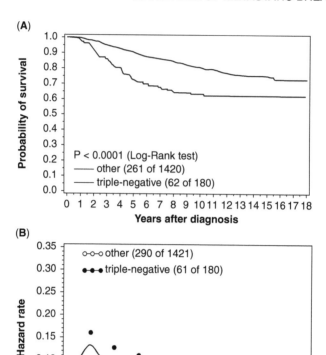

FIGURE 2 Prognosis of triple-negative breast cancer. Triple-negative cancers have a poor prognosis not only due to early relapse, but also as the cancers behave in an aggressive fashion with a short time from relapse to death. **(A)** Overall survival of triple-negative breast cancer compared to cancers expression either the hormone receptors or HER2. **(B)** Risk of relapse after treatment of primary breast cancer expressed as the hazard ratio for relapse in 6-month periods. Triple-negative cancers have a high risk of early relapse, but are less likely to relapse late compared to other cancers. *Source*: Adapted from Ref. 67.

TABLE 1 Metastatic Disease Site Differs According to Molecular Subtype

| | ER+ HER2− | HER2+ | Triple-negative | | p-Value |
			Basal-like	Non- basal	
n[a]	836	253	159	109	
Brain	9%	23%	25%	22%	<0.0001
Liver	30%	45%	21%	32%	<0.0001
Lungs	27%	42%	43%	36%	<0.0001
Bone	69%	62%	39%	43%	<0.0001
Distant nodal	19%	24%	40%	36%	<0.0001
Pleural/periotoneal	31%	33%	30%	28%	0.82

[a]Frequency of sites involved by metastatic disease in patients who developed distant recurrence as observed in a study of 3726 patients, diagnosed between 1986 and 1992, of which 9.8% were basal-like breast cancer and 8.5% triple-negative breast cancer.
Abbreviations: ER+, oestrogen receptor positive; HER2+, HER2 positive; n, number in each group; p value, Chi squared test.
Source: Adapted from Ref. 64.

Brain Metastases and TNBC

Brain metastases are also frequently described in patients with triple-negative disease. In a report where 679 women with TNBC treated at the MD Anderson Cancer Center (69), 200 developed distant recurrences, of whom 42 (21%) developed brain metastases. This was similar to the incidence seen in a study comparing metastatic sites from a Canadian breast cancer database, in which 25.2% of women with distant recurrence from TNBC developed brain metastasis, in numbers similar to that of HER2-enriched breast cancer, whereas women with luminal subtypes and distant recurrence had a lower frequency (7.1%) (64).

The prognosis for women with TNBC brain metastases is particularly poor (69), with a median survival from diagnosis with a brain metastasis of 0.24 years for TNBC compared with 0.8 years for HR^+HER2^-, 1.19 years for HR^-HER^+, and 1.27 years for a HR^+HER^+ group (p = 0.002) (70). This at least in part reflects the observation that extracranial disease is frequently poorly controlled in patients with TNBC and brain metastases. The general poor prognosis of TNBC with brain metastases should be taken into consideration if a surgical resection is planned.

TREATMENT OF HEREDITARY BREAST CANCER
Chemotherapy for Hereditary Breast Cancer

There is substantial pre-clinical evidence that BRCA1/2-deficient cells are sensitive to particular chemotherapy drugs, in particular platinum agents as discussed previously. However, current clinical evidence is limited to small retrospective studies. A retrospective study of 102 Polish women with BRCA1 mutation treated with neoadjuvant chemotherapy reported an overall pathCR rate of 24% (71). Interestingly, 10/12 (83%) patients treated with cisplatin had a pathCR, which was substantially higher than that seen in patients treated with other regimens (1/14 with cyclophosphamide, methotrexate, fluorouracil (CMF), 2/25 with taxane/anthracycline, 11/51 with anthracycline). In an historical cohort of 278 Ashkenazi Jews, patients with BRCA1 deficiency and breast cancer treated with adjuvant chemotherapy had a better prognosis than those not (72). Similarly patients with BRCA1/2-deficient ovarian cancer have an improved outcome with chemotherapy (73) with high sensitivity specifically to platinum-based chemotherapy (74).

There is a lack of evidence on whether patients with metastatic hereditary BRCA1/2-related cancers should be treated with different chemotherapy protocols to sporadic cancers. In the United Kingdom, the BRCA trial (NCT00321633) is attempting to address this, randomising patients between carboplatin and docetaxel as the standard of care. However, recruiting to such studies is challenging. In the absence of definitive evidence the weight of the pre-clinical and clinical evidence supports the use of platinum -based chemotherapy in metastatic hereditary cancer, provided patients have sufficient performance status and lack contraindications such as poor renal function. The optimal timing of platinum-based therapy, versus anthracycline based or taxane based, is unclear.

Synthetic Lethality and PARP Inhibitor

PARP 1 is a nuclear enzyme that is required for the repair of single strand DNA breaks (SSB) (75–77). Multiple PARP inhibitors were initially developed as potentiators of the cytotoxicity of chemotherapy drugs, and radiation, through inhibition of damage repair. Interest in PARP inhibitors as a class of anti-cancer drugs changed dramatically with the demonstration that cancer cell lines with defects in BRCA1 and BRCA2 are highly sensitive to PARP inhibitors *in vitro* (75,77,78) (Fig. 3). Underlying this sensitivity is the shared role of both BRCA1 and BRCA2 in HR, with the sensitivity of BRCA1/2-deficient cancers not reflecting the loss of BRCA1 or BRCA2 *per se* but the resulting defect in HR-based DNA repair (77).

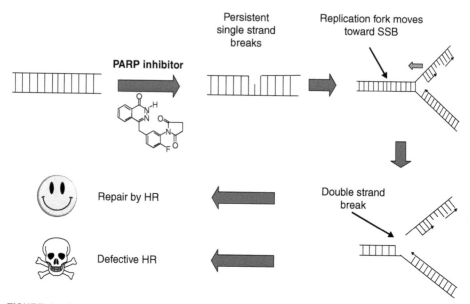

FIGURE 3 Currently established mechanism of action of poly (ADP-ribose) polymerase (PARP) inhibitors. PARP inhibitors inhibitor the PARP1 enzyme that is required for normal DNA single strand break (SSB) repair. Following exposure to a PARP inhibitor, SSBs remain unrepaired, which in themselves are not toxic to the cell. However, during S phase if an SSB collides with a replication form, this collapses the fork creating a double strand break (DSB). DSBs are highly toxic to the cell if not repaired efficiently. DSBs that form at collapsed replication forks can only efficiently be repaired by homologous recombination (HR) DNA repair, and consequently if HR is impaired PARP inhibitors are highly toxic to the cell. Both BRCA1 and BRCA2 are essential for normal HR function, and consequently cancers deficient in either BRCA1 or BRCA2 are highly sensitive to PARP inhibitors (75–77).

The proposed mechanism underlying the sensitivity of HR-defective cancers to PARP inhibitors (discussed in Fig. 3) is often referred to as an example of synthetic lethality (79). This describes a situation where the inhibition of PARP is tolerated by the cell, loss of BRCA1/2 is tolerated by the cell, but loss of PARP and BRCA1/2 together is not tolerated and is "synthetically lethal". Most crucially, loss of BRCA1/2 function is limited to the cancer in women with heterozygous germline BRCA1/2 mutations, as the wild-type allele is lost in cancer cells but retained in normal cells.

Evidence for PARP Inhibitors in Hereditary Breast Cancer

The pre-clinical evidence on PARP inhibitors has translated into substantial efficacy in clinical trials. Fong et al. (80) reported phase I trial results of PARP inhibition with oral olaparib, in 60 patients with solid organ tumours enriched for 22 patients with BRCA1/2 mutations. Olaparib was tolerated well without the usual side effects associated with chemotherapy, with fatigue and thrombocytopenia dose limiting toxicities. Anti-tumour activity was only seen in patients with BRCA1/2 mutations. Of patients with BRCA1/2 mutations, 12 of the 19 patients derived clinical benefit (response or stable disease for 4 or more months) and the remaining 9 had response.

These results led rapidly to the recruitment of a phase II trial of olaparib in women with recurrent and advanced breast cancer and confirmed BRCA1/2 mutation (81). The study investigated two doses of olaparib, and in the high dose cohort the

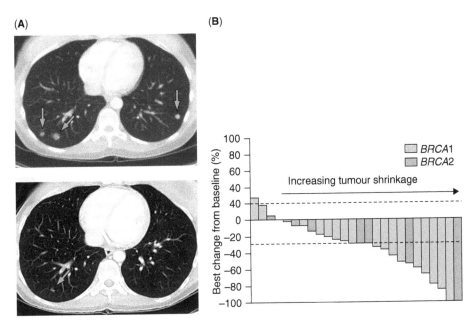

FIGURE 4 Efficacy of poly (ADP-ribose) polymerase (PARP) inhibitors in hereditary breast cancer. (**A**) Response in lung metastases of a patient with triple-negative BRCA1 hereditary breast cancer with CT scan at baseline (top) and after 180 days of treatment with PARP inhibitor olaparib (bottom). (**B**) The best percentage change in the tumour size of a target lesion on olaparib. *Source*: Adapted from Ref. 81.

primary endpoint of objective response rate was 41% (Fig. 4). Lower activity was seen in the lower dose cohort suggesting a dose–response relationship. The most common grade 3 and 4 adverse events were fatigue (15%) and anaemia (11%) in the high dose cohort. Efficacy was seen in both BRCA1- and BRCA2-related cancers, and in both triple-negative and non-triple-negative cancers (81).

Further studies demonstrating the efficacy of PARP inhibitors in hereditary BRCA1/2-related breast cancer have been reported in abstract form with MK4827 monotherapy (82) and with velaparib in combination with temozolomide (83). Therefore, there is now substantial evidence for the efficacy of PARP inhibitors in hereditary breast cancer. However, at the time of writing there are no registration studies running with a PARP inhibitor in hereditary breast cancer, and it is therefore unclear when, and whether, a PARP inhibitor will be licensed for this indication.

Resistance to PARP Inhibitors in Hereditary Breast Cancer
A likely major mechanism of resistance to PARP inhibition is restoration of normal HR-based DNA repair, reversing the reason that cancer cells are sensitive, through re-expression of a functional BRCA1/2 protein (84,85). Revertant mutations in BRCA1 (85) and BRCA2 genes (84,86) that restore the function of the BRCA1/2 protein have been demonstrated *in vitro* and in platinum-resistant hereditary ovarian cancer. It is likely, although not yet proven, that the same mechanism will lead to acquired resistant to PARP inhibition in hereditary breast cancer.

Loss of 53BP1 expression has been identified as a possible mechanism of resistance in BRCA1-related cancers (52,87), which partly rescues the deficiency in HR seen BRCA1-deficient cells *in vitro*. It is unknown whether this is a clinically relevant mechanism of resistance.

TREATMENT OF SPORADIC TNBC
Chemotherapy for TNBC

In the neoadjuvant setting both TNBC and BLBC are highly sensitive to chemotherapy. In one study of 81 patients treated with neoadjuvant paclitaxel followed by fluorouracil, doxorubicin, and cyclophosphamide, patients with basal-like and HER2 overexpressing molecular subtypes had a pathCR of 45%, compared to 6% in the luminal subtype (88). Similarly in a further study 27% of TNBC had pathCR compared with 36% in the HER2-positive group, and 7% in the luminal subgroups (66).

In the metastatic setting patients with TNBC frequently respond to chemotherapy, but unfortunately this does not translate into a longer progression free survival (PFS) in many studies, as responses tend to be of short duration (89). The decision on which chemotherapy to administer depends in part on the chemotherapy administered in the (neo)adjuvant setting and the time from adjuvant chemotherapy to relapse. Rechallenge with the same chemotherapy is rarely performed with a relapse-free interval of less than 1 year, with uncertainty in the benefits of rechallenging with an interval less than 2 years.

The similarity between hereditary BRCA1 mutant carriers and sporadic TNBC has lead to a widespread use of platinum-based chemotherapy in metastatic TNBC, although the evidence to support this general change in oncology practice is weak. A number of retrospective, non-randomised case series have been reported. A report from the Royal Marsden Hospital found a non-significant increase in response rates of TNBC to MVP chemotherapy (mitomycin C, vinblastine, and cisplatin) compared to non-TN cancers (TNBC 41% vs. non-TN 31%, p = 0.3) with a significant improvement in PFS (90). A report from the Institut-Curie in Paris of 143 patients treated with platinum-based chemotherapy found an insignificant increase in response rates (91) (TNBC 33% vs. 22%, p = 0.1), with no difference in PFS and OS. A Korean retrospective analysis of 106 patients with metastatic TNBC treated with platinum-containing chemotherapy in first or second line again showed no significant difference in RR between that of TNBC (39%) and other subtypes (92).

In contrast to this data, neoadjuvant studies suggest a high sensitivity of TNBC to platinum-based chemotherapy. A study of 28 patients with TNBC treated with four cycles of neoadjuvant cisplatin reported a partial response rate of 64% with 22% having a pathCR (93). Tumours with BRCA1 promoter methylation, low BRCA1 mRNA expression, and complex p53 mutations were more likely to respond well to chemotherapy. The findings that low BRCA1 expression correlated with cisplatin response provides support for "BRCAness"; that low BRCA1 expression explains the similar phenotype between TNBC and BRCA-deficient BC, and that this may produce a targetable defect in DNA repair.

It is likely that the heterogeneity of TNBC may explain the findings in these reports. It is likely that only a proportion of TNBC have the defective DNA repair defect that makes them intrinsically highly sensitive to platinum (94), and therefore only a subset would be expected to benefit specifically from platinum-based chemotherapy. However, at present there are no clinically applicable tests to identify this subset.

There is limited evidence to suggest that TNBC may show selective sensitivity to ixabepilone, an epothilone B analogue microtubule stabiliser, in a retrospective analysis of results of five phase II studies of ixabepilone and a prospective pooled analysis of two phase III trials (95). Of 2261 patients included in these studies, 556 (24.5%) had TNBC. Neoadjuvant pathCR was 26% for ixabepilone in TNBC compared with 15% in non-TNBC. However in the metastatic setting, response rate to ixabepilone monotherapy was similar between TNBC and non-TN cancers. The addition of ixabepilone to capecitabine improved PFS compared with capecitabine monotherapy (4.2 months vs. 1.7 months, hazard ratio 0.63 [0.52–0.77]). It should be noted that ixabepilone is not licensed for the treatment of breast cancer in Europe, although is licensed by the Food and Drug Administration.

In conclusion, there is only limited evidence to recommend that metastatic TNBC should be treated with chemotherapy protocols different from that of non-TNBC. In routine clinical practice it is considered that metastatic TNBC is a relative indication for platinum-based chemotherapy, although the lack of high quality evidence to support this practice should be acknowledged. The combination of gemcitabine with carboplatin or cisplatin is a commonly used schedule (96–98).

MOLECULAR THERAPIES
PARP Inhibitors
The shared characteristics of TNBC (especially of the basal subtype) and hereditary BRCA1-related cancers, and the evidence discussed previously that the loss of BRCA1 is frequent in TNBC has led to the investigation of PARP inhibitors in metastatic TNBC.

O'Shaughnessy et al. (99) randomised 123 patients with metastatic TNBC in an open label phase II study, between the chemotherapy doublet gemcitabine/carboplatin given alone and in combination with the PARP inhibitor iniparib (BSI-201). The primary endpoint was the clinical benefit rate (CBR), with the addition of iniparib improving CBR from 34 to 56% (p = 0.01). The most exciting part of the results, however, was the improvement in survival. Patients treated with iniparib and chemotherapy had an improved median PFS (3.6 months lengthened to 5.9 months, hazard ratio 0.59, p = 0.01) and improved median overall survival (7.7 months lengthened to 12.3 months, hazard ratio 0.57, p = 0.01) (Fig. 5). A phase III trial with an adequate statistical power to detect difference in survival endpoints has been performed. Although this has not yet been formally reported, at the time of writing this chapter it had been

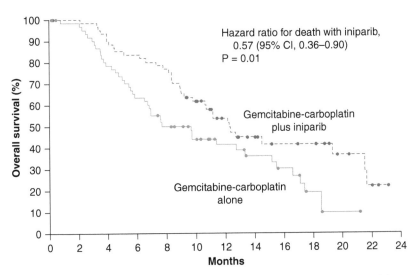

FIGURE 5 Efficacy of poly (ADP-ribose) polymerase (PARP) inhibitors in sporadic triple-negative breast cancer (TNBC). An overall survival analysis of patients with metastatic sporadic TNBC randomised to treatment with gemcitabine/carboplatin chemotherapy alone or the combination of gemcitabine/carboplatin and the PARP inhibitor iniparib. Addition of PAPR inhibitor iniparib improved the overall survival with the median overall survival increasing from 7.7 months to 12.3 months (p = 0.01). *Source*: Adapted from Ref. 99.

announced by press release that this registration phase III study had not achieved the primary endpoint. Therefore, the benefit of PARP inhibitors in sporadic metastatic TNBC is unclear.

There are other ambiguities in the results of O'Shaughnessy et al. (99). The dosing of carboplatin in the study, AUC2 days 1 and 8, is non-standard leading to some uncertainty over the efficacy of the control arm. There was no difference in toxicity between the two groups and although this suggests iniparib was well tolerated, it contrasted markedly with the experience of other PARP inhibitors in combination with chemotherapy, which led to a substantial increase in bone marrow suppression. This has led to a conjecture regarding whether iniparib is actually functioning as a PARP inhibitor, and as to the exact mechanism that explains the observed efficacy.

A number of other trials have reported on PARP inhibitors in TNBC. Dent et al. (100) reported safety and preliminary efficacy data of a single-arm phase I/II trial of olaparib combined with weekly paclitaxel in metastatic TNBC, reporting a response rate of 37%. In addition, a number of negative trials have reported no response to either olaparib given as a single agent in heavily pre-treated sporadic TNBC (101) or velaparib in combination with temozolomide in sporadic TNBC (83). Exactly how one should interpret the negative trials is unclear. Potentially they suggest that PARP inhibitors as a single agent have no efficacy in sporadic cancers, and efficacy is only seen in combination with chemotherapy. However, the negative studies were conducted in heavily pretreated breast cancer, whereas O'Shaughnessy et al. (99) treated predominantly first-line metastatic patients. Whether prior chemotherapy exposure has obscured the efficacy of single agent PARP inhibitors in the negative studies is unclear.

Angiogenesis Targeting
Subgroup analyses of randomised studies of bevacizumab have demonstrated efficacy in TNBC, but do not suggest superior efficacy over other breast cancer subtypes. A subgroup analysis of the E2100 trial showed an improved PFS in the ER$^-$/PR$^-$ group (of which most were triple-negative) for bevacizumab added to chemotherapy, with hazard ratio being 0.53 (0.40–0.70) compared with chemotherapy alone (102), but this benefit was similar to that seen in the ER$^+$/PR$^+$ tumours (hazard ratio 0.54 (0.44–0.70)). Similarly, a subgroup analysis of the Avastin and Docetaxel (AVADO) trial provided no evidence of variation in the efficacy with hormone receptor expression (103). Partly due to lack of other targeted therapies in breast cancer bevacizumab is frequently used in metastatic TNBC. However, with no evidence to prove that bevacizumab improves overall survival (104), at the time of writing this book, the Food and Drug Administration has considered revoking the breast cancer license for bevacizumab. The VEGFR tyrosine kinase inhibitor sunitinib has shown only a limited efficacy in metastatic TNBC with a reported response rate of 11% (105).

Growth Factor Receptor Targeting
A number of growth factor receptors are expressed as part of the basal-like phenotype. EGFR is expressed in approximately 50% of tumours, with EGFR amplifications in very few tumours. Two studies have explored the efficacy of EGFR-targeted therapies in metastatic TNBC. Single-agent cetuximab has very limited efficacy with a response rate of 6% in one study (106). The recently reported BALI-1 trial found that the addition of cetuximab to cisplatin doubled the overall response rate (ORR) (20.0% vs. 10.3%, p = 0.5) and significantly improved the time to progression (hazard ratio 0.675, p = 0.032) (107). This raises the possibility that EGFR may present a target in a minority of TNBCs, potentially those with EGFR amplification, although further work is required to establish biomarkers of sensitivity.

The c-MET receptor is expressed in TNBC, with a strong evidence for an oncogenic role of c-MET in mouse models of basal-like breast cancer (108). A clinical trial of a c-MET antibody in metastatic TNBC in combination with paclitaxel is planned (NCT01186991). The receptor c-KIT is expressed as part of the basal-like phenotype although no responses were observed with c-KIT inhibitor imatinib in breast cancers expressing c-KIT (109). FGFR2 is amplified in a small subset of TNBC, and at least *in vitro*, presents a potential therapeutic target in these cancers (32).

Other Targeted Therapies
In vitro TNBC cell lines are sensitive to inhibitors of Src (110), although only a limited efficacy was seen with dasatinib in heavily pre-treated TNBC (111). The androgen receptor is expressed in a minority of TNBCs, and the potential to target the androgen receptor therapeutically is being explored with the hormonal therapy abiraterone (NCT00755885).

TNBCs frequently show a brisk lymphocytic infiltrate, and the presence of the lymphocytic infiltrate is correlated with a good response. Although it is not possible to draw causal inference from this association, there may be the potential to target TNBC with therapies that enhance the immune response (such as with ligands for toll-like receptors, CTLA4 antibodies, or cancer vaccines).

CONCLUSION
At present the systemic treatment of metastatic TNBC is restricted to the use of chemotherapy, with no targeted therapies other than potentially bevacizumab. Significant progress is being made in the clinical trials of targeted therapies; the most progress being made with PARP inhibitors but also with some potential evidence of efficacy with the EGFR targeting antibody, cetuximab. The major challenge will be identifying biomarkers to predict the optimal therapy for each individual cancer.

REFERENCES
1. Reis-Filho JS, Tutt AN. Triple-negative tumours: a critical review. Histopathology 2008; 52: 108–18.
2. Carey L, Winer E, Viale G, Cameron D, Gianni L. Triple-negative breast cancer: disease entity or title of convenience? Nat Rev Clin Oncol 2010; 7: 683–92.
3. Foulkes WD, Smith IE, Reis-Filho JS. Triple-negative breast cancer. N Engl J Med 2010; 363: 1938–48.
4. Bauer KR, Brown M, Cress RD, Parise CA, Caggiano V. Descriptive analysis of estrogen receptor (ER)-negative, progesterone receptor (PR)-negative, and HER2-negative invasive breast cancer, the so-called triple-negative phenotype: a population-based study from the California cancer Registry. Cancer 2007; 109: 1721–8.
5. Morris GJ, Naidu S, Topham AK, et al. Differences in breast carcinoma characteristics in newly diagnosed African-American and Caucasian patients: a single-institution compilation compared with the National Cancer Institute's Surveillance, Epidemiology, and End Results database. Cancer 2007; 110: 876–84.
6. Rakha EA, El-Sayed ME, Green AR, et al. Prognostic markers in triple-negative breast cancer. Cancer 2007; 109: 25–32.
7. Kyndi M, Sorensen FB, Knudsen H, et al. Estrogen receptor, progesterone receptor, HER-2, and response to postmastectomy radiotherapy in high-risk breast cancer: the Danish Breast Cancer Cooperative Group. J Clin Oncol 2008; 26: 1419–26.
8. Carey LA, Perou CM, Livasy CA, et al. Race, breast cancer subtypes, and survival in the Carolina Breast Cancer Study. JAMA 2006; 295: 2492–502.
9. Dolle JM, Daling JR, White E, et al. Risk factors for triple-negative breast cancer in women under the age of 45 years. Cancer Epidemiol Biomarkers Prev 2009; 18: 1157–66.

10. Perou CM, Sorlie T, Eisen MB, et al. Molecular portraits of human breast tumours. Nature 2000; 406: 747–52.
11. Sorlie T. Molecular portraits of breast cancer: tumour subtypes as distinct disease entities. Eur J Cancer 2004; 40: 2667–75.
12. Weigelt B, Baehner FL, Reis-Filho JS. The contribution of gene expression profiling to breast cancer classification, prognostication and prediction: a retrospective of the last decade. J Pathol 2010; 220: 263–80.
13. Sotiriou C, Pusztai L. Gene-expression signatures in breast cancer. N Engl J Med 2009; 360: 790–800.
14. Herschkowitz JI, Simin K, Weigman VJ, et al. Identification of conserved gene expression features between murine mammary carcinoma models and human breast tumors. Genome Biol 2007; 8: R76.
15. Brenton JD, Carey LA, Ahmed AA, Caldas C. Molecular classification and molecular forecasting of breast cancer: ready for clinical application? J Clin Oncol 2005; 23: 7350–60.
16. Nielsen TO, Hsu FD, Jensen K, et al. Immunohistochemical and clinical characterization of the basal-like subtype of invasive breast carcinoma. Clin Cancer Res 2004; 10: 5367–74.
17. Cheang MC, Voduc D, Bajdik C, et al. Basal-like breast cancer defined by five biomarkers has superior prognostic value than triple-negative phenotype. Clin Cancer Res 2008; 14: 1368–76.
18. Rakha EA, Reis-Filho JS, Ellis IO. Impact of basal-like breast carcinoma determination for a more specific therapy. Pathobiology 2008; 75: 95–103.
19. Rakha EA, Reis-Filho JS, Ellis IO. Basal-like breast cancer: a critical review. J Clin Oncol 2008; 26: 2568–81.
20. Tsuda H, Takarabe T, Hasegawa F, Fukutomi T, Hirohashi S. Large, central acellular zones indicating myoepithelial tumor differentiation in high-grade invasive ductal carcinomas as markers of predisposition to lung and brain metastases. Am J Surg Pathol 2000; 24: 197–202.
21. Foulkes WD, Brunet JS, Stefansson IM, et al. The prognostic implication of the basal-like (cyclin E high/p27 low/p53+/glomeruloid-microvascular-proliferation+) phenotype of BRCA1-related breast cancer. Cancer Res 2004; 64: 830–5.
22. Banerjee S, Reis-Filho JS, Ashley S, et al. Basal-like breast carcinomas: clinical outcome and response to chemotherapy. J Clin Pathol 2006; 59: 729–35.
23. Fulford LG, Easton DF, Reis-Filho JS, et al. Specific morphological features predictive for the basal phenotype in grade 3 invasive ductal carcinoma of breast. Histopathology 2006; 49: 22–34.
24. Lakhani SR, Reis-Filho JS, Fulford L, et al. Prediction of BRCA1 status in patients with breast cancer using estrogen receptor and basal phenotype. Clin Cancer Res 2005; 11: 5175–80.
25. Livasy CA, Karaca G, Nanda R, et al. Phenotypic evaluation of the basal-like subtype of invasive breast carcinoma. Mod Pathol 2006; 19: 264–71.
26. Tsuda H, Takarabe T, Hasegawa T, Murata T, Hirohashi S. Myoepithelial differentiation in high-grade invasive ductal carcinomas with large central acellular zones. Hum Pathol 1999; 30: 1134–9.
27. Niemeier LA, Dabbs DJ, Beriwal S, Striebel JM, Bhargava R. Androgen receptor in breast cancer: expression in estrogen receptor-positive tumors and in estrogen receptor-negative tumors with apocrine differentiation. Mod Pathol 2010; 23: 205–12.
28. Saal LH, Gruvberger-Saal SK, Persson C, et al. Recurrent gross mutations of the PTEN tumor suppressor gene in breast cancers with deficient DSB repair. Nat Genet 2008; 40: 102–7.
29. Park SY, Lee HE, Li H, et al. Heterogeneity for stem cell-related markers according to tumor subtype and histologic stage in breast cancer. Clin Cancer Res 2010; 16: 876–87.
30. Hennessy BT, Giordano S, Broglio K, et al. Biphasic metaplastic sarcomatoid carcinoma of the breast. Ann Oncol 2006; 17: 605–13.
31. Marchio C, Weigelt B, Reis-Filho JS. Adenoid cystic carcinomas of the breast and salivary glands (or 'The strange case of Dr Jekyll and Mr Hyde' of exocrine gland carcinomas). J Clin Pathol 2010; 63: 220–8.

32. Turner N, Lambros MB, Horlings HM, et al. Integrative molecular profiling of triple-negative breast cancers identifies amplicon drivers and potential therapeutic targets. Oncogene 2010; 29: 2013–23.

33. Tan DS, Marchio C, Jones RL, et al. Triple-negative breast cancer: molecular profiling and prognostic impact in adjuvant anthracycline-treated patients. Breast Cancer Res Treat 2008; 111: 27–44.

34. Bertucci F, Finetti P, Cervera N, et al. How basal are triple-negative breast cancers? Int J Cancer 2008; 123: 236–40.

35. Wooster R, Weber BL. Breast and ovarian cancer. N Engl J Med 2003; 348: 2339–47.

36. Rakha EA, El-Sayed ME, Reis-Filho J, Ellis IO. Patho-biological aspects of basal-like breast cancer. Breast Cancer Res Treat 2009; 113: 411–22.

37. Turner NC, Reis-Filho JS. Basal-like breast cancer and the BRCA1 phenotype. Oncogene 2006; 25: 5846–53.

38. Tan DS, Marchio C, Reis-Filho JS. Hereditary breast cancer: from molecular pathology to tailored therapies. J Clin Pathol 2008; 61: 1073–82.

39. Rakha E, Reis-Filho JS. Basal-like breast carcinoma: from expression profiling to routine practice. Arch Pathol Lab Med 2009; 133: 860–8.

40. Lakhani SR, Van De Vijver MJ, Jacquemier J, et al. The pathology of familial breast cancer: predictive value of immunohistochemical markers estrogen receptor, progesterone receptor, HER-2, and p53 in patients with mutations in BRCA1 and BRCA2. J Clin Oncol 2002; 20: 2310–18.

41. Lakhani SR. The pathology of familial breast cancer: morphological aspects. Breast Cancer Res 1999; 1: 31–5.

42. Turner N, Tutt A, Ashworth A. Hallmarks of 'BRCAness' in sporadic cancers. Nat Rev Cancer 2004; 4: 814–19.

43. Liu S, Ginestier C, Charafe-Jauffret E, et al. BRCA1 regulates human mammary stem/progenitor cell fate. Proc Natl Acad Sci USA 2008; 105: 1680–5.

44. Molyneux G, Geyer FC, Magnay FA, et al. BRCA1 basal-like breast cancers originate from luminal epithelial progenitors and not from basal stem cells. Cell Stem Cell 2010; 7: 403–17.

45. Esteller M, Silva JM, Dominguez G, et al. Promoter hypermethylation and BRCA1 inactivation in sporadic breast and ovarian tumors. J Natl Cancer Inst 2000; 92: 564–9.

46. Esteller M. Epigenetics in cancer. N Engl J Med 2008; 358: 1148–59.

47. Turner NC, Reis-Filho JS, Russell AM, et al. BRCA1 dysfunction in sporadic basal-like breast cancer. Oncogene 2007; 26: 2126–32.

48. Hedenfalk I, Duggan D, Chen Y, et al. Gene-expression profiles in hereditary breast cancer. N Engl J Med 2001; 344: 539–48.

49. Esteller M, Fraga MF, Guo M, et al. DNA methylation patterns in hereditary human cancers mimic sporadic tumorigenesis. Hum Mol Genet 2001; 10: 3001–7.

50. Rio PG, Maurizis JC, Peffault de Latour M, Bignon YJ, Bernard-Gallon DJ. Quantification of BRCA1 protein in sporadic breast carcinoma with or without loss of heterozygosity of the BRCA1 gene. Int J Cancer 1999; 80: 823–6.

51. Veeck J, Ropero S, Setien F, et al. BRCA1 CpG island hypermethylation predicts sensitivity to poly (adenosine diphosphate)-ribose polymerase inhibitors. J Clin Oncol 2010; 28: e563–4; author reply e5–6.

52. Richardson AL, Wang ZC, De Nicolo A, et al. X chromosomal abnormalities in basal-like human breast cancer. Cancer Cell 2006; 9: 121–32.

53. Manie E, Vincent-Salomon A, Lehmann-Che J, et al. High frequency of TP53 mutation in BRCA1 and sporadic basal-like carcinomas but not in BRCA1 luminal breast tumors. Cancer Res 2009; 69: 663–71.

54. Holstege H, Horlings HM, Velds A, et al. BRCA1-mutated and basal-like breast cancers have similar aCGH profiles and a high incidence of protein truncating TP53 mutations. BMC Cancer 2010; 10: 654.

55. Rodriguez AA, Makris A, Wu MF, et al. DNA repair signature is associated with anthracycline response in triple-negative breast cancer patients. Breast Cancer Res Treat 2010; 123: 189–96.

56. Konstantinopoulos PA, Spentzos D, Karlan BY, et al. Gene expression profile of BRCAness that correlates with responsiveness to chemotherapy and with outcome in patients with epithelial ovarian cancer. J Clin Oncol 2010; 28: 3555–61.

57. Venkitaraman AR. Cancer susceptibility and the functions of BRCA1 and BRCA2. Cell 2002; 108: 171–82.
58. Kennedy RD, Quinn JE, Johnston PG, Harkin DP. BRCA1: mechanisms of inactivation and implications for management of patients. Lancet 2002; 360: 1007–14.
59. Turner N, Tutt A, Ashworth A. Targeting the DNA repair defect of BRCA tumours. Curr Opin Pharmacol 2005; 5: 388–93.
60. Kennedy RD, Quinn JE, Mullan PB, Johnston PG, Harkin DP. The role of BRCA1 in the cellular response to chemotherapy. J Natl Cancer Inst 2004; 96: 1659–68.
61. Moynahan ME, Cui TY, Jasin M. Homology-directed dna repair, mitomycin-c resistance, and chromosome stability is restored with correction of a Brca1 mutation. Cancer Res 2001; 61: 4842–50.
62. Shafee N, Smith CR, Wei S, et al. Cancer stem cells contribute to cisplatin resistance in Brca1/p53-mediated mouse mammary tumors. Cancer Res 2008; 68: 3243–50.
63. Lafarge S, Sylvain V, Ferrara M, Bignon YJ. Inhibition of BRCA1 leads to increased chemo-resistance to microtubule-interfering agents, an effect that involves the JNK pathway. Oncogene 2001; 20: 6597–606.
64. Kennecke H, Yerushalmi R, Woods R, et al. Metastatic behavior of breast cancer subtypes. J Clin Oncol 2010; 28: 3271–7.
65. Dent R, Hanna WM, Trudeau M, et al. Pattern of metastatic spread in triple-negative breast cancer. Breast Cancer Res Treat 2009; 115: 423–8.
66. Carey LA, Dees EC, Sawyer L, et al. The triple-negative paradox: primary tumor chemo-sensitivity of breast cancer subtypes. Clin Cancer Res 2007; 13: 2329–34.
67. Dent R, Trudeau M, Pritchard KI, et al. Triple-negative breast cancer: clinical features and patterns of recurrence. Clin Cancer Res 2007; 13: 4429–34.
68. Voduc KD, Cheang MC, Tyldesley S, et al. Breast cancer subtypes and the risk of local and regional relapse. J Clin Oncol 2010; 28: 1684–91.
69. Dawood S, Broglio K, Esteva FJ, et al. Survival among women with triple receptor-negative breast cancer and brain metastases. Ann Oncol 2009; 20: 621–7.
70. Anders CK, Deal AM, Miller CR, et al. The prognostic contribution of clinical breast cancer subtype, age, and race among patients with breast cancer brain metastases. Cancer 2011; 117: 1602–11.
71. Byrski T, Gronwald J, Huzarski T, et al. Pathologic complete response rates in young women with BRCA1-positive breast cancers after neoadjuvant chemotherapy. J Clin Oncol 2010; 28: 375–9.
72. Goffin JR, Chappuis PO, Begin LR, et al. Impact of germline BRCA1 mutations and over-expression of p53 on prognosis and response to treatment following breast carcinoma: 10-year follow up data. Cancer 2003; 97: 527–36.
73. Cass I, Baldwin RL, Varkey T, et al. Improved survival in women with BRCA-associated ovarian carcinoma. Cancer 2003; 97: 2187–95.
74. Tan DS, Rothermundt C, Thomas K, et al. "BRCAness" syndrome in ovarian cancer: a case-control study describing the clinical features and outcome of patients with epithelial ovar-ian cancer associated with BRCA1 and BRCA2 mutations. J Clin Oncol 2008; 26: 5530–6.
75. Farmer H, McCabe N, Lord CJ, et al. Targeting the DNA repair defect in BRCA mutant cells as a therapeutic strategy. Nature 2005; 434: 917–21.
76. Ashworth A. A synthetic lethal therapeutic approach: poly(ADP) ribose polymerase inhibitors for the treatment of cancers deficient in DNA double-strand break repair. J Clin Oncol 2008; 26: 3785–90.
77. McCabe N, Turner NC, Lord CJ, et al. Deficiency in the repair of DNA damage by homol-ogous recombination and sensitivity to poly(ADP-ribose) polymerase inhibition. Cancer Res 2006; 66: 8109–15.
78. Bryant HE, Schultz N, Thomas HD, et al. Specific killing of BRCA2-deficient tumours with inhibitors of poly(ADP-ribose) polymerase. Nature 2005; 434: 913–17.
79. Hartwell LH, Szankasi P, Roberts CJ, Murray AW, Friend SH. Integrating genetic approaches into the discovery of anticancer drugs. Science 1997; 278: 1064–8.
80. Fong PC, Boss DS, Yap TA, et al. Inhibition of poly(ADP-ribose) polymerase in tumors from BRCA mutation carriers. N Engl J Med 2009; 361: 123–34.
81. Tutt A, Robson M, Garber JE, et al. Oral poly(ADP-ribose) polymerase inhibitor olaparib in patients with BRCA1 or BRCA2 mutations and advanced breast cancer: a proof-of-concept trial. Lancet 2010; 376: 235–44.

82. RM Wenham SK, Sandhu GW, Sun L, et al. First in human trial of a poly(ADP)-ribose polymerase (PARP) inhibitor MK-4827 in advanced cancer patients (p) with antitumor activity in BRCA-deficient and sporadic ovarian cancers. In: EORTC-NCI-AACR Symposium on Molecular Targets and Cancer Therapeutics. Berlin, 2010.
83. Isakoff SJ, Overmoyer B, Tung NM, et al. A phase II trial of the PARP inhibitor veliparib (ABT888) and temozolomide for metastatic breast cancer. ASCO Meeting Abstracts 2010; 28: 1019.
84. Edwards SL, Brough R, Lord CJ, et al. Resistance to therapy caused by intragenic deletion in BRCA2. Nature 2008; 451: 1111–15.
85. Swisher EM, Sakai W, Karlan BY, et al. Secondary BRCA1 mutations in BRCA1-mutated ovarian carcinomas with platinum resistance. Cancer Res 2008; 68: 2581–6.
86. Sakai W, Swisher EM, Karlan BY, et al. Secondary mutations as a mechanism of cisplatin resistance in BRCA2-mutated cancers. Nature 2008; 451: 1116–20.
87. Foulkes WD. BRCA1 functions as a breast stem cell regulator. J Med Genet 2004; 41: 1–5.
88. Rouzier R, Perou CM, Symmans WF, et al. Breast cancer molecular subtypes respond differently to preoperative chemotherapy. Clin Cancer Res 2005; 11: 5678–85.
89. Kassam F, Enright K, Dent R, et al. Survival outcomes for patients with metastatic triple-negative breast cancer: implications for clinical practice and trial design. Clin Breast Cancer 2009; 9: 29–33.
90. Sirohi B, Arnedos M, Popat S, et al. Platinum-based chemotherapy in triple-negative breast cancer. Ann Oncol 2008; 19: 1847–52.
91. Staudacher L, Cottu PH, Dieras V, et al. Platinum-based chemotherapy in metastatic triple-negative breast cancer: the Institut Curie experience. Ann Oncol 2011; 22: 848–56.
92. Uhm JE, Park YH, Yi SY, et al. Treatment outcomes and clinicopathologic characteristics of triple-negative breast cancer patients who received platinum-containing chemotherapy. Int J Cancer 2009; 124: 1457–62.
93. Silver DP, Richardson AL, Eklund AC, et al. Efficacy of neoadjuvant Cisplatin in triple-negative breast cancer. J Clin Oncol 2010; 28: 1145–53.
94. Graeser M, McCarthy A, Lord CJ, et al. A marker of homologous recombination predicts pathologic complete response to neoadjuvant chemotherapy in primary breast cancer. Clin Cancer Res 2010; 16: 6159–68.
95. Perez EA, Patel T, Moreno-Aspitia A. Efficacy of ixabepilone in ER/PR/HER2-negative (triple-negative) breast cancer.. Breast Cancer Res Treat 2010; 121: 261–71.
96. Chew HK, Doroshow JH, Frankel P, et al. Phase II studies of gemcitabine and cisplatin in heavily and minimally pretreated metastatic breast cancer. J Clin Oncol 2009; 27: 2163–9.
97. Loesch D, Asmar L, McIntyre K, et al. Phase II trial of gemcitabine/carboplatin (plus trastuzumab in HER2-positive disease) in patients with metastatic breast cancer. Clin Breast Cancer 2008; 8: 178–86.
98. Yardley DA, Burris HA 3rd, Simons L, et al. A phase II trial of gemcitabine/carboplatin with or without trastuzumab in the first-line treatment of patients with metastatic breast cancer. Clin Breast Cancer 2008; 8: 425–31.
99. O'Shaughnessy J, Osborne C, Pippen JE, et al. Iniparib plus chemotherapy in metastatic triple-negative breast cancer. N Engl J Med 2011; 364: 205–14.
100. Dent RA, Lindeman GJ, Clemons M, et al. Safety and efficacy of the oral PARP inhibitor olaparib (AZD2281) in combination with paclitaxel for the first- or second-line treatment of patients with metastatic triple-negative breast cancer: results from the safety cohort of a phase I/II multicenter trial. ASCO Meeting Abstracts 2010; 28: 1018.
101. Gelmon KA, Hirte HW, Robidoux A, et al. Can we define tumors that will respond to PARP inhibitors? A phase II correlative study of olaparib in advanced serous ovarian cancer and triple-negative breast cancer. ASCO Meeting Abstracts 2010; 28: 3002.
102. Miller K, Wang M, Gralow J, et al. Paclitaxel plus bevacizumab versus paclitaxel alone for metastatic breast cancer. N Engl J Med 2007; 357: 2666–76.
103. Miles DW, Chan A, Dirix LY, et al. Phase III study of bevacizumab plus docetaxel compared with placebo plus docetaxel for the first-line treatment of human epidermal growth factor receptor 2-negative metastatic breast cancer. J Clin Oncol 2010; 28: 3239–47.
104. Valachis A, Polyzos NP, Patsopoulos NA, et al. Bevacizumab in metastatic breast cancer: a meta-analysis of randomized controlled trials. Breast Cancer Res Treat 2010; 122: 1–7.

105. Burstein HJ, Elias AD, Rugo HS, et al. Phase II study of sunitinib malate, an oral multitar-geted tyrosine kinase inhibitor, in patients with metastatic breast cancer previously treated with an anthracycline and a taxane. J Clin Oncol 2008;26:1810–16.

106. Carey LA, Rugo HS, Marcom PK, et al. TBCRC 001: EGFR inhibition with cetuximab added to carboplatin in metastatic triple-negative (basal-like) breast cancer. ASCO Meeting Abstracts 2008; 26: 1009.

107. Baselga J, Stemmer S, Pego A, et al. Cetuximab + Cisplatin in Estrogen Receptor-Negative, Progesterone Receptor-Negative, HER2-Negative (Triple-Negative) Metastatic Breast Cancer: Results of the Randomized Phase II BALI-1 Trial. In: San Antonio Breast Cancer Symposium. San Antonio, Texas, USA, 2010.

108. Ponzo MG, Lesurf R, Petkiewicz S, et al. Met induces mammary tumors with diverse histologies and is associated with poor outcome and human basal breast cancer. Proc Natl Acad Sci USA 2009; 106: 12903–8.

109. Cristofanilli M, Morandi P, Krishnamurthy S, et al. Imatinib mesylate (Gleevec) in advanced breast cancer-expressing C-Kit or PDGFR-beta: clinical activity and biological correlations. Ann Oncol 2008; 19: 1713–19.

110. Finn RS, Dering J, Ginther C, et al. Dasatinib, an orally active small molecule inhibitor of both the src and abl kinases, selectively inhibits growth of basal-type/"triple-negative" breast cancer cell lines growing in vitro. Breast Cancer Res Treat 2007; 105: 319–26.

111. Finn RS, BC, Ibrahim N, et al. Phase II trial of dasatinib in triple-negative breast cancer: results of study CA180059. In: San Antonio Breast Cancer Symposium. San Antonio, Texas, USA, 2008.

112. Rakha EA, Elsheikh SE, Aleskandarany MA, et al. Triple-negative breast cancer: distinguishing between basal and nonbasal subtypes. Clin Cancer Res 2009; 15: 2302–10.

6

Chemotherapy and metastatic breast cancer

Charles Swanton

INTRODUCTION

As patients with metastatic breast cancer (MBC) cannot be cured, the role of any treatment including cytotoxic chemotherapy is to maximise the duration of time without disease-related symptoms. This should be achieved with minimal toxicity from therapy in order that the quality of life can be maintained. It has been shown that the quality of life in advanced breast cancer is clearly linked with treatment response (1–3) and that chemotherapy can have a significant benefit for patients because of its anti-cancer effects that can reduce or prevent tumour-related symptoms. It has been questionable whether chemotherapy for MBC has any significant benefit in terms of overall survival, and the clinical trials of chemotherapy versus best supportive care have not been undertaken in this setting. However, historical comparisons have shown that the introduction of combination cytotoxic chemotherapy in the late 1970s has produced a modest 9–12 month gain in survival over untreated patients (4,5). Likewise, individual patients with life-threatening visceral disease who have a good clinical response to chemotherapy, will clearly have a survival benefit compared with while not having the therapy. With the recent introduction of effective cytotoxic drugs and combinations, including those with biological agents, significant impacts on survival are now being observed in individual trials compared with previous standard chemotherapy drugs. Therefore, it is likely that patients with MBC will derive significant clinical benefits from modern-day chemotherapy. Finally, the plethora of drugs with non-cross resistant mechanisms of action, has given the oncologist several lines of therapy to offer patients.

This chapter reviews some of the underlying principles in the use of chemotherapy to treat MBC, outlines the major classes of cytotoxic drugs, and highlights some of the recent developments in schedules and combination approaches with new agents available.

PRINCIPLES OF TREATMENT

Patients who relapse with MBC may often present with a single- site of disease (i.e., bone or visceral organs). The decision to start chemotherapy is often complex and involves a careful assessment of the patient's treatment history, biological characteristics of the tumour (estrogen and progesterone receptor status and HER2/neu expression), disease-free interval, anatomical site, extent of the metastatic relapse, tumour-related symptoms, the effect of visceral or bone metastases upon organ function, and performance status (Table 1) (6). Increasingly, prognostic and predictive factors derived from gene expression data or other surrogates of proliferation such as Ki67 are being adopted into clinical trial designs in advanced breast cancer to distinguish biologically relevant patient subgroups, in for example, ER-positive breast cancer, with different clinical outcomes (Chapter 2). Furthermore, the identification of distinct molecular subtypes has led to a change in the focus of clinical trial design in advanced breast cancer from dose escalation and dose-intense chemotherapeutic regimens to target-driven approaches in increasingly smaller patient cohorts (6). Indeed, an increased molecular understanding of this disease has led to the recognition that patients with breast cancer with inherited germline mutations in BRCA2

TABLE 1   The ECOG Performance Status[a]

Grade 0	Fully active, able to carry on all pre-disease performance without restriction
Grade 1	Restricted in physically strenuous activity but ambulatory and able to carry out work of a light and sedentary nature, light house work, office work
Grade 2	Ambulatory and capable of all self-care but unable to carry out any work activities. Up and about more than 50% of waking hours
Grade 3	Capable of only limited self-care, confined to bed or chair more than 50% of waking hours
Grade 4	Completely disabled. Cannot carry on any self-care. Totally confined to bed or chair

[a]The Eastern Cooperative Oncology Group (ECOG) performance status scale acts as a useful unified guide for the clinician to assess the suitability of a patient for chemotherapy and an objective scale by which to measure functional response to treatment (www.ecog.org).

have disease which appears to be more sensitive to first-line anthracycline or cyclophosphamide, methotrexate, and fluorouracil 5FU (CMF)-based chemotherapeutic regimens than sporadic breast cancers (7).

Chemotherapy is usually reserved for patients with disease unresponsive to endocrine agents or patients with the rapidly progressive or life threatening disease. Patients who have relapsed with oestrogen/progesterone receptor-positive disease with long treatment-free interval, soft tissue or bone as the dominant site of metastasis, and good performance status are usually treated with endocrine therapy first (Chapter 3). Equally, oestrogen/progesterone receptor-positive patients with low volume visceral disease and normal organ function assessed biochemically may also be treated with a trial of endocrine therapy. Symptomatic or radiological progression of metastatic disease after a trial of endocrine therapy inevitably leads to the decision to initiate chemotherapy.

Many patients with MBC are above 65 years and may present with life threatening disease requiring chemotherapy. Elderly patients may be at increased risk of myelosuppression induced by cytotoxic agents and co-morbidity; also, drug history should be considered when choosing the appropriate regimen. Thus, agents with lower toxicity may often be considered as preferable for this patient group.

INFLUENCE OF PRIOR THERAPIES

Use of prior adjuvant chemotherapy is not an impediment to the benefit of chemotherapy for MBC (8). However, a disease-free interval of less than 12 months since prior adjuvant treatment implies a degree of resistance to the previous regimen and will influence the choice of first-line chemotherapy for MBC.

The goals of chemotherapy treatment continue to remain the same for all patients with MBC, namely minimising the toxicity of treatment and hospital admissions whilst maximising symptom improvement, quality of life, and survival. Following use of first-line chemotherapy for MBC, at subsequent disease progression, different cytotoxic drugs or combinations may be used. However, further use of sequential chemotherapy needs careful consideration in relation to likelihood of benefit versus risk of toxicity and deteriorating performance status. The extent of prior treatment is one factor that should be considered in estimating the likelihood of clinical benefit derived from further chemotherapy. Tumour response rates are the maximum if patients have previously received one or no prior therapy (40–60% depending on the study and drug combination) but sadly decline as treatment progresses [30% in the third setting (9)]. Likewise, prior lack of response to first-line chemotherapy with or without a short treatment and/or progression-free period is associated with a much lower likelihood of subsequent response to second- or third-line chemotherapy.

TABLE 2 RECIST Criteria[a]

CR	Complete response: disappearance of all target lesions
PR	Partial response: 30% decrease in the sum of the longest diameter of target lesions
PD	Progressive disease: 20% increase in the sum of the longest diameter of target lesions
SD	Stable disease: small changes that do not meet the above criteria

[a]Since 2000, disease response is commonly measured radiologically by unified criteria termed "RECIST" (Response Evaluation Criteria in Solid Tumours).

Indeed, response to previous chemotherapeutic regimens was recently identified as the only independent predictive variable associated with response to third-line chemotherapeutic regimens (9). This needs to be borne in mind when discussing further lines of chemotherapy with patients.

RESPONSE ASSESSMENT

Tumour response assessment usually occurs 8–12 weeks after the start of chemotherapy and comprises a summary of radiological and clinical responses, symptomatic benefit (including any improvement in performance status) balanced against toxicities of treatment. Radiological response (determined by Response Evaluation Criteria in Solid Tumours (RECIST) criteria, Table 2) is an important guide to the clinician in deciding whether to continue or change therapies. While objective tumour responses (i.e., tumour shrinkage by more than 30%; Table 2) set the standard used in clinical trials to judge the efficacy of chemotherapy, stabilisation of disease by RECIST criteria with a symptomatic benefit is an equally important endpoint. In patients with non-measurable disease, (e.g., bone-only disease) treated with chemotherapy, serial tumour markers together with symptomatic benefit are important indicators of response to treatment.

Increasingly, circulating tumour cells are recognised as important surrogates of response to endocrine and cytotoxic regimens with declines in circulating tumour cell number preceding radiographic response by up to 9 weeks (10). Radiological response frequently forms a key endpoint within clinical trial design in advanced breast cancer. However, the correlation of overall survival with response rate or progression-free survival (PFS) has proved a contentious issue. In a recent meta-analysis of 11 randomised trials, neither overall response rate nor PFS or time to progression (TTP) could be demonstrated as a good surrogate for overall survival (11).

Measuring symptomatic benefit from treatment should include an assessment of the patient's main tumour-related complaints and overall functional status as measured by Eastern Cooperative Oncology Group (ECOG) performance status (Table 1). This should be done prior to starting chemotherapy, followed by repeat assessments during treatment that are balanced by treatment-related toxicities (graded according to the ECOG common toxicity criteria scale www.ecog.org/general/ctc.pdf).

CHOICE AND DURATION OF CHEMOTHERAPY REGIMEN (SEQUENTIAL OR COMBINATION THERAPY)

There is considerable debate in the management of MBC as to whether combination or sequential monotherapy strategies should be pursued. In general, response rates tend to be higher with combination regimens when used as first-line therapy, but often at the expense of greater toxicity and short-term deterioration in quality of life. Furthermore, most of the clinical trials that assess new combination strategies have not been adequately structured to address whether long-term outcomes (especially survival) are equivalent or superior to using the same agents administered sequentially. At the 6th European Breast Cancer Conference, the European School of Oncology Metastatic Breast Cancer Task Force, having reviewed available data, recommended that in the absence of rapid clinical progression or life threatening visceral metastases or the need for immediate symptom palliation, sequential chemotherapy regimens should be used (12).

Several clinical trials that have compared a sequential versus combined regimen in a randomised fashion support this concept (Table 3). Combination doxorubicin (A) and paclitaxel (T) therapy leads to improved response rates with no survival benefit over sequential treatment (13). Likewise, equivalent survival and response rates were observed in a trial comparing single-agent mitoxantrone with combination 5-fluorouracil, epirubicin, and cyclophosphamide (FEC) with less toxicity and improved quality of life in the monotherapy arm (14). Joensuu and colleagues demonstrated that there was no survival difference when FEC followed by mitomycin C and vinblastine was compared with monotherapy with epirubicin followed by mitomycin C on disease progression (15). An overview of 106 randomised trials in MBC involving over 17,000 patients suggested only a small, but significant, benefit for combination chemotherapy versus single-agent chemotherapy (16). This was before the widespread introduction of taxanes as first-line chemotherapy.

Despite the lack of impact on long-term outcome, combination strategies may be advisable for patients of good performance status (0/1) with rapidly progressing visceral disease and evidence of organ dysfunction, particularly in the first-line setting. In general, monotherapy is considered best for second- or third-line chemotherapy options when toxicity considerations become paramount, often on the background

TABLE 3 Combination vs. Monotherapy Chemotherapy Studies

Study	Treatment	Results
Sledge 2003 (7) Phase III 739 patients	Doxorubicin [(A), 50 mg/m²] Paclitaxel [(T) 150 mg/m²]/24 hr + GCSF Vs.	Response rate (RR): AT 47% T 34% A 36%
	Sequential doxorubicin (60 mg/m²) On disease progression (or vice versa) Paclitaxel (175 mg/m²)	No survival benefit No difference in quality of life
Heidemann (8) 260 previously untreated patients	Mitoxantrone 12 mg/m² Vs. 5-Fluourouracil (500 mg/m²) Epirubicin (50 mg/m²) Cyclophosphamide 500 mg/m² q. 3 wk 2nd -line mitomycin C (Mmc), vindesine vinblastine (Vinbl), prednisolone	No difference in RRs No survival difference
Joensuu (1998) (9)	FEC, then Mmc (8 mg/m²), Vinbl (6 mg/m²) Vs. Epirubicin 20 mg/m² q.wkly Then Mmc (8 mg/m²/d)	RR FEC 53% Mmc, Vin 6% Epi 44% Mmc 14% No survival difference

Abbreviations: FEC, fluorouracil, epirubicin, and cyclophosphamide; G-CSF, granulocyte-colony stimulating factor.

of worsening performance status in relation to progressive disease. In addition, single-agent treatment is often preferable for women with extensive life-threatening visceral involvement of the liver or bone marrow. In this situation, dose reductions of a single agent are more readily controllable and titrated to organ function. If organ function improves following a successful reduction in tumour burden, the chemotherapy dose can be increased.

One course of chemotherapy encompasses a period of approximately 4–6 months given a satisfactory response at interval assessments. Maintenance chemotherapy has not demonstrated a clear advantage. Indeed, in one study where patients were randomised to maintenance paclitaxel versus control in patients who did not experience disease progression following first-line anthracycline/paclitaxel combination therapy, there was no benefit in terms of PFS in the maintenance arm (17).

In certain cases, chemotherapy regimens may be extended beyond 6 months (taking into account cumulative toxicity of drugs such as the anthracyclines) if patients are continuing to derive benefit from treatment and have symptoms that can be effectively palliated by prolonged chemotherapy.

Anthracyclines

Doxorubicin (Fig. 1) is an anthracycline antibiotic synthesised by the fungus *Streptomyces peucetius*. Anthracycline cytotoxicity is mediated through DNA intercalation and inhibition of DNA and protein synthesis, topoisomerase II inhibition, and free radical generation. Side effects of this class of drug include the risk of cardiac toxicity above a cumulative dose threshold, alopecia, gastrointestinal disturbances (nausea, vomiting, diarrhoea, and stomatitis), and complications of neutropaenia. Patients should also be aware of the risk associated with treatment-related leukaemia. In studies of epirubicin therapy in the adjuvant setting, the cumulative risk of secondary acute myelogenous leukaemia was 0.2% at 2 years and 0.8% at 5 years. Pre-menopausal

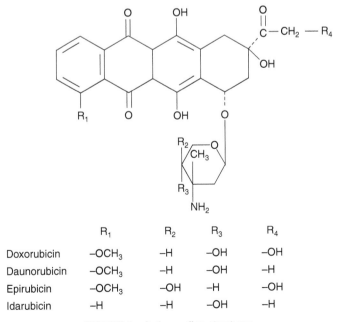

	R_1	R_2	R_3	R_4
Doxorubicin	$-OCH_3$	$-H$	$-OH$	$-OH$
Daunorubicin	$-OCH_3$	$-H$	$-OH$	$-H$
Epirubicin	$-OCH_3$	$-OH$	$-H$	$-OH$
Idarubicin	$-H$	$-H$	$-OH$	$-H$

FIGURE 1 Anthracycline structures.

patients should also be warned of the risks of irreversible amenorrhoea and premature menopause.

In women with MBC who have not received prior adjuvant anthracycline-based chemotherapy, meta-analyses support the view that anthracycline chemotherapy regimens improve response rates, time to disease progression, and survival over non-anthracycline-containing regimens (16,18).

In patients who have relapsed with no prior anthracycline exposure, first-line treatment options include doxorubicin or epirubicin with cyclophosphamide (AC or EC), or with cyclophosphamide and 5-FU (FAC or FEC) or single-agent epirubicin or doxorubicin. The anthracenediones such as mitoxantrone are less toxic than anthracyclines, but have been deemed less effective.

In recent years, however, most patients who relapse with MBC have received anthracycline chemotherapy as part of an adjuvant treatment protocol. Cumulative exposure and cardiac risk have made re-treatment with anthracycline difficult. The cumulative dose of anthracycline should not exceed 450–550 mg/m² for doxorubicin or 700–900 mg/m² for epirubicin (Table 4). Retrospective studies demonstrated an incidence of symptomatic cardiac failure of 6–10% of adults who had received cumulative bolus doses above 550 mg/m² of doxorubicin, with elderly patients at increased risk.

Therefore, factors such as age (>70 years) and co-morbidity such as diabetes, hypertension, and ischaemic, valvular, or myocardial heart disease should be taken into account prior to the use of these agents. Previous chest wall radiotherapy particularly has been shown to increase the risk of cardiac damage. Furthermore, doxorubicin is considered unsafe in combination with trastuzumab due to the higher risk of cardiotoxicity (19).

A baseline ECG is recommended for all patients prior to initiation of anthracycline therapy. Left ventricular ejection fraction should be assessed by multi-gated radionuclide angiography (MUGA) or by echocardiography. A repeat assessment of left ventricular ejection fraction is recommended for patients treated with higher cumulative doses of anthracycline. In patients with a high-risk cardiac profile or those with a prior history of chest wall radiotherapy in need of anthracycline therapy, consideration may be given to the use of liposomal anthracyclines or anthracyclines with less cardiotoxicity such as epirubicin. The pegylated liposomal formulation of Liposomal doxorubicin (Caelyx®, Schering-Plough) has been shown to have comparable efficacy with reduced cardiotoxicity, myelosuppression, vomiting, and alopecia in comparison to standard doxorubicin in the first-line treatment of MBC (20). Recent evidence also supports the utility of re-challenging patients with liposomal doxorubicin plus cyclophosphamide in patients >12 months since completion of an adjuvant anthracycline regimen. In a phase II multicentre trial, this regimen was associated with an ORR of 38% and a median TTP of 12.2 months (21).

Dexrazoxane hydrochloride (Cardioxane® Novartis Pharmaceuticals) is a cardioprotective agent used in patients requiring anthracycline therapy. Its active metabolite is thought to act through iron chelation thereby reducing doxorubicin-induced free-radical generation. Several studies have demonstrated the

TABLE 4 Incidence of Cardiomyopathy by Cumulative Epirubicin Dose

Cumulative dose (mg/m²)	Incidence (%)
550	0.9
700	1.6
900	3.3

cardioprotective role of dexrazoxane in anthracycline-treated patients. A study of patients randomised to doxorubicin (as part of a FAC regimen) and placebo versus doxorubicin and dexrazoxane after a total dose of 300 mg/m² revealed a 3% incidence of congestive cardiac failure in the dexrazoxane-treated patients compared with 22% in the placebo arm (22). Twenty-six per cent of patients treated with dexrazoxane were able to receive 15 courses of therapy versus only 5% of the placebo group. Furthermore, median survival for those receiving doxorubicin and placebo was 460 days as opposed to 882 days in those receiving both doxorubicin and dexrazoxane. Therefore, dexrazoxane may limit the cardiotoxic side effects of anthracyclines allowing potentially effective treatment to continue beyond the maximum tolerated dose limit. The American Society of Clinical Oncology has issued guidelines regarding the use of this agent: Cardioxane/dexrazoxane is not routinely recommended for patients with MBC who receive doxorubicin-based chemotherapy but may be considered in those who have received a cumulative dose of more than 300 mg/m² who may benefit from the continued use of doxorubicin.

There are some practical considerations in the use of anthracyclines. Anthracyclines should not be given to patients with a baseline neutrophil count <1500 cells/mm³, recent myocardial infarction or history of cardiac failure, severe arrhythmias, or significant hepatic dysfunction. Previous anthracycline exposure up to a maximum cumulative dose is a contraindication to further use. Lower starting doses should be considered in patients with pre-existing bone marrow depression (and malignancy-related marrow infiltration).

Patients with a bilirubin level between 1.2 and 3 mg/dL (20–51 µmol/dL) or an aspartate aminotransferase (AST) 2–4 times the upper limit of normal (ULN) should receive a 50% dose reduction of epirubicin. Patients with bilirubin >3 mg/dL (>51 µmol/dL) or AST >4 times the ULN should receive a 75% dose reduction of epirubicin. There is evidence that epirubicin toxicity correlates better with AST values than with bilirubin levels. The schedule with the most extensive data in patients with liver metastases and organ dysfunction is weekly epirubicin (25 mg/m²) with further dose reductions made according to liver function tests (23,24).

Dose adjustments should also be made if doxorubicin is to be considered in patients with liver dysfunction. The risk of haematological and mucosal toxicity is increased with significant liver dysfunction. The manufacturers suggest a 50% dose reduction of doxorubicin with a bilirubin level of 1.2–3 mg/dL (20–51 µmol/dL) with no clear recommendation according to AST rise. A 75% dose reduction is advisable if the bilirubin rises above 3 mg/dL (51 µmol/dL). Lower doses should also be considered for patients with severe renal impairment.

Taxanes

Taxanes stabilise the microtubule through interaction with beta tubulin thereby preventing normal chromosomal segregation at mitosis (Fig. 2). An intricate molecular process activates the spindle checkpoint leading to cellular proliferation arrest at the metaphase–anaphase transition. Following cell cycle arrest, sensitive cancer cells may activate a conserved death pathway (apoptosis) or die by necrosis. Alternatively, cells may remain in a permanent state of arrest, failing to segregate chromosomes faithfully. Evidence suggests that cells with a defective spindle checkpoint are more resistant to microtubule inhibitors and that ensuing chromosomal instability that may result from defective spindle checkpoint activity is associated with taxane resistance (25,26).

Taxanes are now considered one of the most active compounds in clinical use for MBC. A recent Cochrane meta-analysis confirmed a statistically significant overall survival benefit in favour of taxane-containing regimens (hazard ratio for survival 0.90) (27). The two most commonly used taxanes in clinical practice are paclitaxel and docetaxel (Fig. 3).

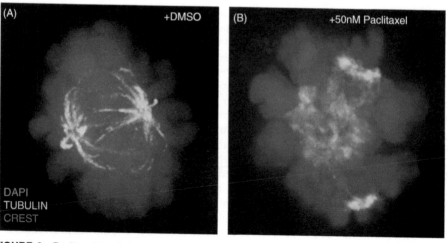

FIGURE 2 Paclitaxel treatment causes gross mitotic spindle abnormalities. HCT116 cells treated with either (**A**) DMSO or (**B**) 50nM paclitaxel. Cells were fixed in methanol and stained with antibodies for tubulin and kinetochores (CREST serum). DMSO-treated cells show normal bipolar mitotic spindles, while paclitaxel treated cells display gross mitotic spindle abnormalities, due to hyper-stabilisation of microtubules. *Source*: Courtesy of Rebecca Burrell and Sarah Mcclelland.

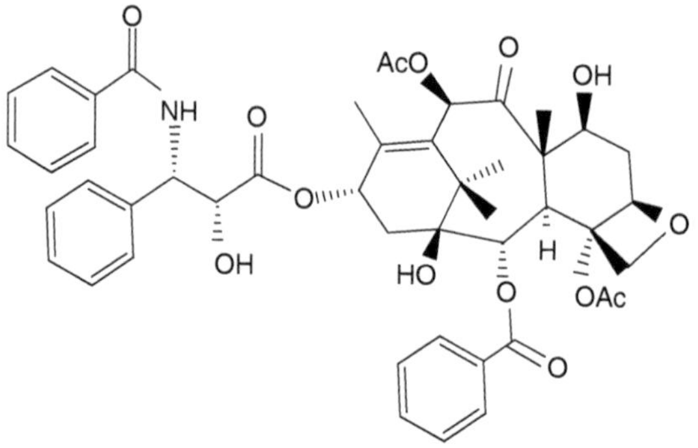

FIGURE 3 Structure of paclitaxel.

Side effects associated with paclitaxel given in a 3-weekly schedule are neutropaenia, alopecia, myalgia, and neurosensory impairment. Weekly schedules of paclitaxel cause significantly less myelosuppression and hair loss, but may still be associated with neurosensory side effects associated with cumulative long-term exposure. Weekly schedules of docetaxel are also associated with less myelosuppression, but a greater incidence of myocutaneous toxicity, fatigue, and asthenia.

Docetaxel side effects are otherwise similar to paclitaxel with neutropaenia usually occurring slightly earlier (days 5–7 as opposed to day 11 with paclitaxel). Asthenia and stomatitis are also common adverse events. In addition early studies of the drug encountered problems with fluid retention, oedema, and pleural effusions. This side effect has been largely overcome with the 3-day dexamethasone course (8 mg bd) starting the day before chemotherapy. Other side effects include nail changes, nausea, and diarrhoea.

Docetaxel should not be given to patients with bilirubin higher than the ULN or alkaline phosphatase > 2.5× ULN or AST/ALT >1.5× ULN. Patients with neutrophil counts less than $1500\,cells/mm^3$ should not receive docetaxel or paclitaxel. Patients with a history of hypersensitivity to docetaxel or other drugs formulated in polysorbate 80 should not receive docetaxel.

Dose adjustments of paclitaxel should be considered in patients with moderate to severe hepatic impairment. Concerning paclitaxel administered every 3 weeks in a 3-hour infusion at the standard dose of $175\,mg/m^2$, the manufacturer recommends a dose reduction to $135\,mg/m^2$ with baseline bilirubin levels between 1.26 and $2\,mg/dL$ (21–34 µmol/dL) and to $90\,mg/m^2$ for patients with bilirubin between 2.0–5.0 (34–85 µmol/dL). Modified doses of weekly paclitaxel may be appropriate for patients with liver dysfunction due to its reduced myelosuppressive effects compared with the 3-weekly schedule (which can be exacerbated by liver function impairment).

Paclitaxel is contraindicated in patients who have a history of hypersensitivity to paclitaxel or other drugs formulated in Cremaphor EL® (BASF Corp).

Anthracycline-Naive Patients
First-Line Paclitaxel Monotherapy
Response rates to paclitaxel monotherapy in the first-line setting range from 15% to 60% depending on the study and dosing schedule. The two most commonly used dosing schedules are weekly paclitaxel (80–$90\,mg/m^2$) and paclitaxel $175\,mg/m^2$ every 3 weeks. Doses higher than $175\,mg/m^2$ have failed to consistently demonstrate improved response rates or overall survival (28). Weekly paclitaxel is often the treatment of choice for elderly patients or those with poor performance status owing to the reduced myelosuppression associated with this schedule. However, weekly paclitaxel is associated with more neurotoxicity than the 3-weekly schedule (29). Recent data have demonstrated the superiority of a weekly paclitaxel to the traditional 3-weekly schedule in terms of response rate and overall survival. The drug is commonly administered at a dose of 80–$90\,mg/m^2$ per week continuously although treatment for 3 weeks followed by a 1-week break may reduce the incidence of neurotoxicity. The CALGB 9840 study confirmed higher treatment response rates and longer TTP and survival for weekly paclitaxel as opposed to the 3-weekly schedule in patients treated with 0 or 1 chemotherapy regimens (29). Further studies are required to find out whether weekly paclitaxel is equivalent to 3-weekly docetaxel.

First-Line Docetaxel Monotherapy
The usual docetaxel dose used in the advanced disease setting is between 75–$100\,mg/m^2$. A randomised phase III trial demonstrated higher toxicity with no survival benefit for $100\,mg/m^2$ vs. $75\,mg/m^2$ docetaxel in the second-line setting (30). In this study, however, there was a dose–response relationship with superior response rates with $100\,mg/m^2$ than the lower two doses (29.8% vs. 22.3% vs. 19.9%, $p = 0.026$). Therefore, $100\,mg/m^2$ is still recommended for patients with a performance status of 0 or 1 with aggressive visceral disease, in whom immediate disease control is a priority, with or without granulocyte-colony stimulating factor (G-CSF) support and/or prophylactic antibiotics. A dose of $75\,mg/m^2$ is recommended for heavily pre-treated patients, patients of poorer performance status, or with mild impairment of liver function.

Reported response rates to first-line 3-weekly docetaxel monotherapy appear superior to 3-weekly paclitaxel. Studies with docetaxel (dose $100\,mg/m^2$) have demonstrated response rates between 54 and 68% and 40 and 52% with the lower dose of $75\,mg/m^2$. Previous indirect evidence has suggested superiority for docetaxel over paclitaxel monotherapy in studies comparing docetaxel or paclitaxel to doxorubicin. A phase III study revealed superior response rates for $100\,mg/m^2$ docetaxel over $75\,mg/m^2$ doxorubicin (47.8% vs. 33.3%; $P = 0.008$) in patients who had received prior alkylating agent-based treatment although overall survival was same in both the groups (31). In addition, a recently reported phase III trial reported higher response rates for 60 mg/m² docetaxel versus doxorubicin and cyclophosphamide (41% vs. 30%) in the first-line setting (32). In contrast, a trial of 3-weekly paclitaxel versus doxorubicin showed no difference in disease and symptom control in the first-line treatment of metastatic disease (33). Likewise, an intergroup phase III study that compared single-agent doxorubicin or paclitaxel versus the combination of doxorubicin and paclitaxel with growth factor support in the first-line setting revealed equivalent response rates for patients receiving doxorubicin or paclitaxel (13). A recent randomised trial confirmed that 100 mg/m² docetaxel was superior to 175 mg/m² paclitaxel with superior response rates (32% vs. 25%), prolonged TTP (5.7 months vs. 3.6 months, hazard ratio 1.64) and overall survival (15.4 vs. 12.7 months, hazard ratio 1.41) (34). In this study, there were four treatment-related deaths in the docetaxel group (1.8%) and none in the paclitaxel-treated patients.

In clinical practice, therefore, docetaxel monotherapy (75–100 mg/m²) may lead to improved response rates when compared with doxorubicin in anthracycline-naïve patients. This is the standard taxane schedule of choice for patients of good performance status. In addition, previous trials have shown it to be superior to other cytotoxic regimens in anthracycline pre-treated patients, in particular those with anthracycline-resistant disease (35,36). These studies demonstrated the superiority of docetaxel to either mitomycin with vinblastine or methotrexate with 5-fluoruracil in patients who have previously received anthracycline therapy. Nabholtz and colleagues provided data demonstrating higher response rates with docetaxel in patients previously resistant to anthracycline-containing regimens. Weekly paclitaxel (80–90 mg/m²) is the most effective schedule for delivering paclitaxel and is an important alternative taxane option for patients of poorer performance status, extensive visceral disease, or heavy pre-treatment.

First-Line Nab-Paclitaxel (Abraxane) Monotherapy

Pre-clinical data established that nab-paclitaxel, a derivative of paclitaxel complexed with albumin, has been shown to have better tumour penetration in mouse tumour models compared with conventional paclitaxel. Furthermore, nab-paclitaxel does not require Cremaphor as the drug vehicle which has been implicated in some of the toxic effects seen with paclitaxel (including myelosuppression and neuropathy). A phase III trial of nab-paclitaxel and paclitaxel revealed superior response rates and less myelosuppression with ABI-007 (37) and the drug is approved in the United States for treatment of MBC.

In a randomised phase II trial comparing weekly nab-paclitaxel with 3-weekly docetaxel 100 mg/m², weekly nab-paclitaxel 150 mg/m² demonstrated an improved safety and efficacy with a greater PFS (12.9 months vs. 7.5 months) (38). In this study the incidence of sensory neuropathy was equivalent although the recovery was faster in the nab-paclitaxel-treated patients.

First-Line Taxane Combinations

Taxane/Anthracycline Combinations

For chemotherapy naïve patients, trials were initiated to see whether combined anthracycline/taxane chemotherapy would be superior to taxane monotherapy. Nabholtz and colleagues demonstrated the superiority of docetaxel/doxorubicin combination versus doxorubicin/cyclophosphamide in the first-line treatment of MBC (39) with improved overall response rates (59% vs. 47%) and TTP in the taxane combination arm. There was no overall survival difference in the taxane arm although there was a higher rate of grade 3/4 neutropaenia (33% vs. 10%) and febrile neutropaenia (8% vs. 2%). Likewise, docetaxel/anthracycline/cyclophosphamide (TAC) combinations may also lead to higher response rates than FAC combinations but with a greater toxicity (40).

Combination strategies encompassing an anthracycline (doxorubicin) with paclitaxel produced higher response rates than with either drug alone but with no difference in quality of life observed between the treatment arms (response rate 36% anthracycline vs. 34% paclitaxel vs. 47% doxorubicin combined with paclitaxel) (13). Response rates were superior with combination therapy; however, this study failed to demonstrate a survival benefit. Although one study demonstrated an overall survival superiority of doxorubicin/paclitaxel to FAC (41) there was no difference in terms of response rate, PFS, and overall survival in a European Organization for Research and Treatment of Cancer (EORTC) phase III study comparing doxorubicin/paclitaxel with doxorubicin/cyclophosphamide (42). A further phase III study investigating paclitaxel/epirubicin combinations failed to show superiority over epirubicin/cyclophosphamide (43).

In agreement with these data, a meta-analysis of eight randomised combination trials comparing anthracycline/taxane combinations with anthracycline/cyclophosphamide combinations demonstrated that PFS was worse with anthracycline combinations but this was not the case for overall survival (44).

Taxane Combinations with Other Cytotoxics

As other active cytotoxic drugs have been developed, trials have assessed whether these can be added safely to taxanes in order to further enhance their efficacy. An overall survival benefit (Table 5) was reported for the combination of gemcitabine

TABLE 5 Clinical Trials Demonstrating Survival Benefits in MBC

Study	Regimen	Number	Results
Anthracycline Naïve			
Nabholtz 1999 {Nabholtz, 1999}	Docetaxel vs. mitomycin+vinblastine	392	11.4 mon D vs. 8.7 mon M+V
Anthracycline Pre-Treated			
O'Shaughnessy {O'Shaughnessy, 2002}	Docetaxel + capecitabine vs. docetaxel	511	14.5 D+C vs. 11.5 mon D RR 42% vs. 30%
Jones {Jones, 2005}	Docetaxel (100) vs. paclitaxel (175 q.3 wk)	449	15.4 D vs. 12.7 P (p = 0.03) RR 32% vs. 25% (p = 0.1)
Albain {Albain, 2008}	Gemcitabine + paclitaxel vs. paclitaxel	266	18.6 mon GP vs. 15.8 P RR 41.4% vs. 26.2%
Trastuzumab			
Slamon {Slamon, 2001}	Dox + cyclophosphamide vs. Dox + cyclophosphamide + trastuzumab Anthracycline pre-treated: paclitaxel vs. paclitaxel + trastuzumab	469	25.1 mon vs. 20.3 mon
Marty{Marty, 2005}	Docetaxel + trastuzumab vs. docetaxel No prior chemotherapy for metastatic dx	186	OS 31.2 mon vs. 22.7 RR 61% vs. 34%
Eribulin			
Cortes J (2011)	Eribulin vs. physician's choice		13.1 mon vs. 10.6 mon

Abbreviations: mon, month/s; OS, overall survival; RR, response rate.

and paclitaxel (compared with paclitaxel alone) in patients with MBC, pre-treated with an anthracycline in the adjuvant setting (45). Median overall survival was 18.6 months in the combination arm versus 15.8 months for paclitaxel alone. Early quality of life parameters were not adversely affected by the combination strategy.

The efficacy of gemcitabine and docetaxel compared to capecitabine with docetaxel was recently assessed in a phase III trial. There was no difference in overall survival or PFS between the arms (46).

Similarly, the capecitabine/taxane combination has attracted much interest. In the first-line setting, treatment with capecitabine (850 mg/m^2 bd days 1–14) and paclitaxel (175 mg/m^2 q.3 wk) achieved response rates of 51% (47). A similar response rate was seen with this combination (higher dose of capecitabine 1000 mg/m^2 bd) in anthracycline pre-treated patients (48). Docetaxel in combination with capecitabine (docetaxel 75 mg/m^2 and capecitabine 1250 mg/m^2 days 1–14 q.3 wk) leads to improved survival and response rates (overall survival 14.5 months vs. 11.5 months, response rate 42% vs. 30%) when compared to docetaxel alone (100 mg/m^2) (49) (Table 2). However, in this study following failure of docetaxel monotherapy, 35% of patients did not receive further chemotherapy. Interestingly, in an updated analysis of the patients who were randomised to docetaxel monotherapy, those patients who received post-study capecitabine experienced a significantly improved survival over other cytotoxic agents (50). Thus, the question of whether combined taxane/capecitabine treatment is superior overall to sequential use of both drugs has not been answered. A prospective phase III clinical trial is required to address whether sequential docetaxel with capecitabine monotherapy at subsequent progression is equivalent to the upfront combination in terms of survival, toxicity, and quality of life.

Novel Therapeutics in Combination with Taxane-Based Therapy

Trastuzumab is a monoclonal antibody targeting the epidermal growth factor receptor, HER2 that is overexpressed in 20% of breast carcinomas. Combinations of either paclitaxel and trastuzumab, or docetaxel and trastuzumab are significantly superior to the use of taxane chemotherapy alone in these patients (19,51). The rationale and clinical data for use of trastuzumab are discussed in greater detail in Chapter 4.

Recent trial results indicate that the combination of the vascular endothelial growth factor (VEGF) monoclonal antibody, Bevacizumab, Avastin® (Genentech/Roche) with taxanes improves response rates and PFS; however, a meta-analysis of bevacizumab trials in breast cancer has not demonstrated an improvement in overall survival (52) (Chapter 8).

Results of an independent review of 722 patients randomised into the E2100 open-label trial of paclitaxel alone or paclitaxel with bevacizumab were recently reported (53). A majority of patients had received prior chemotherapy and were HER2 negative and had hormone receptor-positive disease. The combination of paclitaxel with bevacizumab significantly improved PFS compared to paclitaxel alone (11.3 months vs. 5.8 months; HR 0.48; p < 0.0001) with a more than doubling of the response rate. However in this trial, the overall survival was the same in both treatment arms (54). Similarly, the combination of Bevacizumab 15 mg/kg (but not 7.5 mg/kg) with docetaxel improved PFS when compared with docetaxel alone in a randomised placebo-controlled trial in HER2-negative MBC (10.1 months vs. 8.2 months) (55). However, overall survival was similar across all the arms of this trial.

Treatment Options Following Prior Anthracycline- and Taxane-Based Chemotherapy

Inevitably, patients with MBC develop resistance to both anthracyclines and taxanes. Common therapeutic options in the third-line setting are single-agent treatment with capecitabine, vinorelbine, or gemcitabine. Combination therapy with platinum-based therapies may also be an effective third -line option. More recent anti-mitotic drugs such as the epothilones also demonstrate activity in this setting. There is very little data comparing the relative efficacy of these agents with each other and therefore treatment should be selected for patients balanced on the knowledge of the risks in terms of side effect profile and potential quality of life benefits offered by chemotherapy.

Capecitabine

Capecitabine is an oral fluoropyrimidine carbamate that is converted to 5-Fluoroura-cil by the enzyme thymidine phosphorylase that is overexpressed in tumour tissue. Capecitabine is active in taxane and anthracycline refractory patients and generally well tolerated with the benefits such as minimal hair loss and limited bone marrow suppression (Fig. 4). Therefore, its use should also be considered in elderly patients or patients of poorer performance status. A 20% response rate was reported in a phase II study with 163 patients, all of whom had received prior paclitaxel, 91% had received an anthracycline, and 82% had received prior bolus 5-fluorouracil treatment (56). Importantly for this patient group, capecitabine was well tolerated with diarrhoea (14%) and hand and foot syndrome (10%) as the only grade 3 and 4 events reported in more than 10% of patients. Both these events were managed successfully with dose adjustment or dose interruption. A further phase II study confirmed that capecitabine is active and well tolerated in patients who have disease that is resistant to taxane therapy with response rates of 26% reported (57). Fumoleau and colleagues reported a 28% response rate in patients with anthracycline and taxane pre-treated disease with an improvement of the mean Global Health Score quality of life score (58). Finally, in an analysis of 631 patients who had received a taxane-based regimen and at least one other treatment line for MBC the ORR was 35% with a median TTP of 6.6 months with no grade 3 or 4 alopecia and only rare grade 3 or 4 myelosuppression (59).

In patients with HER2-positive breast cancer who have progressed on trastu-zumab regimen, continuation of trastuzumab beyond progression in combination with capecitabine has been proven to be more efficacious in terms of TTP and response rate than capecitabine monotherapy (median TTP 8.2 months vs. 5.6 months) (60).

However, bevacizumab (a monoclonal antibody targeting the VEGF receptor) in combination with capecitabine improves response rates (with no overall survival difference) in comparison to capecitabine monotherapy in patients with anthracy-cline and taxane pre-treated disease (61).

The main toxicities associated with oral capecitabine administration are muco-sitis, hand and foot syndrome (plantar palmar erythema), nausea, vomiting, and diarrhoea. Patients should be instructed to stop treatment and seek medical advice in the event of grade 2 diarrhoea (an increase of 4–6 stools/day or stools at night),

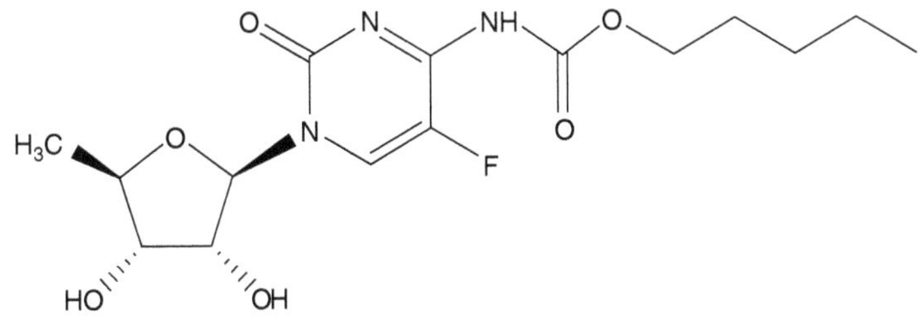

FIGURE 4 Structure of capecitabine.

nausea and vomiting (2-5 episodes/24hours), hand and foot syndrome (painful erythema), stomatitis (painful erythema, oedema, or ulcers of thee mouth or tongue). Patients should also stop treatment and seek medical support in the event of fever >38°C.

Contraindications for Capecitabine Use and Dose Adjustments
The most commonly used dose is 1000–1250 mg/m² bd swallowed with water 30 minutes after a meal for 14 days followed by 7 days' rest. Patients should be aware that capecitabine is supplied as 150 mg and 500 mg tablets. Capecitabine and its metabolic products are predominantly excreted in the urine and is therefore contra-indicated in patients with severe renal impairment (creatinine clearance (CrCl) <30 mL/min). Patients with a CrCl of 30–50 mL/min should receive a 25% dose reduction. The drug is also contraindicated in patients with known dihydropyrimi-dine dehydrogenase deficiency (DPD) and in patients with a known hypersensitiv-ity to 5-fluorouracil. Capecitabine may induce myocardial ischaemia/infarction, angina, cardiac arrest, arrhythmias, cardiomyopathy, and sudden death. Patients with a history of coronary artery disease or cardiac failure should not take capecitabine. Capecitabine may cause severe diarrhoea necessitating urgent intrave-nous re-hydration and careful fluid balance. If grade 2, 3, or 4 diarrhoea develops, treatment should be stopped immediately and not re-introduced until symptoms have subsided when a dose reduction should be considered (Table 6). Capecitabine may provoke hyperbilirubinemia (7–15% grade 3, 1.5–3× ULN and 2–3.9% >3× ULN) and is more likely to occur in those patients with hepatic metastases. If the serum bilirubin increases to >1.5× ULN, treatment should be interrupted immedi-ately until the episode resolves and a dose reduction is initiated. The manufacturers do not recommend a dose adjustment for mild to moderate hepatic dysfunction at baseline. Neutropaenia is a rare event with capecitabine monotherapy but may occur in approximately 3% patients. Thrombocytopenia and anemia have been reported in 1.7% and 2.4% respectively. Capecitabine decreases the clearance of war-farin and the INR should be more frequently monitored and warfarin dose adjusted appropriately whilst on treatment. Some oncologists would recommend switching to low-molecular-weight heparin during the course of treatment. The phenytoin dose may also need to be reduced in patients treated with capecitabine.

TABLE 6   Dose Adjustment in Capecitabine Monotherapy (Manufacturer's Advice)

NCIC toxicity	During treatment	Dose adjustment
Grade 1	Maintain dose level	Maintain dose
Grade 2		
1st event	Interrupt until grade 0–1	100%
2nd event	Interrupt until grade 0–1	75%
3rd event	Interrupt until grade 0–1	50%
4th event	Discontinue	
Grade 3		
1st event	Interrupt until grade 0–1	75%
2nd event	Interrupt until grade 0–1	50%
3rd event	Discontinue	
Grade 4		
1st event	Discontinue on physician's discretion; interrupt until grade 0–1; 50% dose adjustment	

Vinorelbine

Vinorelbine is a vinca alkaloid that interferes with microtubule assembly (Fig. 5). Reminiscent of the taxanes, vinorelbine also induces a cell cycle arrest at mitosis due to its microtubule targeting activity. Vinorelbine may induce neutropaenia as its dose limiting side effect, and patients should be warned in advance of the complications and management of febrile neutropaenia. Severe constipation, paralytic ileus, and intestinal obstruction and perforation have also been reported. Diarrhoea is a recognised complication of therapy. Rarely, cases of interstitial pulmonary changes and acute respiratory distress have been reported with single-agent vinorelbine use. Patients with recent onset dyspnoea, cough, or hypoxia following vinroelbine use should be evaluated immediately. Use of vinorelbine in patients who have received prior radiotherapy may result in radiation recall reactions. Patients with a history of neuropathy should be monitored for an exacerbation during treatment (severe neuropathy <1% of patients). Women of childbearing potential should be advised against becoming pregnant during treatment due to its genotoxic potential. Vinorelbine is a moderate vesicant and pain at the injection site is common. Vinorelbine is not a potent emetogenic drug and therefore prophylaxis with serotonin antagonists is not required. Fatigue is a common side effect and increases with cumulative dosing.

The common dose range of vinorelbine is 25–30 mg/m² administered on day 1 and day 8 of a 3-week cycle. Vinorelbine use is contraindicated in patients with neutrophil counts less than 1500 cells/mm³. Neutrophil nadirs usually occur at 7–10 days. Vinorelbine undergoes hepatic metabolism mediated by the CYP3A cytochrome complex. Although data regarding vinorelbine use in patients with hepatic dysfunction are limited, patients with deranged liver function should undergo dose modification (Table 7). A careful drug history should be taken to avoid concurrent use of cytochrome enzyme inhibitors.

No dose modification is suggested for renal impairment. Vinorelbine should be discontinued if neurotoxicity occurs at grade 2 or above. There are no established guidelines for vinorelbine extravasation events, and local policies should be followed.

Vinorelbine is an attractive agent due to its limited toxicity profile with minimal alopecia and low emetogenic potential. Although vinorelbine is active in patients with previously untreated MBC (62) in practice, its use tends to be reserved for anthracycline-resistant disease in the second or third-line setting with pooled response rates from phase II trials of 19% (CI 14–24%). One study demonstrated a

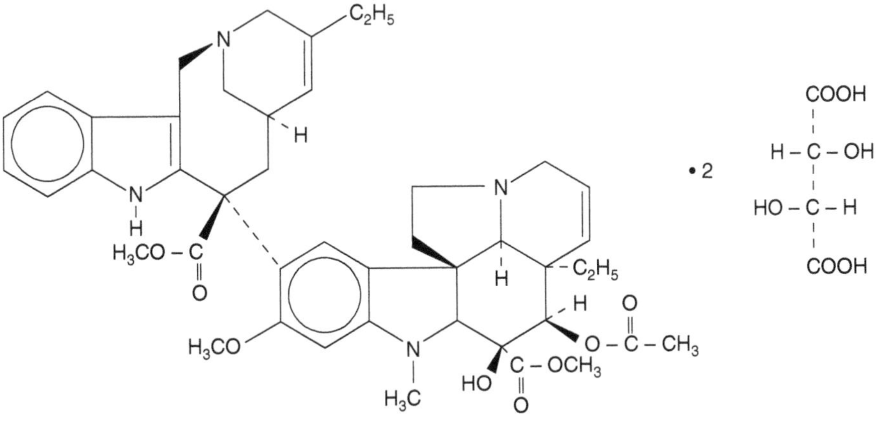

FIGURE 5 Vinorelbine tartrate structure.

survival benefit for vinorelbine (over melphalan) in patients who had failed to respond to an anthracycline regimen with no difference in the quality-of-life scores between the two treatment arms (63).

An exception to this practice is in the HER2 3+ or 2+/FISH+ patient group who may warrant treatment with vinorelbine and trastuzumab in the first-line setting due to the impressive response rates in phase II studies with this combination. Vinorelbine/trastuzumab combination approaches are effective as first-line treatment of MBC with response rates of 61–78% reported (64,65). A small phase II study reported impressive response rates of 42% with vinorelbine/trastuzumab in the second or third-line setting following relapse after trastuzumab or trastuzumab/taxane therapy (66).

Vinorelbine has been combined with other active drugs in MBC. A phase III randomised study in patients who have not received prior chemotherapy reported the comparable activity of the combination of vinorelbine and doxorubicin (75% response rate) to FAC (74% response rate) with no survival difference and similar toxicities in each arm (67). A separate phase III randomised study demonstrated no survival benefit and similar efficacy of the combination of 5-fluoruracil and vinorelbine compared with docetaxel monotherapy (100 mg/m²) in patients who had received prior anthracycline therapy (68). Docetaxel monotherapy appeared to be less toxic than the vinorelbine combination with five possible treatment-related deaths in the combination arm and 1 with docetaxel. Finally, a phase III study has revealed that the combination of doxorubicin and vinorelbine does not appear to offer a survival benefit over doxorubicin alone in vinca alkaloid and anthracycline naive patients (69). Therefore, the combination of vinorelbine with either doxorubicin or docetaxel does not offer any significant advantage over anthracycline or taxane monotherapy. Thus the utility of this drug is likely to be in combination with trastuzumab or as monotherapy in patients with anthracycline-resistant disease. However, oral derivatives of vinorelbine are in development which may be attractive in combination with other active oral agents such as capecitabine.

Platinum Combinations

Mitomycin C/vinblastine and cisplatin (MVP) is an active combination regimen in pre-treated patients with MBC. In a recently reported phase II study, the response rates associated with this regimen were approximately 30% with no statistically significant difference in response rates when MVP was given as the first, second, or

TABLE 7 Dose Modification for Vinorelbine

Granulocytes on day of treatment (cells/mm³)	Percentage of starting dose of NAVELBINE
≥1500	100%
1000–1499	50%
<1000	Do not administer. Repeat granulocyte count in 1 wk. If 3 consecutive weekly doses are held because granulocyte count is <1000 cells/mm³, discontinue NAVELBINE

Note: For patients who, during treatment with NAVELBINE, experienced fever and/or sepsis while granulocytopenic or had 2 consecutive weekly doses held due to granulocytopenia, subsequent doses of NAVELBINE should be:

≥1500	75%
1000 to 1499	37.5%
<1000	See above

Source: Table from prescribing information, GSK/Pierre Fabre.

subsequent line of treatment (70). The toxicity profile is also mild with this regimen with minimal hair loss. MVP may, therefore, be appropriate for use in the third-line setting after anthracycline and taxane relapse.

The combination of cisplatin or carboplatin with 5FU may be well suited to the treatment of patients with significant liver dysfunction but normal renal function with response rates of 40–60% in the first-line setting.

Synergy between trastuzumab, platinum salts, and taxanes has been demonstrated in pre-clinical studies. Two multicentre phase II studies have recently reported activity of this combination in MBC in patients with HER2 overexpressing disease. Response rates were impressive, ranging between 58% and 79% (71).

Gemcitabine

Gemcitabine is a nucleoside analogue that is metabolised within the cell by nucleoside kinases to the active diphosphate and triphosphate nucleosides. The cytotoxic effects of this drug are thought to be due to these two products of nucleoside phosphorylation by inhibiting ribonucleotide reductase and competing with dCTP for incorporation into DNA leading to inhibition of further DNA synthesis.

The most frequent adverse events associated with gemcitabine are bone marrow suppression with neutropaenia occurring more frequently than thromobocytopenia and anemia. Nausea, vomiting, and fatigue are also recognised side effects. A macular or maculopapular rash is common with gemcitabine (30% patients). Reversible elevation of liver transaminases may also occur with serious hepatotoxicity reported rarely, either alone or in combination with other hepatotoxic drugs. Mild proteinuria and haematuria were commonly reported in clinical trials. Haemolytic uremic syndrome (HUS) (0.25%) and renal failure have been reported in patients treated with one or more doses of gemcitabine. HUS should be suspected if a patient develops evidence of microangiopathic haemolysis, a raised bilirubin or LDH, severe thrombocytopenia, anemia, or renal failure. Pulmonary toxicity has also been observed and discontinuation of therapy should proceed immediately. Anaphylaxis and bronchospasm may also occur. Supraventricular arrythmias, congestive heart failure, and myocardial infarction have been reported rarely with gemcitabine. Hair loss is usually minimal.

Gemcitabine is contraindicated in patients with a known hypersensitivity to the drug. Clearance of the drug is reduced in women and the elderly. There is limited information available for the treatment of patients with severe hepatic or renal impairment and gemcitabine should be used cautiously in patients with hepatic and renal insufficiency. A starting dose of $800\,mg/m^2$ is recommended for patients with hyperbilirubinemia (with normal renal function). Routine evaluation of hepatic and renal function should be obtained prior to initiating and during therapy. There are reports of fatal cholestatic liver failure associated with gemcitabine.

Gemcitabine dose adjustments are indicated for haematological toxicity, and a full blood count and differential should be taken prior to each cycle of therapy (Tables 8 and 9).

TABLE 8 Gemcitabine Monotherapy Dose Adjustments: Haematological Toxicity

Absolute granulocyte count $\times 10^6/L$		Platelet count $\times 10^6/L$	% of full dose
≥1000	And	≥100,000	100
500–999	Or	50,000–99,000	75
<500	Or	<50,000	Hold

TABLE 9 Day-8 Dose Adjustments for Gemcitabine in Combination with Paclitaxel

Absolute granulocyte count $\times 10^6$/L		Platelet count $\times 10^6$/L	Percentage of full dose
≥1200	And	>75,000	100
1000–1199	Or	50,000–75,000	75
700–999	And	≥50,000	50
<700	Or	<50,000	Hold

Gemcitabine is active as a single agent in MBC with response rates between 14 and 37%. Phase II studies in anthracycline and taxane refractory patients have documented response rates of 22–30%. Several phase II trials have studied the combination of docetaxel with gemcitabine. One small second-line phase II trial revealed response rates of 79% with this combination (72). However, grade 4 neutropaenia occurred in over 90% of patients with febrile neutropaenia occurring in 3 of 39 patients. Grade 3 or 4 thrombocytopenia may be less frequent than with gemcitabine alone, indicating a possible platelet sparing effect with the taxane combination. A similar activity has also been reported for paclitaxel/gemcitabine combination strategies with toxicity of myelosuppression, neuropathy, and nausea and vomiting (paclitaxel 175 mg/m² q.3 wk and gemcitabine 1250 mg/m² days 1 and 8 of a 3-weekly cycle) (Table 8). In December 2004, the Medicines and Healthcare Products Regulatory Agency awarded the licence for the combination of paclitaxel and gemcitabine for the treatment of MBC in patients who have been treated with an anthracycline. Interim phase III trial data for gemcitabine/paclitaxel versus paclitaxel alone have shown a 41% response rate for the doublet compared with 22% for single-agent paclitaxel (73). TTP was also improved with the combination (5.2 months vs. 2.9 months) and interim median survival analysis was also superior in the combination arm (18.5 months vs. 15.8 months). As expected in the combination arm, the incidence of febrile neutropaenia was higher (5% vs. 1%). Nevertheless, the important question as to whether combination therapy is superior to sequential (paclitaxel-gemcitabine) treatment remains to be answered before this regimen becomes a new standard of care.

Novel Anti-Mitotics Ixabepilone and Eribulin Mesylate

Pre-clinical data suggest that the epothilones may overcome taxane-drug resistance associated with p-glycoprotein expression and tubulin mutations (74) although the *in vivo* relevance of these observations remains unclear (75). Ixabepilone is a semi-synthetic analogue of epothilone B. In patients who have not previously been exposed to taxanes, ixabepilone achieved a response rate of 57% with a median TTP of 5.5 months (76). A phase II study of ixabepilone in patients previously treated with a taxane in either the adjuvant or metastatic setting demonstrated tumour control (PR, CR, and SD) in over 50% of the patients treated (77). In a trial of ixabepilone in patients who had progressed on prior taxane therapy (73% had progressed within 1 month of prior taxane therapy) the response rate was 12% (78). In a large phase II trial of 1221 patients, there was no overall survival benefit with the combination of ixabepilone with capecitabine compared with capecitabine alone (79). Toxicities experienced with epothilones are neurotoxicity, diarrhoea, and febrile neutropaenia.

Eribulin mesylate is a microtubule inhibitor and a synthetic analogue of hali-chondrin B derived from the marine sponge *Halichondria okadai*. Pre-clinical work has established the efficacy of this compound in taxane-resistant cell lines. A phase II trial of Eprirubin mesylate in patients pre-treated with both anthracycline and taxanes (and a median of four prior chemotherapy regimens) resulted in a response rate of 11.5% and a median PFS of 2.6 months (80). A phase III open-label clinical trial of Eribulin Mesylate was recently reported to demonstrate a superior overall survival for the use of this agent compared with physicians' choice (13.1 months vs. 10.6 months) (81). Remarkably, this was a clinical trial in heavily pre-treated patients with MBC who had progressed through 2–5 lines of prior chemotherapy including an anthracycline and a taxane. These results demonstrate that a positive impact upon overall survival, even in advanced stages of the disease course, is achievable with the addition of novel cytotoxics.

Early-Phase Clinical Trials
Once all treatment lines have been exhausted in patients with MBC or if patients have derived minimal benefit from cytotoxic regimens, patients with good performance status and organ function may want to consider phase I clinical trial options. A recent review of National Cancer Institute-sponsored phase I studies in the United States between 1991 and 2002 documented an overall response rate of 10.6% with an overall death rate due to toxic events of 0.49% (82). This response rate is similar to the 11.4% response rate observed specifically in patients with breast cancer enrolled at the Royal Marsden Hospital phase I unit over a 7-year period in 30 clinical trials (83).

SPECIAL TREATMENT CONSIDERATIONS
Elderly Patients
Elderly patients generally tolerate chemotherapy that does not seem to be at the expense of a deterioration in quality of life (84). Therefore, chronological age should not influence the decision to commence palliative chemotherapy. Physiological age with attention to co-morbidity, and pharmacological, nutritional, and psychosocial issues should have more influence over the choice of chemotherapy regimen. Unfortunately, as most of the clinical studies preclude entry to patients older than 75, the evidence is too little to make the appropriate decisions. Furthermore, as most studies have strict entry criteria, results with regards to toxicity and quality of life benefit may not necessarily translate to the management of MBC in the elderly.

Patients over the age of 70 may suffer from increased chemotherapy-related myelosuppression and growth factor support should be considered in this high risk group (85). Capecitabine monotherapy in the elderly population (>80 years) can cause significant morbidity with over half of patients experiencing a grade 3 or 4 adverse event. Grade 3 and 4 thrombocytopenia is more common in elderly patients treated with gemcitabine.

Caution should be taken with trastuzumab combinations in elderly patients at risk of cardiac toxicity and liposomal anthracycline formulations should be considered in those at risk of cardiomyopathy. Declining renal function with age necessitates appropriate chemotherapy dose adjustments with reference to the patient's glomerular filtration rate (discussed next).

Renal Impairment
Special consideration should be given to patients with renal impairment and cytotoxic dose adjustments should be made appropriately. For example, capecitabine is contraindicated in patients with a CrCl less than 30 mL/min. A 25% dose reduction is indicated for patients with a CrCl of 30–50 mL/min as grade 3 and 4 toxicities are increased. Cisplatin is nephrotoxic and it is contraindicated in patients with renal impairment [glomerular filtration rate (GFR) <40 mL/min] and dose reductions

should be considered with a GFR 40–60 mL/min. Carboplatin use is preferable in patients with a GFR <60 mL/min. There are no recommended dose adjustments for docetaxel or paclitaxel in renal impairment. Mitoxantrone dose adjustments are not necessary in patients with renal impairment. Epirubicin and Doxorubicin should be given at a reduced dose in patients with severe renal impairment. Vinorelbine dose modifications in renal impairment are recommended.

The Diabetic Patient
Glucocorticoid-induced hyperglycemia is common in diabetic patients treated with chemotherapy where steroids form part of the anti-emetic regimen and patients should be advised to monitor blood glucose levels more frequently. Diabetic neuropathy can be exacerbated by treatment with Taxane or vinca alkaloid-based chemotherapy. Patients with diabetic cardiomyopathy may be more sensitive to the cardiac toxicity of anthracyclines.

Cutaneous Metastasis and Topical Miltefosine
A small patient group may present with an isolated cutaneous metastatic disease with no organ involvement. A trial of topical miltefosine may be considered in this group prior to initiating systemic chemotherapy. A randomised double blind placebo controlled trial using a topical 6% solution demonstrated an increased time to treatment failure with the use of miltefosine over placebo (86).

Central Nervous System Disease and Intrathecal Chemotherapy
The management of cerebral metastatic disease requires a multi-disciplinary approach. For some patients of good performance status with disease well controlled at other sites and a solitary cerebral metastasis, neurosurgical intervention may be appropriate (Chapter 13). For patients with multi-focal disease, palliative whole brain radiotherapy (Chapter 12), or stereotactic approaches may improve the quality of life. There is limited, randomised, prospectively collected data for the management of cerebral metastasis. Meningeal disease may be managed with intrathecal chemotherapy. In a retrospective analysis, high-dose intrathecal methotrexate may improve neurological function over conventional-dose methotrexate (87). However, treatment with intrathecal chemotherapy is controversial with other studies demonstrating no improvement in relief from clinical symptoms associated with leptomeningeal

TABLE 10 Suggested Dose Modifications According to Liver Function (see Mano et al. 2005 for review)

Drug	Bilirubin (μmole/dL)	ALK PHOS	AST	Suggested DR (%) or dose
Epirubicin	20–51		or 2–4× ULN	50%
	>51		or 4× ULN	75%
Doxorubicin	20–51			50%
	>51			75%
Paclitaxel (175 mg/m² q.3 wk)	21–34		<10× ULN	135 mg/m²
	34–85		>10× ULN	90 mg/m²
	>85			Not recommended
Docetaxel 100 mg/m²	>ULN	Or >2.5 ULN	or >1.5× ULN	Not recommended
Vinorelbine	36–51			50%
	>51			75%

Abbreviation: ULN, upper limit of normal.

metastasis. Indeed a recent, small randomised trial demonstrated no survival benefit and increased risk of neurotoxicity associated with the addition of intraventricular therapy.

Liver Dysfunction
Patients with liver metastases with deranged liver function tests are frequently encountered in the management of MBC. Dose reductions are required according to the bilirubin and AST levels with anthracyclines, taxanes, the vinca alkaloids, and gemcitabine (Table 10). Even in patients treated with these agents with appropriate dose reductions, unexpected toxicities may occur. Particular care should be taken with the elderly, patients with poor performance status, patients on warfarin or other drugs metabolised by the liver, and those with limited bone marrow reserve (88). Consideration should be given to the use of drugs with predominant renal excretion, such as platinum agents or capecitabine. In patients with normal renal function, no dose reductions are required for platinum agents and as noted previously the combination of cisplatin or carboplatin with 5FU may be appropriate in the first-line setting.

CONCLUSIONS
Progress in the field of MBC has been rapid over the last 5 years. Improved therapy in the adjuvant setting has led to fewer relapses with metastatic disease and improved survival. The chapter has presented substantial evidence to support these points: the overall survival remains a valid clinical endpoint in clinical trials for advanced breast cancer, and even in heavily pre-treated patients, improvements in overall survival are still achievable. Ultimately, the greatest advance in MBC will derive from optimising adjuvant therapy to prevent relapse. The sad reality is that advanced breast cancer remains an incurable disease in a vast majority of cases, with the rapid acquisition of multi-drug resistance that occurs through sequential lines of therapy. The major challenge and unmet clinical need is to establish the mechanisms through which multi-drug resistance is acquired in MBC and how to specifically target this process. It is likely that with advances in next-generation sequencing technologies and genomics profiling of tumour somatic events, progress will be made in our understanding of how to integrate cytotoxic therapies with targeted agents in patient cohorts with molecularly defined tumour somatic aberrations and how to predict a sub-population of patients most likely to benefit from current treatment regimens.

REFERENCES
1. Tannock IF, Boyd NF, DeBoer G, et al. A randomized trial of two dose levels of cyclophosphamide, methotrexate, and fluorouracil chemotherapy for patients with metastatic breast cancer. J Clin Oncol 1988; 6: 1377–87.
2. Carlson RW. Quality of life issues in the treatment of metastatic breast cancer. Oncology (Huntingt) 1998; 12(3 Suppl 4): 27–31.
3. Ramirez AJ, Towlson KE, Leaning MS, Richards MA, Rubens RD. Do patients with advanced breast cancer benefit from chemotherapy? Br J Cancer 1998; 78: 1488–94.
4. Cold S, Jensen NV, Brincker H, Rose C. The influence of chemotherapy on survival after recurrence in breast cancer - a population based study of patients treated in the 1950s, 1960s and 1970s. Eur J Cancer 1993; 29A: 1146–52.
5. Ross MB, Buzdar AU, Smith TL, et al. Improved survival of patients with metastatic breast cancer receiving combination chemotherapy. Cancer 1985; 55: 341–6.
6. Andreopoulou E, Hortobagyi GN. Prognostic factors in metastatic breast cancer: successes and challenges toward individualized therapy. J Clin Oncol 2008; 26: 3660–2.

7. Kriege M, Seynaeve C, Meijers-Heijboer H, et al. Sensitivity to first-line chemotherapy for metastatic breast cancer in BRCA1 and BRCA2 mutation carriers. J Clin Oncol 2009; 27: 3764–71.
8. Buzdar AU, Legha SS, Hortobagyi GN, et al. Management of breast cancer patients failing adjuvant chemotherapy with adriamycin-containing regimens. Cancer 1981; 47: 2798–802.
9. Banerji U, Kuciejewska A, Ashley S, et al. Factors determining outcome after third line chemotherapy for metastatic breast cancer. Breast (Edinburgh, Scotland) 2007; 16: 359–66.
10. Liu MC, Shields PG, Warren RD, et al. Circulating tumor cells: a useful predictor of treatment efficacy in metastatic breast cancer. J Clin Oncol 2009; 27: 5153–9.
11. Burzykowski T, Buyse M, Piccart-Gebhart MJ, et al. Evaluation of tumor response, disease control, progression-free survival, and time to progression as potential surrogate end points in metastatic breast cancer. J Clin Oncol 2008; 26: 1987–92.
12. Cardoso F, Bedard PL, Winer EP, et al. International guidelines for management of metastatic breast cancer: combination vs sequential single-agent chemotherapy. J Natl Cancer Inst 2009; 101: 1174–81.
13. Sledge GW, Neuberg D, Bernardo P, et al. Phase III trial of doxorubicin, paclitaxel, and the combination of doxorubicin and paclitaxel as front-line chemotherapy for metastatic breast cancer: an intergroup trial (E1193). J Clin Oncol 2003; 21: 588–92.
14. Heidemann E, Stoeger H, Souchon R. Is first line single-agent mitoxantrone in the treatment of high-risk metastatic breast cancer patients as effective as combination chemotherapy? No difference in survival but higher quality of life were found in a multicenter randomized trial. Ann Oncol 2002; 11: 1717–29.
15. Joensuu H, Holli K, Heikkinen M. Combination chemotherapy versus single agent therapy as first and second line treatment in metastatic breast cancer: a prospective randomized trial. J Clin Oncol 1998; 16: 3270–730.
16. Fossati R, Confalonieri C, Torri V, et al. Cytotoxic and hormonal treatment for metastatic breast cancer: a systematic review of published randomized trials involving 31,510 women. J Clin Oncol 1998; 16: 3439–60.
17. Gennari A, Amadori D, De Lena M, et al. Lack of benefit of maintenance paclitaxel in first-line chemotherapy in metastatic breast cancer. J Clin Oncol 2006; 24: 3912–8.
18. A'Hern RP, Smith IE, Ebbs SR. Chemotherapy and survival in advanced breast cancer: the inclusion of doxorubicin in Cooper type regimens. Br J Cancer 1993; 4: 801–5.
19. Slamon DJ, Leyland-Jones B, Shak S, et al. Use of chemotherapy plus a monoclonal antibody against HER2 for metastatic breast cancer that overexpresses HER2. N Engl J Med 2001; 344: 783–92.
20. O'Brien ME, Wigler N, Inbar M, et al. Reduced cardiotoxicity and comparable efficacy in a phase III trial of pegylated liposomal doxorubicin HCL (Caelyx/Doxil) versus conventional doxorubicin as first-line treatment of metastatic breast cancer. Ann Oncol 2004; 15: 440–9.
21. Trudeau ME, Clemons MJ, Provencher L, et al. Phase II multicenter trial of anthracycline rechallenge with pegylated liposomal doxorubicin plus cyclophosphamide for first-line therapy of metastatic breast cancer previously treated with adjuvant anthracyclines. J Clin Oncol 2009; 27: 5906–10.
22. Swain SM, Whaley FS, Gerber MC, et al. Delayed administration of dexrazoxane provides cardioprotection for patients with advanced breast cancer treated with doxorubicin-containing therapy. J Clin Oncol 1997; 15: 1333–40.
23. Twelves CJ, O'Reilly SM, Coleman RE, Richards MA, Rubens RD. Weekly epirubicin for breast cancer with liver metastases and abnormal liver biochemistry. Br J Cancer 1989; 60: 938–41.
24. Twelves CJ, Richards MA, Smith P, Rubens RD. Epirubicin in breast cancer patients with liver metastases and abnormal liver biochemistry: initial weekly treatment followed by rescheduling and intensification. Ann Oncol 1991; 2: 663–6.
25. Swanton C, Nicke B, Schuett M, et al. Chromosomal instability determines taxane response. Proc Natl Acad Sci USA 2009; 106: 8671–6.

26. Swanton C, Marani M, Pardo O, et al. Regulators of mitotic arrest and ceramide metabolism are determinants of sensitivity to paclitaxel and other chemotherapeutic drugs. Cancer Cell 2007; 11: 498–512.
27. Ghersi D, Wilcken N, Simes J, Donoghue E. Taxane containing regimens for metastatic breast cancer. Cochrane Database Syst Rev (Online) 2003; (3): CD003366.
28. Winer EP, Berry DA, Woolf S, et al. Failure of higher-dose paclitaxel to improve outcome in patients with metastatic breast cancer: cancer and leukemia group B trial 9342. J Clin Oncol 2004; 22: 2061–8.
29. Seidman AD, Berry D, Cirrincione C, et al. Randomized phase III trial of weekly compared with every-3-weeks paclitaxel for metastatic breast cancer, with trastuzumab for all HER-2 overexpressors and random assignment to trastuzumab or not in HER-2 nonoverexpressors: final results of Cancer and Leukemia Group B protocol 9840. J Clin Oncol 2008; 26: 1642–9.
30. Mouridsen H, ed. Phase III study of docetaxel 100 vs 75 vs 60mg/m^2 as second line chemotherapy in advanced breast cancer. San Antonio Breast Cancer Symposium, 2002.
31. Chan S, Friedrichs K, Noel D, et al. Prospective randomized trial of docetaxel versus doxorubicin in patients with metastatic breast cancer. J Clin Oncol 1999; 17: 2341–54.
32. Katsumata N, Minami K, Aogi T, Tabei K. Phase III trial of doxorubicin (A)/cyclophosphamide (C), docetaxel (D), and alternating AC and D (AC-D) as front line chemotherapy for metastatic breast cancer (MBC): Japan Clinical Oncology Group trial (JCO G9802). Proc ASCO 2005.
33. Paridaens R, Biganzoli L, Bruning P, et al. Paclitaxel versus doxorubicin as first-line single-agent chemotherapy for metastatic breast cancer: a European Organization for Research and Treatment of Cancer Randomized Study with cross-over. J Clin Oncol 2000; 18: 724–33.
34. Jones SE, Erban J, Overmoyer B, et al. Randomized phase III study of docetaxel compared with paclitaxel in metastatic breast cancer. J Clin Oncol 2005; 23: 5542–51.
35. Nabholtz JM, Senn HJ, Bezwoda WR, et al. Prospective randomized trial of docetaxel versus mitomycin plus vinblastine in patients with metastatic breast cancer progressing despite previous anthracycline-containing chemotherapy. 304 Study Group. J Clin Oncol 1999; 17: 1413–24.
36. Sjostrom J, Blomqvist C, Mouridsen H, et al. Docetaxel compared with sequential methotrexate and 5-fluorouracil in patients with advanced breast cancer after anthracycline failure: a randomised phase III study with crossover on progression by the Scandinavian Breast Group. Eur J Cancer 1999; 35: 1194–201.
37. Gradishar WJ, Tjulandin S, Davidson N, et al. Phase III trial of nanoparticle albumin-bound paclitaxel compared with polyethylated castor oil-based paclitaxel in women with breast cancer. J Clin Oncol 2005; 23: 7794–803.
38. Gradishar WJ, Krasnojon D, Cheporov S, et al. Significantly longer progression-free survival with nab-paclitaxel compared with docetaxel as first-line therapy for metastatic breast cancer. J Clin Oncol 2009; 27: 3611–19.
39. Nabholtz JM, Falkson C, Campos D, et al. Docetaxel and doxorubicin compared with doxorubicin and cyclophosphamide as first-line chemotherapy for metastatic breast cancer: results of a randomized, multicenter, phase III trial. J Clin Oncol 2003; 21: 968–75.
40. Mackey J, ed. Final results of the phase III radnomized trial comparing docetaxel (T), doxorubicin (A) and cyclophosphamide (C) to FAC as first line chemotherapy (CT) for patients (pts) with metastatic breast cancer. Proc Am Soc Clin Oncol 2002.
41. Jassem J, Pienkowski T, Pluzanska A, et al. Doxorubicin and paclitaxel versus fluorouracil, doxorubicin, and cyclophosphamide as first-line therapy for women with metastatic breast cancer: final results of a randomized phase III multicenter trial. J Clin Oncol 2001; 19: 1707–15.
42. Biganzoli L, Cufer T, Bruning P, et al. Doxorubicin and paclitaxel versus doxorubicin and cyclophosphamide as first-line chemotherapy in metastatic breast cancer: The European Organization for Research and Treatment of Cancer 10961 Multicenter Phase III Trial. J Clin Oncol 2002; 20: 3114–21.

43. Langley RE, Carmichael J, Jones AL, et al. Phase III trial of epirubicin plus paclitaxel compared with epirubicin plus cyclophosphamide as first-line chemotherapy for metastatic breast cancer: United Kingdom National Cancer Research Institute trial AB01. J Clin Oncol 2005; 23: 8322–30.

44. Piccart-Gebhart MJ, Burzykowski T, Buyse M, et al. Taxanes alone or in combination with anthracyclines as first-line therapy of patients with metastatic breast cancer. J Clin Oncol 2008; 26: 1980–6.

45. Albain KS, Nag SM, Calderillo-Ruiz G, et al. Gemcitabine plus Paclitaxel versus Paclitaxel monotherapy in patients with metastatic breast cancer and prior anthracycline treatment. J Clin Oncol 2008; 26: 3950–7.

46. Chan S, Romieu G, Huober J, et al. Phase III study of gemcitabine plus docetaxel compared with capecitabine plus docetaxel for anthracycline-pretreated patients with metastatic breast cancer. J Clin Oncol 2009; 27: 1753–60.

47. Gradishar WJ, Meza LA, Amin B, et al. Capecitabine plus paclitaxel as front-line combination therapy for metastatic breast cancer: a multicenter phase II study. J Clin Oncol 2004; 22: 2321–7.

48. Batista N, Perez-Manga G, Constenla M, et al. Phase II study of capecitabine in combination with paclitaxel in patients with anthracycline-pretreated advanced/metastatic breast cancer. Br J Cancer 2004; 90: 1740–6.

49. O'Shaughnessy J, Miles D, Vukelja S, et al. Superior survival with capecitabine plus docetaxel combination therapy in anthracycline-pretreated patients with advanced breast cancer: phase III trial results. J Clin Oncol 2002; 20: 2812–23.

50. Miles D, Vukelja S, Moiseyenko V, et al. Survival benefit with capecitabine/docetaxel versus docetaxel alone: analysis of therapy in a randomized phase III trial. Clin Breast Cancer 2004; 5: 273–8.

51. Marty M, Cognetti F, Maraninchi D, et al. Randomized phase II trial of the efficacy and safety of trastuzumab combined with docetaxel in patients with human epidermal growth factor receptor 2-positive metastatic breast cancer administered as first-line treatment: the M77001 study group. J Clin Oncol 2005; 23: 4265–74.

52. Valachis A, Polyzos NP, Patsopoulos NA, et al. Bevacizumab in metastatic breast cancer: a meta-analysis of randomized controlled trials. Breast Cancer Res Treat 2010; 122: 1–7.

53. Gray R, Bhattacharya S, Bowden C, Miller K, Comis RL. Independent review of E2100: a phase III trial of bevacizumab plus paclitaxel versus paclitaxel in women with metastatic breast cancer. J Clin Oncol 2009; 27: 4966–72.

54. Miller K, Wang M, Gralow J, et al. Paclitaxel plus bevacizumab versus paclitaxel alone for metastatic breast cancer. N Engl J Med 2007; 357: 2666–76.

55. Miles DW, Chan A, Dirix LY, et al. Phase III study of bevacizumab plus docetaxel compared with placebo plus docetaxel for the first-line treatment of human epidermal growth factor receptor 2-negative metastatic breast cancer. J Clin Oncol 2010; 28: 3239–47.

56. Blum JL, Jones SE, Buzdar AU, et al. Multicenter phase II study of capecitabine in paclitaxel-refractory metastatic breast cancer. J Clin Oncol 1999; 17: 485–93.

57. Blum JL, Dieras V, Lo Russo PM, et al. Multicenter, Phase II study of capecitabine in taxane-pretreated metastatic breast carcinoma patients. Cancer 2001; 92: 1759–68.

58. Fumoleau P, Largillier R, Clippe C, et al. Multicentre, phase II study evaluating capecitabine monotherapy in patients with anthracycline- and taxane-pretreated metastatic breast cancer. Eur J Cancer 2004; 40: 536–42.

59. Venturini M, Paridaens R, Rossner D, et al. An open-label, multicenter study of outpatient capecitabine monotherapy in 631 patients with pretreated advanced breast cancer. Oncology 2007; 72: 51–7.

60. von Minckwitz G, du Bois A, Schmidt M, et al. Trastuzumab beyond progression in human epidermal growth factor receptor 2-positive advanced breast cancer: a german breast group 26/breast international group 03-05 study. J Clin Oncol 2009; 27: 1999–2006.

61. Miller KD, Chap LI, Holmes FA, et al. Randomized phase III trial of capecitabine compared with bevacizumab plus capecitabine in patients with previously treated metastatic breast cancer. J Clin Oncol 2005; 23: 792–9.

62. Fumoleau P, Delgado FM, Delozier T, et al. Phase II trial of weekly intravenous vinorelbine in first-line advanced breast cancer chemotherapy. J Clin Oncol 1993; 11: 1245–52.

63. Jones S, Winer E, Vogel C, et al. Randomized comparison of vinorelbine and melphalan in anthracycline-refractory advanced breast cancer. J Clin Oncol 1995; 13: 2567–74.
64. Jahanzeb M, Mortimer JE, Yunus F, et al. Phase II trial of weekly vinorelbine and trastuzumab as first-line therapy in patients with HER2(+) metastatic breast cancer. Oncologist 2002; 7: 410–17.
65. Chan A, Untch M, Petruzelka L, eds. Navelbine and Herceptin combination as first line therapy for HER2-overexpressing metastatic breast cancer is a highly active and safe regimen. 26th Annual San Antonio Breast Cancer Symposium, 2003.
66. Suzuki Y, Tokuda Y, Saito Y, Ohta M, Tajima T. Combination of trastuzumab and vinorelbine in metastatic breast cancer. Jpn J Clin Oncol 2003; 33: 514–17.
67. Blajman C, Balbiani L, Block J, et al. A prospective, randomized Phase III trial comparing combination chemotherapy with cyclophosphamide, doxorubicin, and 5-fluorouracil with vinorelbine plus doxorubicin in the treatment of advanced breast carcinoma. Cancer 1999; 85: 1091–7.
68. Bonneterre J, Roche H, Monnier A, et al. Docetaxel vs 5-fluorouracil plus vinorelbine in metastatic breast cancer after anthracycline therapy failure. Br J Cancer 2002; 87: 1210–15.
69. Norris B, Pritchard KI, James K, et al. Phase III comparative study of vinorelbine combined with doxorubicin versus doxorubicin alone in disseminated metastatic/recurrent breast cancer: National Cancer Institute of Canada Clinical Trials Group Study MA8. J Clin Oncol 2000; 18: 2385–94.
70. Urruticoechea A, Archer CD, Assersohn LA, et al. Mitomycin C, vinblastine and cisplatin (MVP): an active and well-tolerated salvage regimen for advanced breast cancer. Br J Cancer 2005; 92: 475–9.
71. Pegram MD, Pienkowski T, Northfelt DW, et al. Results of two open-label, multicenter phase II studies of docetaxel, platinum salts, and trastuzumab in HER2-positive advanced breast cancer. J Natl Cancer Inst 2004; 96: 759–69.
72. Laufman LR, Spiridonidis CH, Pritchard J, et al. Monthly docetaxel and weekly gemcitabine in metastatic breast cancer: a phase II trial. Ann Oncol 2001; 12: 1259–64.
73. Albain KS, Nag S, Calderillo-Ruiz G, eds. Global phase III study of gemcitabine plus paclitaxel (GT) vs paclitaxel (T) as frontline therapy for metastatic breast cancer (MBC) : First report of overall survival. Proc Am Soc Clin Oncol 2004.
74. Goodin S, Kane MP, Rubin EH. Epothilones: mechanism of action and biologic activity. J Clin Oncol 2004; 22: 2015–25.
75. Harrison M, Swanton C. Epothilones and new analogues of the microtubule modulators in taxane-resistant disease. Expert Opin Investig Drugs 2008; 17: 523–46.
76. Denduluri N, Low JA, Lee JJ, et al. Phase II trial of ixabepilone, an epothilone B analog, in patients with metastatic breast cancer previously untreated with taxanes. J Clin Oncol 2007; 25: 3421–7.
77. Low JA, Wedam SB, Lee JJ, et al. Phase II clinical trial of ixabepilone (BMS-247550), an epothilone B analog, in metastatic and locally advanced breast cancer. J Clin Oncol 2005; 23: 2726–34.
78. Thomas E, Tabernero J, Fornier M, et al. Phase II clinical trial of ixabepilone (BMS-247550), an epothilone B analog, in patients with taxane-resistant metastatic breast cancer. J Clin Oncol 2007; 25: 3399–406.
79. Sparano JA, Vrdoljak E, Rixe O, et al. Randomized phase III trial of ixabepilone plus capecitabine versus capecitabine in patients with metastatic breast cancer previously treated with an anthracycline and a taxane. J Clin Oncol 2010; 28: 3256–63.
80. Vahdat LT, Pruitt B, Fabian CJ, et al. Phase II study of eribulin mesylate, a halichondrin B analog, in patients with metastatic breast cancer previously treated with an anthracycline and a taxane. J Clin Oncol 2009; 27: 2954–61.
81. Cortes J, O'Shaughnessy J, Loesch D, et al.; EMBRACE (Eisai Metastatic Breast Cancer Study Assessing Physician's Choice Versus E7389) investigators. Eribulin monotherapy versus treatment of physician's choice in patients with metastatic breast cancer (EMBRACE): a phase 3 open-label randomised study. Lancet 2011; 377: 914–23.
82. Horstmann E, McCabe MS, Grochow L, et al. Risks and benefits of Phase I Oncology Trials, 1991 through 2002. N Engl J Med 2005; 352: 895–904.

83. Brunetto AT, Sarker D, Papadatos-Pastos D, et al. A retrospective analysis of clinical outcome of patients with chemo-refractory metastatic breast cancer treated in a single institution phase I unit. Br J Cancer 2010; 103: 607–12.
84. Chen H, Cantor A, Meyer J, et al. Can older cancer patients tolerate chemotherapy? A prospective pilot study. Cancer 2003; 97: 1107–14.
85. Balducci L, Carreca I. Supportive care of the older cancer patient. Crit Rev Oncol Hematol 2003; 48(Suppl): S65–70.
86. Leonard R, Hardy J, van Tienhoven G, et al. Randomized, double-blind, placebo controlled, mutlicenter trial of 6% miltefosine solution, a topical chemotherapy in cutaneous metastases from breast cancer. J Clin Oncol 2001; 19: 4150–9.
87. Fizazi K, Asselain B, Vincent-Salomon A, et al. Meningeal carcinomatosis in patients with breast carcinoma. Clinical features, prognostic factors, and results of a high-dose intrathecal methotrexate regimen. Cancer 1996; 77: 1315–23.
88. Mano MS, Cassidy J, Canney P. Liver metastases from breast cancer: management of patients with significant liver dysfunction. Cancer Treat Rev 2005; 31: 35–48.

7 | Bisphosphonates and their role in metastatic breast cancer

David A. Cameron

Metastatic breast cancer remains a challenge for the patients and their clinician. The advent of new therapies that can successfully target cancer cells has led to a welcome improvement in survival (1). Patients therefore live longer with metastatic disease, but do not necessarily avoid the morbidity it causes. This chapter will address the role of bisphosphonates in treating and preventing the skeletal morbidity, including pain, which patients have to face when they develop bone metastases.

INTRODUCTION

The fact why breast cancer has such a propensity to spread to bone is not fully established, but almost certainly it dynamically depends on the microenvironment of bone, and the biological characteristics of breast cancer cells. Bone is a dynamic organ, actively maintained in a healthy state to permit a good quality life. Traditionally, bone metastases were seen as less important than visceral disease, with a low-key palliative approach often being taken in terms of endocrine therapy and occasional radiotherapy. However, the degree of dysfunction, pain, and loss of motility that can be consequent upon bone metastases is considerable. Bone is a common site of disease. Bone metastasis occurs in up to 75% of all patients with advanced breast cancer, and eventually appearing in at least a quarter of all patients presenting with early, operable breast cancer. While more common in patients with ER positive disease, it can also develop in patients with ER negative HER2+ve disease, as well as triple-negative cancers. It could be considered less important as rapid progression is less common than in visceral disease, but as systemic treatments get better, more patients live longer with bone metastases, so that to an extent they can become the major source of morbidity and resource utilisation for some patients with metastatic breast cancer.

PATHOPHYSIOLOGY OF BONE METASTASES

Normal bone is in a constant state of turnover, with osteoclasts resorbing the old bone and osteoblasts synthesising a new bone. By finely balancing these two opposing processes of bone destruction and synthesis, bone health is maintained. A key cytokine in this normal homeostasis is RANKL (receptor activator of NF-kB ligand), which is essential for the formation and activation of osteoclasts (2). Expressed on the surface of osteoblasts, it binds to and activates the RANK receptor, expressed in turn on osteoclasts and their precursor cells. It promotes osteoclast formation and prolongs osteoclast life span (3). It has a natural antagonist, OPG (osteoprotegerin) which acts as a decoy receptor for RANKL (4). Alterations in the ratio of RANKL to OPG are critical in the pathogenesis of bone disease that results from increased bone resorption.

In many disease states the balance between bone resorption and synthesis is altered, for example, as a normal consequence of fracture repair, in benign conditions such as Paget's disease, and of course in bone metastases from any primary site. Under normal circumstances, the cross-talk between the osteoclasts and osteoblasts contributes to the maintenance of bone homeostasis. In addition, the bone matrix acts as a repository for many growth-regulating factors, of which one of the most abundant is TGFβ.

The relevance of the normal bone turnover in metastatic bone disease becomes clear when one considers the potential for metastatic cancer cells to disrupt the cross-talk between osteoclasts and osteoblasts. Micrometastatic disease leads to local bone destruction by the stimulation of osteoclasts; production of factors like parathormone-related peptide (PTHrP) (5) can enhance RANKL production, and the increased bone resorption can release factors from the bone matrix that in turn encourage further tumour growth (6). It has been clearly shown, for example, that TGFβ, released from the resorbed bone matrix, can increase the production of PTHrP through tumour cells in the vicinity, leading to a vicious cycle of increased bone resorption resulting in yet more PTHrP and subsequent osteolysis (7).

Both the loss of normal bone through increased osteolysis and the presence of soft-tissue metastases lead to weakened bone and neural compression. This gives rise to the clinical manifestations of bone metastases such as pathological fractures, pain, and nerve compression syndromes like spinal cord compression (8). The increased release of calcium from the inorganic bone matrix may exceed clearance mechanisms and give rise to hypercalcaemia, although the relative contributions to this process of local and systemically produced PTHrP remain unclear.

BISPHOSPHONATES

The bisphosphonates are a family of compounds based on the structure of pyrophosphate, which have a high affinity for trabecular bone. They have a basic P-C-P structure which promotes their binding to mineralized bone matrix, and the remainder of the molecule determines potency, side effects etc. It appears that their main mechanism of action is the inhibition of osteoclast activity, and thus they can significantly reduce bone resorption by interrupting the vicious cycle of increased bone destruction discussed earlier.

However, not all bisphosphonates are the same, as can be seen from the molecular structures (Table 1). The main distinction lies in whether or not they contain nitrogen, as this relates to their mechanism of action. Nitrogen-containing amino-bisphosphonates such as pamidronate, ibandronate, and zoledronate are capable of interfering with mevalonate metabolism, acting as farnesyl transferase inhibitors, downstream of the Ras protein (9). There is good evidence that their efficacy as farnesyl transferase inhibitors directly correlates with their potency in inhibiting osteoclasts (10). In contrast, the non-aminobisphosphonate clodronate induces cell death after it has been metabolised to a non-hydrolysable ATP analogue, adenosine 5-triphsophate.

There is increasing experimental evidence that these agents have direct effects on tumour cells as well as osteoclasts. They appear to be able to induce tumour-cell apoptosis on their own (9,11), but possibly more importantly, in synergy with both cytotoxics and tamoxifen (12,13). Whether these experimental observations are relevant to their clinical benefits remains unclear.

Clinical Experience of Using Bisphosphonates in Advanced Disease

Bisphosphonates have been effectively used for many years to treat hypercalcaemia of malignancy. Early studies with the intravenous compound pamidronate showed an efficacy of around 90% (14), and thus in the United Kingdom as well as the United States, this drug became the most widely used agent (15), although other drugs, such as intravenous clodronate are also active. Therefore, it was in this setting that the first studies with the new, more potent aminobisphosphonates like ibandronate and zoledronate were conducted (16). For example, 4 mg of zoledronate has been shown in a

TABLE 1 Bisphosphonates Used in Breast Cancer

	Dose hypercalcaemia	Maintenance	Nitrogen-containing?	Structure
Clodronate	600mg i.v.	1600 mg p.o./day	No	
Pamidronate	90 mg i.v.	90 mg i.v. q 28 days	Yes	
Ibandronate		6 mg i.v. q 28 days or 50 mg daily p.o.	Yes	
Zoledronate	4–8 mg i.v.	4 mg i.v. q 28 days	Yes	

randomised trial to restore calcium levels faster and more effectively than the previous standard of 90 mg pamidronate (17).

Once the pathophysiology of bone metastases was understood, their potent anti-osteoclast activity made the preventive approach in patients with bone metastases a logical development. Early studies suggested efficacy (18), but the most convincing data came from two large randomised trials of the intravenous bisphosphonate pamidronate given in conjunction with systemic therapy for patients with osteolytic bone metastases. Table 2 gives a summary of the benefits, and it is clear from the more recent updates that this effect lasts at least for the 2 years of therapy (19–22). Similar studies were conducted with the more potent compound ibandronate, including both oral and intravenous formulations (23,24). It is clear that this agent is also active, as compared with placebo. In contrast, studies have also been reported with the oral bisphosphonates like clodronate (18), etidronate, and pamidronate (25). Although benefits were clearly seen, in general it is clear from the data that less activity has been observed (26). Whether this is due to variable oral bioavailability, or a difference in activity is not clear, but based on indirect comparisons, the oral agent with the most convincing efficacy data is ibandronate at a dose of 50 mg daily (27).

Only one bisphosphonate has to date shown superiority over another in a head to head comparison, and that is 4-mg zoledronate given over 15 minutes as

TABLE 2 Benefits from Bisphosphonates in Advanced Breast Cancer
(in Combination with Systemic Therapy)

	Pamidronate in Combination with		Zoledronate vs. Pamidronate
	Chemotherapy[a]	Hormonal Therapy[a]	
Bone pain	Significant reduction	Significant reduction	No data
Radiation to bone	45% reduction	30% reduction	No significant differences were seen in these individual endpoints, but a multiple event analysis showed a significant 20% further improvement for zoledronate over pamidronate
Hypercalcaemia	55% reduction	60% reduction	
Cord compression	N/A	(50% reduction n.s.)	
Surgery to bone	65% reduction	(35% reduction n.s.)	
	50 mg/day Oral Ibandronate vs. Placebo		6 mg i.v. Ibandronate vs. Placebo
Bone pain	Significant reduction		Significant reduction
Radiation to bone	26% reduction		17% reduction
Vertebral fractures	8% reduction		13% reduction
Surgery to bone	11% reduction		8% reduction
Overall event rate	38% reduction		40% reduction

[a]End-point definitions are different for the Ibandronate studies as compared with the Pamidronate studies so cross-agent comparisons from these data are NOT meaningful.

compared with pamidronate 90 mg given over 90–120 minutes. This large phase III trial included patients with both multiple myeloma and breast cancer, and demonstrated a 20% *further* reduction in skeletal morbidity, based on a multiple event analysis (28). However, a retrospective subgroup analysis suggests that the benefit is confined largely to patients with breast cancer, by virtue of their higher baseline rates of bone resorption.

In addition to their ability to prevent skeletal complications, there are good data on their efficacy in reducing bone pain in patients with skeletal metastases, and therefore one area of debate lies in whether all patients with bone metastases should receive these drugs in a prophylactic manner, or just those with symptoms. A detailed cost–benefit analysis for the United Kingdom has not been published—that from the United States is not relevant because the base cost of pamidronate is much higher. Treatment was given for 24 months in the two pivotal pamidronate studies, and the data suggest that the benefit, if anything, increased with the longer duration of therapy. The data suggest that they are associated with excellent long-term tolerability (22,29). Furthermore, there are good data to prove that the risk of skeletal events, and even death, is directly proportional to the level of bone resorption (30,31). A recent analysis of patients not treated with bisphosphonates suggests that only skull metastases do not give rise to significant levels of morbidity (32). Therefore, the U. K. practice is to give bisphosphonates increasingly to all breast cancer patients with bone metastases, and to continue them until patients are either too unwell to receive them, or too close to the end to benefit.

Similarly, there is the dilemma as to whether patients should receive bisphosphonates intravenously at the hospital, or as an oral preparation in the community. Some clinicians compromise by giving them intravenously while they are on chemotherapy (since the patients are already attending the hospital regularly), and then switch to oral therapy once there is no need for 3- or 4-weekly visits to the hospital. However, it must be borne in mind that at present the one drug, zoledronate, which has been shown to be superior to any other bisphosphonate is available only as an intravenous drug. Direct comparisons with oral ibandronate have been conducted in terms of bone marker effects, but not yet in terms of skeletal events.

UNANSWERED QUESTIONS

While it is very clear from the data that bisphosphonates reduce the skeletal morbidity for patients with bone metastases, important questions such as these remain unanswered:

- Do all patients need to be treated?

The clinical trials only included patients with lytic disease; yet the pathophysiology suggests that any bone metastasis is associated with increased bone resorption, which can be reversed by administration of bisphosphonates. Defining a group of patients with bone metastases who do not benefit from their use is not therefore possible at the present time, other than perhaps isolated skull lesions (vide supra).

- Which is the best drug?

Current data suggest that zoledronate is the most effective drug, being the only one to be shown to be superior to another agent. However, important randomised trials comparing it with the other third-generation amino-bisphosphonate, ibandronate, are yet to complete and/or report. Therefore, it is not possible to precisely define the group which can be equally well treated with a less potent agent. Recent data suggest that the actual level of bone resorption may be important, such that those with persisting high levels of resorption, despite the use of a bisphosphonate, do worse (30).

- Which is the best schedule?

Also, the optimal schedule has not been defined. For patients with persisting osteolysis, despite standard dosing, we do not know whether a more intense schedule might help. Similarly, for those whose bone resorption is well controlled, less frequent administration might well be as effective. This is the approach that was tested in the BISMARK trial (cost effectiveness of BISphosphonates in metastatic bone disease, a comparison of bone MARKer-directed zoledronic acid therapy with a standard schedule). However, despite the importance of this question, it did not recruit the planned number of patients, so it may not have the power to answer the question.

Finally, newer agents that inhibit bone resorption are being developed, of which the most important is denosumab, a fully human monoclonal antibody against RANKL. It has already been approved for use in treating osteoporosis, and the results of a pivotal phase III trial against zoledronate have reported its superior efficacy (33). Thus, although bisphosphonates remain a key component of the treatment of bone metastases, alongside systemic anti-cancer treatment, it is highly likely that denosumab will replace at least some of the use of bisphosphonates in the near future.

TOXICITY

Bisphosphonates are in general well tolerated. There are toxicities common to all those used in clinical practice, but there is considerable variation between them. All are capable of causing GI side effects, although they appear to be worse with the oral route of administration, especially with oral clodronate (18). An acute phase response, consisting of chills or flu-like symptoms, is seen in a proportion of patients treated with intravenous bisphosphonates, although tachyphylaxis does occur with repeated administrations (34).

Two important toxicities deserve a more detailed discussion, as there are suggestions that there may be key differences between agents.

Renal Dysfunction

There is evidence, particularly with the intravenous drugs pamidronate and zoledronate, that chronic administration can cause deterioration in renal function (35). This can in rare cases give rise to acute renal failure, leading in some cases to death. An important paper related this to the use of zoledronate in the United States, particularly in patients with multiple myeloma (36). However, it has to be acknowledged that the actual manner in which the drug was given, including the degree of monitoring of renal function, is not clear.. It must be recognised that the rate of infusion may be important in determining renal toxicity, such that giving a drug more slowly may reduce renal toxicity. The early data with zoledronate point to this, in that during the trial which compared zoledronate with pamidronate in breast cancer and multiple myeloma, two substantial protocol modifications had to be made, due to an initial higher rate of renal toxicity with zoledronate. First the higher dose, 8 mg given over 5 minutes, was discontinued, and then the 4-mg dose was given over 15 rather than 5 minutes (28). As a result of these changes, in the final analysis, the renal toxicity with zoledronate 4 mg was not significantly worse than with the comparator of pamidronate given over 2 hours. Pre-clinical data are consistent with this (37,38). Therefore apparent differences in renal toxicity when using ibandronate 6 mg given over 1 hour could be due not to fundamental differences in pharmacology, but just the rate of infusion.

In practice, if there is any suggestion of deterioration in renal function with an intravenous bisphosphonate, the first thing is to reduce the rate of infusion. Recent guidance data from the manufacturer of zoledronate have suggested that lower doses (to be given over the same time) be given to patients with lower initial creatinine clearance, though they have not been confirmed in a phase III trial to be either safer or as efficacious. Nonetheless, caution and a regular monitoring of renal function is needed along with bisphosphonates and zoledronate in particular.

Osteonecrosis of the Jaw

This is another rare side effect which was not initially recognised. It appears to be a class effect, but has been most commonly reported with zoledronate. This is a painful condition, and in the past may have been under-reported, being mistaken as mandibular bone metastases. The incidence appears higher in patients with dental problems, recent dental history, and those with cancer, receiving chemotherapy, radiotherapy, and/or steroids.

Optimal management or prevention strategies have not been defined, but clinicians need to be aware of this, particularly in patients who develop jaw pain. It is good practice therefore to require patients to be reviewed by a dentist before starting bisphosphonates, and in the event of suspected osteonecrosis of the jaws (ONJ), to be reviewed by a maxillofacial surgeon, or a dentist with experience in the diagnosis and management of ONJ (39,40).

CONCLUSIONS

For patients with advanced breast cancer, regular bisphosphonate therapy, whether administered orally or intravenously, is well tolerated and has been shown to reduce skeletal morbidity, including bone pain and hypercalcaemia and the need for other therapeutic interventions. Although one cannot mandate which patient should get a particular drug or schedule, the extensive phase III data clearly show their efficacy, and therefore the use of a bisphosphonate should be considered for any patient with breast cancer that has metastasised to bones.

REFERENCES

1. Andre F, Slimane K, Bachelot T, et al. Breast cancer with synchronous metastases: trends in survival during a 14 year period. J Clin Oncol 2004; 22: 3302–8.
2. Kong YY, et al. OPGL is a key regulator of osteoclastogenesis, lymphocyte development and lymph-node organogenesis. Nature 1999; 397: 315–23.
3. Khosla S. Minireview: the OPG/RANKL/RANK system. Endocrinology 2001; 142: 5050–5.
4. Teitelbaum SL. Bone resorption by osteoclasts. Science 2000; 289: 1504–8.
5. Kakonen SM, Mundy GR. Mechanisms of osteolytic bone metastases in breast carcinoma [review]. Cancer 2003; 97: 834–9.
6. Orr FW, Lee J, Duivenvoorden WCM, Singh G. Pathophysiologic interactions in skeletal metastases. Cancer 2000; 88: 2912–18.
7. Guise TA. Molecular mechanisms of osteolytic bone metastases. Cancer 2000; 88: 2892–8.
8. Coleman RE. Metastatic bone disease: clinical features, pathophysiology and treatment strategies [review]. Cancer Treat Rev 2001; 27: 165–76.
9. Green JR, Clezardin P. Mechanisms of bisphosphonate effects on osteoclasts, tumor cell growth, and metastasis [review]. Am J Clin Oncol 2002; 25: S3–9.
10. Dunford JE, et al. Structure-activity relationships for inhibition of farnesyl diphosphate synthase in vitro and inhibition of bone resorption in vivo by nitrogen-containing bisphosphonates. J Pharmacol Exp Ther 2001; 296: 235–42.
11. Fromigue O, Lagneaux L, Body JJ. Bisphosphonates induce breast cancer cell death in vitro. J Bone Miner Res 2000; 15: 2211–21.
12. Jagdev SP, et al The bisphosphonate, zoledronic acid, induces apoptosis of breast cancer cells: evidence for synergy with paclitaxel. Br J Cancer 2001; 84: 1126–34.
13. Neville-Webbe HL, et al. Sequence- and schedule-dependent enhancement of zoledronic acid induced apoptosis by doxorubicin in breast and prostate cancer cells. Int J Cancer 2005; 113: 364–71.
14. Possinger K. From laundry product to cancer drug--history of a drug class [German]. Medizinische Klinik 2000; 95(Suppl 2): 3–7.
15. Lorusso P. Analysis of skeletal-related events in breast cancer and response to therapy [review]. Semin Oncol 2001; 28: 22–7.
16. Body JJ, et al. A dose-finding study of zoledronate in hypercalcemic cancer patients. J Bone Miner Res 1999; 14: 1557–61.
17. Major PP, et al. Zoledronic acid is suerpior to pamidronate in the treatment of hypercalcaemia of malignancy: a pooled analysis of two randomized, controlled clinical trials. J Clin Oncol 2001; 19: 558–67.
18. Paterson AH, et al. Double-blind controlled trial of oral clodronate in patients with bone metastases from breast cancer. J Clin Oncol 1993; 11: 59–65.
19. Hortobagyi GN, et al. Efficacy of pamidronate in reducing skeletal complications in patients with breast cancer and lytic bone metastases. Protocol 19 Aredia Breast Cancer Study Group [see comments]. N Engl J Med 1996; 335: 1785–91.
20. Theriault RL, et al. Pamidronate reduces skeletal morbidity in women with advanced breast cancer and lytic bone lesions: a randomized, placebo-controlled trial. Protocol 18 Aredia Breast Cancer Study Group. J Clin Oncol 1999; 17: 846–54.
21. Lipton A, et al. Pamidronate prevents skeletal complications and is effective palliative treatment in women with breast carcinoma and osteolytic bone metastases: long term follow-up of two randomized, placebo-controlled trials. Cancer 2000; 88: 1082–90.
22. Ali SM, et al. Safety and efficacy of bisphosphonates beyond 24 months in cancer patients. J Clin Oncol 2001; 19: 3434–7.
23. Body JJ, et al. Intravenous ibandronate reduces the incidence of skeletal complications in patients with breast cancer and bone metastases [see comment]. Ann Oncol 2003; 14: 1399–405.
24. Body JJ, et al. Oral ibandronate reduces the risk of skeletal complications in breast cancer patients with metastatic bone disease: results from two randomised, placebo-controlled phase III studies. Br J Cancer 2004; 90: 1133–7.

25. Vinholes J, et al. Assessment of bone response to systemic therapy in an EORTC trial: preliminary experience with the use of collagen cross-link excretion. European Organization for Research and Treatment of Cancer. Br J Cancer 1999; 80: 221–8.

26. Major PP, et al. Oral bisphosphonates: A review of clinical use in patients with bone metastases [review]. Cancer 2000; 88: 6–14.

27. Tripathy D, et al. Oral ibandronate for the treatment of metastatic bone disease in breast cancer: efficacy and safety results from a randomized, double-blind, placebo-controlled trial [see comment]. Ann Oncol 2004; 15: 743–50.

28. Rosen LS, et al. Long-term efficacy and safety of zoledronic acid compared with pamidronate disodium in the treatment of skeletal complications in patients with advanced multiple myeloma or breast carcinoma: a randomized, double-blind, multicenter, comparative trial. Cancer 2003; 98: 1735–44.

29. Maclachlan SA, et al. Safety of oral ibandronic acid (ibandronate) in bone metastases from breast cancer: long-term follow-up experience. European Breast Cancer Conference IV 2004 (abstract).

30. Brown JE, et al. Bone resorption predicts for skeletal complications in metastatic bone disease. Br J Cancer 2003; 89: 2031–7.

31. Brown JE, et al. Bone turnover markers as predictors of skeletal complications in prostate cancer, lung cancer, and other solid tumors. J Natl Cancer Inst 2005; 97: 59–69.

32. Major PP, et al. Natural history of malignant bone disease in breast cancer and the use of cumulative mean functions to measure skeletal morbidity. BMC Cancer 2009; 9: 272.

33. Stopeck AT, et al. Denosumab compared with zoledronic acid for the treatment of bone metastases in patients with advanced breast cancer: a randomized, double-blind study. J Clin Oncol 2011 (on-line ahead of print publication).

34. Coleman RE, Seaman JJ. The role of zoledronic acid in cancer: clinical studies in the treatment and prevention of bone metastases [review]. Semin Oncol 2001; 28: 11–16.

35. Smetana S, et al. Pamidronate-induced nephrotoxic tubular necrosis - a case report. Clin Nephrol 2004; 61: 63–7.

36. Chang JT, Green L, Beitz J. Renal failure with the use of zoledronic acid. N Engl J Med 2003; 349: 1676–9.

37. Pecherstorfer M, Diel IJ. Rapid administration of ibandronate does not affect renal functioning: evidence from clinical studies in metastatic bone disease and hypercalcaemia of malignancy [review]. Support Care Cancer 2004; 12: 877–81.

38. Pfister T, Atzpodien E, Bauss F. The renal effects of minimally nephrotoxic doses of ibandronate and zoledronate following single and intermittent intravenous administration in rats [see comment]. Toxicology 2003; 191: 159–67.

39. Khan AA, et al Canadian consensus practice guidelines for bisphosphonate associated osteonecrosis of the jaw. J Rheumatol 2008; 35: 1391–7.

40. Khan AA, et al. Bisphosphonate associated osteonecrosis of the jaw. J Rheumatol 2009; 36: 478–90.

8

Targeting angiogenesis in metastatic breast cancer

David Miles

ANGIOGENESIS

In 2000, Hanahan and Weinberg described six hallmarks of cancer-biochemical and molecular traits that enable cells to become tumourigenic and eventually malignant (1,2). One of these hallmarks is the induction of angiogenesis, the formation of new blood vessels. Angiogenesis is a complex process that is essential for the growth and progression of tumours (Fig. 1) (3). It is involved at all stages, from the initial cancer formation through to the growth of distant metastases (4). The concept of targeting blood vessel formation to prevent tumour growth and metastasis was first proposed by Judah Folkman in the 1970s (5). Theoretically, it was thought that inhibiting angiogenesis could become a universal approach to the treatment of all types of cancer. Targeting a non-mutating host response offered the potential to replace other modalities, such as chemotherapy. This hypothesis led to extensive research to identify pathways for the induction of angiogenesis and methods of inhibiting this process to treat cancer. As our understanding of angiogenesis has improved, three key mechanisms of action of anti-angiogenic treatment approaches have emerged. It has been proposed that anti-angiogenic therapy may lead to:

• Regression of existing tumour vasculature
• Normalisation of surviving vasculature
• Inhibition of vessel regrowth and neovascularisation.

Evidence for these mechanisms of action is derived primarily from preclinical models exploring a range of different anti-angiogenic agents.

Preclinical studies of the anti-vascular endothelial growth factor (VEGF) antibody in mouse xenograft models indicated that vascular permeability was reduced after antibody administration (6). Furthermore, vessel diameter was reduced, the vessels became less tortuous, and after four administrations, vessels disappeared from the tumour surface in one of the models. In addition, administration of a small molecule inhibitor of VEGF receptor 1 (VEGFR-1) and VEGFR-2 in a rat corneal model of angiogenesis resulted in a significant reduction in the number and length of vascular sprouts (7).

The second mechanism is normalisation of surviving vasculature (8–11). Preclinical observations are supported by data derived from patients with rectal cancer treated with a single dose of a monoclonal antibody against VEGF, bevacizumab. Tumour vascular density and interstitial fluid pressure were significantly reduced following administration of bevacizumab, supporting the hypothesis that anti-angiogenic therapy leads to vascular normalisation (9). In addition, treatment with an anti-VEGF antibody significantly increased delivery of chemotherapy in a preclinical study (12).

Finally, anti-angiogenic therapy is thought to inhibit vessel regrowth and neovascularisation. Administration of a receptor tyrosine kinase inhibitor (TKI) in a "vascular window" mouse model prevented the migration of endothelial cells and blood vessel formation (13).

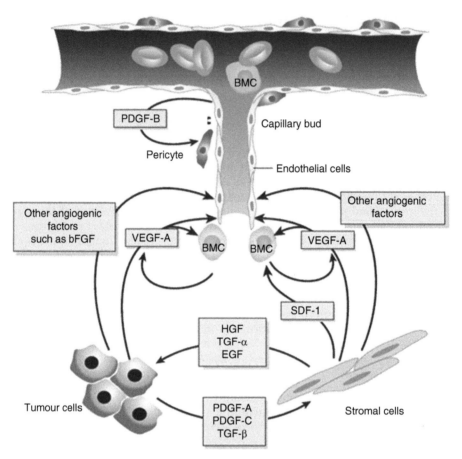

FIGURE 1   Angiogenesis is a complex process. *Abbreviations*: bFGF, basic fibroblast growth factor; BMC, blood mononuclear cell; EGF, epidermal growth factor; HGF, hepatocyte growth factor; PDGF, platelet-derived growth factor; SDF, stromal-derived factor; TGF, transforming growth factor; VEGF-A, vascular endothelial growth factor A. *Source*: Adapted from Ref. 3.

Endostatin/Angiostatin

Several endogenous anti-angiogenic factors are produced by tumour and host cells, including nitric oxide, thrombospondin, angiostatin, and endostatin. Among the first and most potent to be explored as a treatment for cancer were angiostatin and endostatin (14–16). Angiostatin, a plasminogen fragment, is produced in association with primary Lewis lung tumour growth and disappears after the resection of the primary tumour, leading to neovascularisation and growth of micrometastases (14,16). Angiostatin demonstrated high dose-dependent activity in preclinical models (17). Endostatin, a collagen VIII fragment, demonstrated anti-angiogenic activity in preclinical renal cell cancer models (18) and has shown activity in combination with chemotherapy in several solid tumour types (19–21).

Vascular Disrupting Agents

Another early strategy to target angiogenesis was vascular disruption, using agents that target the rapidly proliferating endothelial cells of established tumour vasculature (22). The principal mechanism of action of vascular disrupting agents (VDAs) is to trigger vascular collapse and the development of acute tumour necrosis (23). The selectivity of these agents results from differences between tumour and normal

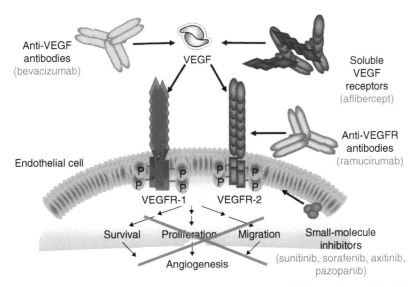

FIGURE 2   Approaches to targeting angiogenesis. *Abbreviations*: VEGF, vascular endothelial growth factor; VEGFR, vascular endothelial growth factor receptor. *Source*: Adapted from Ref. 40.

endothelium, although the side-effect profiles suggest that normal vascular endothelium is also disrupted. VDAs include three major classes of drug: flavonoids, tubulin-binding agents, and N-cadherin antagonists (22). The flavonoid in the most advanced stage of clinical development is 5,6-dimethylxanthenone-4-acetic acid (DMXAA). Randomised phase II trials have demonstrated improvement in some efficacy endpoints when DMXAA is combined with chemotherapy for the treatment of prostate and non-small-cell lung cancers (24,25). Combretastatin A4 phosphate (CA4P), a tubulin-binding agent, has been evaluated in a series of phase I studies in patients with advanced solid tumours (26–29). A CA4P derivative, ombrabulin, demonstrated encouraging activity in a phase I study including 18 patients with breast cancer (30). Development of several other tubulin-binding agents, including ABT-751, MN-029, and ZD6126 has not progressed beyond phase I/II studies. No data are available from trials investigating VDAs specifically in breast cancer.

VASCULAR ENDOTHELIAL GROWTH FACTOR
VEGF, originally termed vascular permeability factor, is one of the key drivers of angiogenesis, and was identified in the 1980s (31,32). VEGF is a heparin-binding growth factor that binds to capillary endothelial cell receptors, generating a downstream signal cascade and promoting angiogenesis (33). VEGF is upregulated in many types of solid tumour, including breast cancer (34,35). Overexpression of VEGF leads to formation of abnormal, leaky blood vessels (36,37). High VEGF levels are associated with poor prognosis and shorter overall survival (38,39). Following identification of this critical player in angiogenesis, the search began for new strategies to target angiogenesis in the treatment of cancer (32). Several approaches have been explored, including antibodies to VEGF and VEGFRs, soluble VEGFRs, small molecules that inhibit tyrosine kinases and anti-sense oligonucleotides targeting VEGF (Fig. 2; Table 1) (40,41).

BEVACIZUMAB
Bevacizumab is a humanised monoclonal antibody that targets the VEGF-A ligand. In preclinical studies, bevacizumab inhibited the growth of human tumour cell lines in nude mice (42). The clinical evaluation of bevacizumab in metastatic breast cancer

TABLE 1 Strategies for Targeting Angiogenesis

Strategy	Agent	Target	Developmental stage in breast cancer
Anti-VEGF antibodies	Bevacizumab	VEGF	Regulatory approval as first-line therapy with paclitaxel or capecitabine (EU and other countries, excluding US)
Soluble VEGF receptors	Aflibercept	VEGF	Development abandoned
Anti-VEGFR antibodies	Ramucirumab (IMC-1121b)	VEGFR-2	Phase III evaluation ongoing
Small-molecule inhibitors	Sorafenib	VEGFR-1, -2, and -3; PDGFR-β, Flt3, c-Kit, Raf	Phase III evaluation ongoing
	Sunitinib	VEGFR-2, PDGFR-β, Flt3, c-Kit	Development abandoned
	Axitinib	VEGFR-1, -2, and -3; PDGFR, c-Kit	Development abandoned
	Pazopanib	VEGFR-1, -2, and -3; PDGFR-α/β, c-Kit	–
	Vatalanib	VEGFR-1, -2, and -3; PDGFR, c-Kit, c-Fos	–
	Cediranib	VEGFR-1, -2, and -3; PDGFR, c-Kit	–
	Vandetanib	VEGFR-2, EGFR, Ret	–
	Motesanib (AMG 706)	VEGFR-1, -2, and -3; PDGFR-β, c-Kit	Phase II evaluation ongoing

Abbreviations: EGFR, epidermal growth factor receptor; PDGFR, platelet-derived growth factor receptor; VEGFR, vascular endothelial growth factor receptor. *Source*: Adapted from Ref. 41.

(mBC) began with a phase I/II dose-finding study of single-agent bevacizumab in 75 patients previously treated with at least one chemotherapy regimen for mBC (43). The principal side effects of bevacizumab were headache, hypertension, and proteinuria, none of which is typical of chemotherapy agents used in mBC. The activity of bevacizumab in this study, particularly in the cohort receiving 10 mg/kg every 2 weeks, was sufficient to warrant further investigation. Therefore, phase III evaluation of bevacizumab in combination with chemotherapy agents was initiated using a dose of 10 mg/kg every 2 weeks or 15 mg/kg every 3 weeks, depending on the schedule of the chemotherapy regimen.

Phase III clinical trials of bevacizumab began simultaneously in colorectal and breast cancers in 2002. In the AVF2107g trial in patients with previously untreated advanced colorectal cancer, bevacizumab significantly improved overall survival when combined with irinotecan and 5-fluorouracil compared with the same chemotherapy alone (44). Subsequent trials in the first- and second-line settings confirmed the efficacy of combining bevacizumab with chemotherapy (45,46).

In mBC, two randomised phase III trials (AVF2119g and E2100) were initiated, differing in both the treatment setting and the chemotherapy regimen given in combination with bevacizumab. In the first, the placebo-controlled AVF2119g trial, patients with mBC who had previously received both an anthracycline and a taxane were treated with capecitabine alone or in combination with bevacizumab (47).

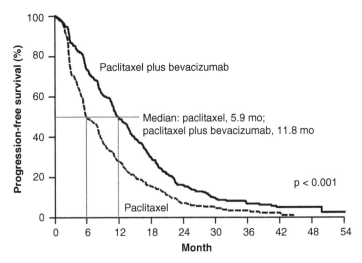

FIGURE 3 Progression-free survival in E2100 (first-line weekly paclitaxel with or without bevacizumab). *Source*: From Ref. 49.

Although bevacizumab demonstrated a biological effect in the study, significantly improving the overall response rate in combination with capecitabine compared with capecitabine alone, there was no significant difference in progression-free survival (PFS). In contrast to the lack of PFS improvement with bevacizumab in the AVF2119g trial in heavily pre-treated refractory/resistant mBC, a subsequent trial in pre-treated disease (RIBBON-2) demonstrated significantly improved PFS in patients receiving bevacizumab in combination with second-line chemotherapy compared with those treated with chemotherapy alone (48). The different outcomes between the RIBBON-2 trial and AVF2119g may be attributable at least in part to differences between the patient populations in the two trials.

While the AVF2119g was being conducted in heavily pre-treated patients, an open-label trial, E2100, led by the Eastern Cooperative Oncology Group, evaluated bevacizumab in combination with weekly paclitaxel as first-line therapy for mBC. This trial showed a substantial effect on PFS and objective response rate (Fig. 3) (49). This led to US and European regulatory approval of bevacizumab in combination with weekly paclitaxel for the treatment of patients with previously untreated mBC.

The contrasting findings of the AVF2119g and E2100 trials led investigators to suggest that targeting VEGF is most effective earlier in the course of disease, when fewer anti-angiogenic pathways are activated. Therefore, subsequent phase III trials [AVADO (50) and RIBBON-1 (51)] were conducted in patients with previously untreated mBC. The primary endpoint of all three trials in the first-line setting was PFS. Both AVADO and RIBBON-1 were double-blind, placebo-controlled randomised trials. AVADO evaluated docetaxel in combination with either placebo or bevacizumab. Two dose levels of bevacizumab were investigated (7.5 mg/kg and 15 mg/kg, both administered every 3 weeks). AVADO was designed to compare each bevacizumab arm with placebo but was not powered to detect a difference in efficacy between the two bevacizumab doses. The RIBBON-1 trial had an "investigator's choice" design: before randomisation to bevacizumab or placebo, the physician selected the preferred chemotherapy for each patient (either capecitabine monotherapy, or anthracycline-based combination or taxane therapy). The two

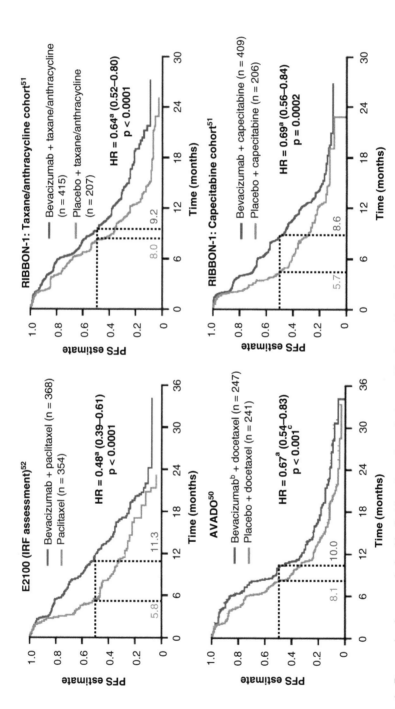

FIGURE 4 Progression-free survival with first-line bevacizumab in combination with chemotherapy regimens: E2100, AVADO, and RIBBON-1 trials. *Abbreviations*: HR, hazard ratio; IRF, independent review facility; PFS, progression-free survival. *Source*: Adapted from Refs. 50,51,54. [a]Censored for non-protocol therapy before disease progression. [b]15 mg/kg q3w. [c]Exploratory p-value.

cohorts (capecitabine or anthracycline/taxane) were independently powered to detect a PFS benefit and therefore RIBBON-1 was essentially two parallel trials.

As shown in Figure 4, bevacizumab significantly improved the PFS in both trials, including both cohorts of the RIBBON-1 trial. The hazard ratios were consistent between the trials, although differences in median PFS were less marked in the AVADO and RIBBON-1 trials than in the E2100 trial. Both trials demonstrated a significant improvement in the overall response rate with bevacizumab (50,51). Neither of the trials showed a difference in overall survival between the treatment arms, although they were neither designed nor powered to detect survival differences. The 1-year overall survival rate, a pre-specified endpoint, was significantly superior in the bevacizumab 15 mg/kg arm versus the chemotherapy-alone arm in AVADO (50).

The most notable side effects of bevacizumab therapy in these trials were hypertension, proteinuria, and epistaxis (49–51). Generally these side effects can be managed effectively with standard medical intervention or temporary suspension of bevacizumab therapy. The incidences of these adverse events were quite consistent across the randomised clinical trials and a safety study (ATHENA) in more than 2000 patients with MBC treated with first-line bevacizumab in combination with chemotherapy in routine oncology practice (53). Subgroup analyses of safety in patients aged ≥70 years treated in the ATHENA study indicated good tolerability, even in these older patients typically at increased risk of side effects (54). Importantly, wound-healing complications, bleeding, and bowel perforation do not seem to be significant issues in these populations of patients with mBC.

TYROSINE KINASE INHIBITORS

An alternative approach to anti-angiogenic therapy is tyrosine kinase inhibition. This has a broader effect, targeting numerous pathways. Several TKI have been evaluated in mBC. While some of these agents have demonstrated benefit in other solid tumour types, results in mBC have been generally disappointing, with toxicity outweighing any benefit in most cases (Table 2) (55–65).

Sunitinib

Clinical evaluation of sunitinib in mBC included a programme of four randomised phase III trials exploring the effect of sunitinib in settings very similar to the phase III evaluation of bevacizumab. Unlike bevacizumab, none of the trials demonstrated an improvement in PFS (the primary endpoint) with sunitinib, as summarised in Table 2 (55–58).

Sunitinib was also explored as maintenance therapy in a randomised trial in patients who had responded to previous taxane-based therapy (66). The proportion of patients with PFS ≥5 months was no higher in the sunitinib arm than in the placebo arm. Furthermore, there was substantial toxicity in the sunitinib arm.

As a result of these trial findings, sunitinib is no longer being developed as a treatment for mBC.

Sorafenib

Sorafenib, an oral multikinase inhibitor, targets VEGFR-1, VEGFR-2, VEGFR-3, platelet-derived growth factor receptor (PDGFR)-β, Raf, c-Kit, and Flt-3. Sorafenib has shown some promise in mBC in randomised phase II trials, although no data from phase III trials are available to date. A randomised phase II trial showed a significant improvement in PFS when sorafenib was combined with capecitabine as first- or second-line therapy (60). A second randomised phase II trial failed to show a statistically significant difference in PFS (59), although time to progression, which excludes non-disease-related deaths, was significantly improved and the investigators speculated

TABLE 2 Summary of Randomised Phase II and III Trials Evaluating Anti-Angiogenic Therapy in Breast Cancer. All are Phase III Trials Unless Otherwise Indicated

Chemotherapy regimen	Setting	Bevacizumab	Sunitinib	Sorafenib	Motesanib	Axitinib	Vandetanib	AMG 386
Paclitaxel	Untreated MBC	E2100: paclitaxel ± bevacizumab HR = 0.48 (52)	SUN1094: paclitaxel + sunitinib vs. paclitaxel + bevacizumab HR = 1.63 (55)	NU07B1 phase II: paclitaxel ± sorafenib HR = 0.79 (59)	TORI phase II: paclitaxel ± motesanib vs. paclitaxel + bevacizumab HR = 0.95 (62)			Paclitaxel + bevacizumab vs. paclitaxel + AMG 386 vs. paclitaxel + bevacizumab + AMG 386 HR = 0.98, 1.12, 1.28 (65)
Docetaxel		AVADO: docetaxel ± bevacizumab HR = 0.67 (50)	SUN1064: docetaxel ± sunitinib HR = 0.92 (56)			Phase II: HR (TTP) = 0.81 (63)[a]		
Capecitabine		RIBBON-1: capecitabine ± bevacizumab cohort HR = 0.69 (51)						
Various		RIBBON-1: anthracycline/taxane ± bevacizumab cohort HR = 0.64 (51)						
Capecitabine	Untreated and pre-treated (mixed)			SOLTI phase II: capecitabine ± sorafenib HR = 0.58 (60)				

Docetaxel

Docetaxel ±
vandetanib,
phase II
HR = 1.19 (64)

Various

Pre-treated
MBC

RIBBON-2:
chemotherapy ±
bevacizumab
HR = 0.78 (48)

Capecitabine

AVF2119g:
capecitabine ±
bevacizumab
HR = 0.98 (47)

SUN1099:
capecitabine ±
sunitinib
HR = 1.22 (57)

None

SUN1107:
capecitabine vs.
sunitinib
HR = 1.47 (58)

Bevacizumab-
pre-treated

AC01B07:
chemotherapy
(gemcitabine
or
capecitabine)
± sorafenib
HR 0.65 (61)

[a]Reported as 1.24 with investigational arm as reference.
Abbreviations: HR, hazard ratio for progression-free survival, primary endpoint, unless otherwise stated; MBC, metastatic breast cancer; TTP, time to progression.

that deaths due to meningitis and tuberculosis-related complications among patients treated in India might have contributed to the lack of PFS benefit. In a third randomised phase II trial (AC01B07), comparing sorafenib plus chemotherapy (gemcitabine or capecitabine) versus chemotherapy alone after progression on or after bevacizumab therapy, PFS was significantly improved in the sorafenib-containing arm (61). The fourth randomised phase II trial that completes the TIES (Trials to Investigate the Efficacy of Sorafenib in breast cancer) programme has not yet been reported. An ongoing phase III trial (RESILIENCE) is comparing sorafenib plus capecitabine versus placebo plus capecitabine in patients with taxane- and anthracycline-pre-treated mBC.

Motesanib

Motesanib is an antagonist of VEGFR-1, VEGFR-2, and VEGFR-3 and inhibits PDGFR and KIT. A randomised, placebo-controlled phase II trial evaluated motesanib in combination with paclitaxel in 282 patients with HER2-negative mBC (62). Patients randomised to the control arm received weekly paclitaxel and placebo, those randomised to the investigational arm received weekly paclitaxel and motesanib, and those randomised to a third arm received weekly paclitaxel and bevacizumab. The study aimed to recruit a similar population to the E2100 trial of bevacizumab plus weekly paclitaxel (49). The trial failed to demonstrate any significant difference between the treatment regimens in overall response rate (the primary endpoint) or PFS. In addition, the incidences of nausea, diarrhoea, hypertension, and hepatobiliary disorders were more frequent with motesanib treatment than with either placebo or bevacizumab in combination with paclitaxel. In summary, the results of the trial do not support further investigation of motesanib in mBC.

Axitinib

Another oral TKI, axitinib, which inhibits VEGFR-1, VEGR-2, and VEGFR-3 (67), was evaluated in combination with docetaxel in a placebo-controlled randomised phase II trial in 168 patients with previously untreated mBC (63). Although overall response rate was significantly higher in the axitinib–docetaxel arm than the placebo–docetaxel arm, there was no difference in time to disease progression, the primary endpoint. Axitinib resulted in significantly more grade 3/4 febrile neutropenia, fatigue, stomatitis, diarrhoea, and hypertension compared with chemotherapy alone, leading to frequent docetaxel and axitinib dose reductions. Axitinib development in breast cancer has been discontinued.

Other Tyrosine Kinase Inhibitors

Vandetanib showed no effect on efficacy in combination with docetaxel in a randomised phase II trial (64). Pazopanib has shown modest activity in a phase II study in mBC, which was prematurely terminated (68). Neither vatalanib nor cediranib has been evaluated in mBC.

Safety of Tyrosine Kinase Inhibitors

The most commonly observed grade 3/4 adverse events with TKIs are fatigue, asthenia, hand-foot syndrome, and gastrointestinal effects (56–61,63). These effects may be attributable to their less specific multi-targeted mechanism of action and can limit delivery of chemotherapy, leading to frequent dose reductions, treatment interruptions, and discontinuations.

Grade 3 hand-foot syndrome was reported in 45% of patients in the SOLTI randomised phase II trial of sorafenib in combination with capecitabine (60) and 39% of patients receiving sorafenib with either gemcitabine or capecitabine in the AC01B07 randomised phase II trial (61). Hand-syndrome is a characteristic side effect of capecitabine and thus a regimen combining these two agents presents challenges for the management of this side effect. The ongoing phase III trial includes guidelines for prophylactic and symptomatic treatment of hand-foot syndrome.

OTHER ANGIOGENIC TARGETS

Other key players in angiogenesis that may represent targets for anti-cancer therapy include basic fibroblast growth factors, transforming growth factor β1, PDGF, placental growth factor (PlGF), angiopoietin 1 and 2, and mTOR. Research into novel agents disrupting the activity of these angiogenic factors continues, as described below.

Angiopoietin Inhibitors

AMG 386 is a peptide-Fc fusion protein that inhibits angiogenesis by neutralising the interaction between the Tie2 receptor and angiopoietin-1 and -2. A randomised phase II trial evaluated paclitaxel plus AMG 386, with or without bevacizumab. There was no apparent prolongation of PFS with the addition of AMG 386 to paclitaxel and bevacizumab (65). Exposure-response analyses indicated that any future evaluation should use an AMG 386 dose >10 mg/kg.

mTOR Inhibitors

mTOR is a downstream protein kinase of the PI3k/Akt pathways. It is thought that aberrant activation of this pathway is important in breast cancer cell proliferation and resistance to treatment (41). mTOR activation also leads indirectly to increased VEGF. mTOR inhibitors currently under investigation as treatment for breast cancer are temsirolimus (CCI-779), everolimus (RAD001), and ridaforolimus (previously deforolimus). To date, activity in breast cancer has been modest. Everolimus combined with docetaxel was considered infeasible in a phase I trial because of unpredictable changes in docetaxel clearance coupled with no activity (69). Furthermore, a randomised phase III trial of temsirolimus plus letrozole versus letrozole alone for advanced breast cancer was prematurely terminated because of excessive toxicity and no improvement in response rate or PFS (70).

Placental Growth Factor Inhibitors

Another approach to targeting angiogenesis is inhibition of PlGF, which selectively binds to VEGF-1 and its co-receptors neuropilin-1 and -2. A neutralising murine anti-VEGF antibody, TB-403, has entered clinical development (41) but to date, no results are available.

ANTI-ANGIOGENIC EFFECTS OF CHEMOTHERAPY

While all of the agents described above have been developed specifically to target angiogenesis, another anti-angiogenic strategy has involved schedule modification of older, conventional chemotherapy agents. Anti-angiogenic activity has been observed with several chemotherapy agents, particularly when administered "metronomically". For example, anti-angiogenic properties are prominent when oral cyclophosphamide is administered at a low dose for extended periods compared with cyclic administration at the maximum tolerated dose (71). In the clinical setting, metronomic cyclophosphamide and oral methotrexate treatment for mBC resulted in a substantial decrease in the levels of circulating VEGF (72). Similarly, paclitaxel appears to have anti-angiogenic properties (73). This chemotherapy strategy may increase the anti-angiogenic activity of certain agents, while reducing both toxicity and the risk of drug-resistant tumour cells compared with conventional administration (74). The combination of metronomic cyclophosphamide and capecitabine with bevacizumab demonstrated high activity and prolonged disease control in a single-arm phase II study in mBC (75).

ROLE OF ANTI-ANGIOGENIC THERAPY IN CLINICAL PRACTICE

The translation of anti-angiogenic therapy from preclinical theory to clinical practice has had very varied success, ranging from widespread regulatory approval and recommendation in clinical guidelines to consistent failure in phase III trials and, ultimately, abandoned clinical development. This disparity may be attributable at least in part to the different targets and mechanisms of action of the various agents, which not surprisingly results in contrasting effects on both efficacy and safety. It appears that targeting a single angiogenic factor (e.g., bevacizumab targeting VEGF-A) is a more effective, better-tolerated strategy in breast cancer than targeting multiple pathways through tyrosine kinase inhibition (e.g., sunitinib).

While the precise targeting approach of bevacizumab has consistently demonstrated improved PFS in several randomised clinical trials (48–52), the overall effect appears to be relatively transient and to date, no anti-angiogenic therapy has significantly improved the median overall survival in mBC. While it is important to note that none of the trials was powered to demonstrate an overall survival benefit, the lack of effect on survival, together with a less dramatic effect on PFS in AVADO, ultimately led to regulatory authorities in many countries restricting the approval of bevacizumab to first-line combination with weekly paclitaxel (as evaluated in the E2100 trial) but not in combination with docetaxel (as evaluated in AVADO). Recognising the need for treatment options in patients in whom taxane therapy may not be preferred or appropriate, the European regulatory authorities have also approved first-line bevacizumab in combination with capecitabine (as evaluated in RIBBON-1). In the US, regulatory authorities recently decided to withdraw approval of bevacizumab for mBC, although few countries in the rest of the world adopted such a stance.

Several hypotheses have been proposed for the lack of overall survival benefit with anti-angiogenic therapy. Preclinical studies suggested that tumour regrowth may be accelerated after exposure to sunitinib and concern was expressed over a potential "rebound" effect. However, extrapolation of these findings from preclinical studies of a TKI into the clinical setting with agents that have a different mechanism of action is not straightforward, and findings from preclinical studies of bevacizumab contradicted these results (76). In addition, analyses of clinical trials evaluating outcomes after discontinuation of bevacizumab did not support this hypothesis (77).

Another potential explanation is the relatively long life expectancy of patients with breast cancer, which means that many patients receive several lines of therapy after their first line of treatment for mBC. This gradual improvement in outlook complicates the use of overall survival as an endpoint in trials evaluating first-line therapy for mBC. Although a patient may not be treated with a specific agent in a randomised trial in the first-line setting, they may subsequently receive this agent in later lines of therapy. For example, in the RIBBON-1 trial, more than half of patients initially randomised to placebo subsequently received bevacizumab as second-line or later therapy (51). As bevacizumab improves PFS in the second-line setting (48), this crossover to bevacizumab may be expected to confound overall survival analyses.

The implications of post-progression survival on determination of the clinical benefit of new treatments have been discussed intensely in recent years (78,79). The opportunity to use several lines of therapy together with the wide array of treatments available for mBC makes it increasingly unlikely that modification of disease at the time of diagnosis will influence the overall outcome for these patients. While clinical trials suggest that overall survival is increasing for patients with breast cancer, this effect appears to be attributable to small incremental improvements across all lines of therapy rather than a dramatic improvement in first-line therapy.

Although no significant improvement in overall survival has been observed when bevacizumab is combined with chemotherapy, improvements in 1-year overall survival rates have been demonstrated in both E2100 and AVADO (49,50). This suggests that bevacizumab may have an effect on survival at least in patients with a particularly short life expectancy. It might be expected, therefore, that if patients with an especially poor prognosis can be identified, it may be possible to select those subsets of patients deriving a substantially greater benefit from bevacizumab. Exploratory analyses of data from the three first-line trials of bevacizumab (E2100, AVADO, and RIBBON-1) have been performed and demonstrated an overall survival benefit in the subgroup of patients with taxane-pre-treated mBC who received bevacizumab in combination with a taxane (80). A trend towards an overall survival benefit was also seen in patients with negative oestrogen receptor, progesterone receptor, and HER2 status ("triple negative") disease both in a meta-analysis of the three first-line trials (81) and in a subgroup analysis of the RIBBON-2 trial in the second-line setting (82). However, such observations require prospective validation, particularly as positive findings among multiple exploratory analyses may be observed by chance.

Traditional efficacy endpoints, such as PFS and overall survival, are not the only considerations for determining the benefit of a treatment in breast cancer. Quality of life and tolerability have an obvious impact on patients, yet quality of life in particular is notoriously difficult to quantify. The majority of patients with advanced breast cancer will be treated with chemotherapy, associated with numerous side effects affecting a patient's quality of life. Hair loss, neuropathy, fatigue, nausea, vomiting, and diarrhoea are all well-known and distressing side effects that typically reduce the quality of life of patients. When biological agents are combined with chemotherapy, the overriding impact of chemotherapy side effects on quality of life still remains. Therefore, even if symptom improvement associated with biological therapy lessens the detrimental effect of chemotherapy, the overall effect is still a deterioration in quality of life. Available instruments for measuring quality of life typically involve questionnaires that ask patients about their symptoms. These questionnaires usually focus on the known side effects of traditional chemotherapy and the impact of biological agents is difficult to detect.

WHERE DO WE GO FROM HERE?
Predicting Benefit and Patient Selection
The phase III trials of bevacizumab provide clear evidence of biological activity, but identification of the patients deriving the most substantial benefit from bevacizumab has been a challenge. Although bevacizumab is sometimes referred to as a targeted therapy, the target remains unclear and understanding of the mechanism of action is far from complete. Numerous subgroup analyses of the individual trials and pooled results of all three trials in the first-line setting have failed to reveal a particular group of patients with a more pronounced improvement in efficacy with bevacizumab (Fig. 5) (83).

Extensive translational research has been undertaken but to date, no biomarker predicting the efficacy of bevacizumab has been identified. Analysis of the E2100 trial suggested that short nucleotide polymorphisms (SNPs) may provide some indication of outcome with bevacizumab therapy (84). SNPs in the promoter region of VEGF-A (VEGF-A -2578, VEGF-A -1154) appeared to correlate with overall survival in patients receiving bevacizumab-containing therapy for mBC. However, data were reported from the bevacizumab arm but not the control arm, and therefore a prognostic role cannot be ruled out. To date, these findings have not been corroborated in analyses of other bevacizumab trials in mBC.

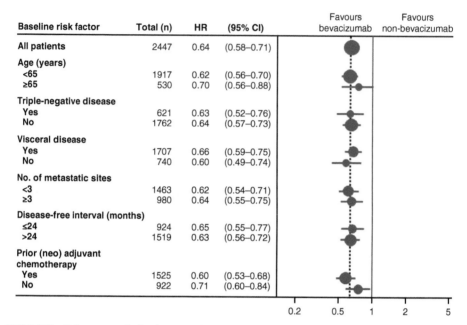

Baseline risk factor	Total (n)	HR	(95% CI)
All patients	2447	0.64	(0.58–0.71)
Age (years)			
<65	1917	0.62	(0.56–0.70)
≥65	530	0.70	(0.56–0.88)
Triple-negative disease			
Yes	621	0.63	(0.52–0.76)
No	1762	0.64	(0.57–0.73)
Visceral disease			
Yes	1707	0.66	(0.59–0.75)
No	740	0.60	(0.49–0.74)
No. of metastatic sites			
<3	1463	0.62	(0.54–0.71)
≥3	980	0.64	(0.55–0.75)
Disease-free interval (months)			
≤24	924	0.65	(0.55–0.77)
>24	1519	0.63	(0.56–0.72)
Prior (neo) adjuvant chemotherapy			
Yes	1525	0.60	(0.53–0.68)
No	922	0.71	(0.60–0.84)

FIGURE 5   Subgroup analysis of progression-free survival: pooled analysis of three trials evaluating first-line bevacizumab in combination with chemotherapy. *Abbreviations*: CI, confidence interval; HR, hazard ratio. *Source*: From Ref. 83.

More promising findings were reported recently from analyses of plasma VEGF-A in the AVADO trial of docetaxel in combination with either bevacizumab or placebo. VEGF-A, the assumed target for bevacizumab, is a logical candidate biomarker and these analyses suggested both a predictive and a prognostic role for bevacizumab efficacy. High baseline levels of plasma VEGF-A and VEGFR-2 may be associated with improved PFS (85). These findings require prospective valida-tion and a randomised trial with VEGF-A as a stratification factor should be a high priority.

Ongoing Evaluation of Anti-Angiogenic Therapies
Although clinical development of several of the agents described above has been abandoned in mBC, bevacizumab has shown a benefit and additional phase III trials in different settings will report in the near future, as shown in Table 3. For example, although most of these agents have been evaluated in patients with HER2-negative disease, upregulation of VEGF by HER2 overexpression (86) and clinical observa-tions of combined antibody therapy (87) provide a rationale for the combination of HER2- and VEGF-directed therapy. Ongoing translational research will play a critical role in determining how this therapy should be used to best effect in patients with breast cancer. Phase III evaluation of sorafenib as a treatment for breast cancer contin-ues and, as described above, alternative approaches to anti-angiogenic therapy are under investigation.

ACKNOWLEDGEMENT
The author is grateful to the Kemp-Lane Fellowship for providing funding for the preparation of this chapter.

TABLE 3 Ongoing Phase III Trials of Anti-VEGF Therapies of MBC

Trial name (number)	Anti-angiogenic regimen	Control arm	Patient population
AVEREL (NCT00391092)	Bevacizumab + trastuzumab + docetaxel	Trastuzumab + docetaxel	Previously untreated HER2-positive mBC
E1105 (NCT00520975)	Bevacizumab + trastuzumab + paclitaxel (± carboplatin)	Trastuzumab + paclitaxel (± carboplatin)	Previously untreated HER2-positive mBC
LEA (NCT00545077)	Bevacizumab + endocrine therapy	Endocrine therapy	Previously untreated hormone receptor-positive mBC
TURANDOT (NCT00600340)	Bevacizumab + capecitabine	Bevacizumab + paclitaxel	Previously untreated HER2-negative mBC
SAKK 24/09 (NCT01131195)	Bevacizumab + metronomic cyclophosphamide + capecitabine	Bevacizumab + paclitaxel	Previously untreated HER2-negative mBC
TABEA (NCT01200212)	Bevacizumab + taxane + capecitabine	Bevacizumab + taxane	Previously untreated HER2-negative mBC
GINECO BR107 (NCT01303679)	Bevacizumab + paclitaxel → bevacizumab + exemestane	Bevacizumab + paclitaxel to disease progression	Hormone receptor-positive HER2-negative mBC, receiving first-line bevacizumab + paclitaxel for mBC
TANIA (NCT01250379)	Bevacizumab + chemotherapy	Chemotherapy	HER2-negative bevacizumab-pre-treated mBC
RESILIENCE (NCT01234337)	Sorafenib + capecitabine	Placebo + capecitabine	Anthracycline- and taxane-pre-treated HER2-negative mBC (first- or second-line setting)
NCT00703326	Ramucirumab + docetaxel	Placebo + docetaxel	Previously untreated HER2-negative mBC

REFERENCES

1. Hanahan D, Weinberg RA. The hallmarks of cancer. Cell 2000; 100: 57–70.
2. Hanahan D, Weinberg RA. Hallmarks of cancer: the next generation. Cell 2011; 144: 646–74.
3. Ferrara N, Kerbel RS. Angiogenesis as a therapeutic target. Nature 2005; 438: 967–74.
4. Poon RT, Fan ST, Wong J. Clinical implications of circulating angiogenic factors in cancer patients. J Clin Oncol 2001; 19: 1207–25.
5. Folkman J. Tumor angiogenesis: therapeutic implications. N Engl J Med 1971; 285: 1182–6.
6. Yuan F, Chen Y, Dellian M, et al. Time-dependent vascular regression and permeability changes in established human tumor xenografts induced by an anti-vascular endothelial growth factor/vascular permeability factor antibody. Proc Natl Acad Sci U.S.A. 1996; 93: 14765–70.
7. Patel N, Sun L, Moshinsky D, et al. A selective and oral small molecule inhibitor of vascular epithelial growth factor receptor (VEGFR)-2 and VEGFR-1 inhibits neovascularization and vascular permeability. J Pharmacol Exp Ther 2003; 306: 838–45.
8. Jain RK. Normalizing tumor vasculature with anti-angiogenic therapy: a new paradigm for combination therapy. Nat Med 2001; 7: 987–9.

9. Willett CG, Boucher Y, di Tomaso E, et al. Direct evidence that the VEGF-specific antibody bevacizumab has antivascular effects in human rectal cancer. Nat Med 2004; 10: 145–7.
10. Tong RT, Boucher Y, Kozin SV, et al. Vascular normalization by vascular endothelial growth factor receptor 2 blockade induces a pressure gradient across the vasculature and improves drug penetration in tumors. Cancer Res 2004; 64: 3731–6.
11. Inai T, Mancuso M, Hashizume H, et al. Inhibition of vascular endothelial growth factor (VEGF) signaling in cancer causes loss of endothelial fenestrations, regression of tumor vessels, and appearance of basement membrane ghosts. Am J Pathol 2004; 165: 35–52.
12. Wildiers H, Guetens G, De Boeck G, et al. Effect of antivascular endothelial growth factor treatment on the intratumoral uptake of CPT-11. Br J Cancer 2003; 88: 1979–86.
13. Osusky KL, Hallahan DE, Fu A, et al. The receptor tyrosine kinase inhibitor SU11248 impedes endothelial cell migration, tubule formation, and blood vessel formation in vivo, but has little effect on existing tumor vessels. Angiogenesis 2004; 7: 225–33.
14. O'Reilly MS, Holmgren L, Shing Y, et al. Angiostatin: a novel angiogenesis inhibitor that mediates the suppression of metastases by a Lewis lung carcinoma. Cell 1994; 79: 315–28.
15. O'Reilly MS, Boehm T, Shing Y, et al. Endostatin: an endogenous inhibitor of angiogenesis and tumor growth. Cell 1997; 88: 277–85.
16. Cao Y. Therapeutic potentials of angiostatin in the treatment of cancer. Haematologica 1999; 84: 643–50.
17. O'Reilly MS, Holmgren L, Chen C, et al. Angiostatin induces and sustains dormancy of human primary tumors in mice. Nat Med 1996; 2: 689–92.
18. Dhanabel M, Ramchandran R, Volk R, et al. Endostatin: yeast production, mutants, and antitumor effect in renal cell carcinoma. Cancer Res 1999; 59: 189–97.
19. Han B, Xiu Q, Wang H, et al. A multicenter, randomized, double-blind, placebo-controlled study to evaluate the efficacy of paclitaxel-carboplatin alone or with endostar for advanced non-small cell lung cancer. J Thorac Oncol 2011; 6: 1104–9.
20. Cui C, Chi Z, Yuan X, et al. Endostatin combined with chemotherapy as first-line therapy for stage IV melanoma patients: a phase II clinical study. J Clin Oncol 2009; 27(15S): e20003.
21. Kulke MH, Bergsland EK, Ryan DP, et al. Phase II study of recombinant human endostatin in patients with advanced neuroendocrine tumors. J Clin Oncol 2006; 24: 3555–61.
22. Hinnen P, Eskens FA. Vascular disrupting agents in clinical development. Br J Cancer 2007; 96: 1159–65.
23. Kanthou C, Tozer GM. Tumour targeting by mictrotubule-depolymerizing vascular disrupting agents. Expert Opin Ther Targets 2007; 11: 1443–57.
24. McKeage MJ, Von Pawel J, Reck M, et al. Randomised phase II study of ASA404 combined with carboplatin and paclitaxel in previously untreated advanced non-small cell lung cancer. Br J Cancer 2008; 99: 2006–12.
25. Pili R, Rosenthal MA, Mainwaring PN, et al. Phase II study on the addition of ASA404 (vadimezan; 5,6-dimethylxanthenone-4-acetic acid) to docetaxel in CRMPC. Clin Cancer Res 2010; 16: 2906–14.
26. Rustin GJ, Galbraith SM, Anderson H, et al. Phase I clinical trial of weekly combretastatin A4 phosphate: clinical and pharmacokinetic results. J Clin Oncol 2003; 21: 2815–22.
27. Rustin GJ, Shreeves G, Nathan PD, et al. A Phase Ib trial of CA4P (combretastatin A-4 phosphate), carboplatin, and paclitaxel in patients with advanced cancer. Br J Cancer 2010; 102: 1355–60.
28. Stevenson JP, Rosen M, Sun W, et al. Phase I trial of the antivascular agent combretastatin A4 phosphate on a 5-day schedule to patients with cancer: magnetic resonance imaging evidence for altered tumor blood flow. J Clin Oncol 2003; 21: 4428–38.
29. Dowlati A, Robertson K, Cooney M, et al. A phase I pharmacokinetic and translational study of the novel vascular targeting agent combretastatin A-4 phosphate on a single-dose intravenous schedule in patients with advanced cancer. Cancer Res 2002; 62: 3408–16.
30. Tresca P, Tosi D, van Doorn L, et al. Phase I and pharmacologic study of the vascular disrupting agent ombrabulin (Ob) combined with docetaxel (D) in patients (pts) with advanced solid tumors. J Clin Oncol 2010; 28(15S Suppl): 3023 (Abstract).
31. Senger DR, Galli SJ, Dvorak AM, et al. Tumor cells secrete a vascular permeability factor that promotes accumulation of ascites fluid. Science 1983; 219: 983–5.

32. Ferrara N, Henzel WJ. Pituitary follicular cells secrete a novel heparin-binding growth factor specific for vascular endothelial cells. Biochem Biophys Res Commun 1989; 161: 851–8.
33. Leung DW, Cachianes G, Kuang WJ, et al. Vascular endothelial growth factor is a secreted angiogenic mitogen. Science 1989; 246: 1306–9.
34. Brown LF, Berse B, Jackman RW, et al. Expression of vascular permeability factor (vascular endothelial growth factor) and its receptors in breast cancer. Hum Pathol 1995; 26: 86–91.
35. Relf M, LeJeune S, Scott PA, et al. Expression of the angiogenic factors vascular endothelial cell growth factor, acidic and basic fibroblast growth factor, tumor growth factor beta-1, platelet-derived endothelial cell growth factor, placenta growth factor, and pleiotrophin in human primary breast cancer and its relation to angiogenesis. Cancer Res 1997; 57: 963–9.
36. Thurston G, Suri C, Smith K, et al. Leakage-resistant blood vessels in mice transgenically overexpressing angiopoietin-1. Science 1999; 286: 2511–14.
37. Carmeliet P, Jain RK. Angiogenesis in cancer and other diseases. Nature 2000; 407: 249–57.
38. Linderholm B, Grankvist K, Wilking N, et al. Correlation of vascular endothelial growth factor content with recurrences, survival, and first relapse site in primary node-positive breast carcinoma after adjuvant treatment. J Clin Oncol 2000; 18: 1423–31.
39. Foekens JA, Peters HA, Grebenchtchikov N, et al. High tumor levels of vascular endothelial growth factor predict poor response to systemic therapy in advanced breast cancer. Cancer Res 2001; 61: 5407–14.
40. Ferrara N. Vascular endothelial growth factor as a target for anticancer therapy. Oncologist 2004; 9(Suppl 1): 2–10.
41. Nielsen DL, Andersson M, Andersen JL, et al. Antiangiogenic therapy for breast cancer. Breast Cancer Res 2010; 12: 209.
42. Presta LG, Chen H, O'Connor SJ, et al. Humanization of an anti-vascular endothelial growth factor monoclonal antibody for the therapy of solid tumors and other disorders. Cancer Res 1997; 57: 4593–9.
43. Cobleigh MA, Langmuir VK, Sledge GW, et al. A phase I/II dose-escalation trial of bevacizumab in previously treated metastatic breast cancer. Semin Oncol 2003; 30(5 Suppl 16): 117–24.
44. Hurwitz H, Fehrenbacher L, Novotny W, et al. Bevacizumab plus irinotecan, fluorouracil, and leucovorin for metastatic colorectal cancer. N Engl J Med 2004; 350: 2335–42.
45. Saltz LB, Clarke S, Díaz-Rubio E, et al. Bevacizumab in combination with oxaliplatin-based chemotherapy as first-line therapy in metastatic colorectal cancer: a randomized phase III study. J Clin Oncol 2008; 26: 2013–19. Erratum in: J Clin Oncol 2009; 27: 653. J Clin Oncol 2008; 26: 3110.
46. Giantonio BJ, Catalano PJ, Meropol NJ, et al. Bevacizumab in combination with oxaliplatin, fluorouracil, and leucovorin (FOLFOX4) for previously treated metastatic colorectal cancer: results from the Eastern Cooperative Oncology Group Study E3200. J Clin Oncol 2007; 25: 1539–44.
47. Miller KD, Chap LI, Holmes FA, et al. Randomized phase III trial of capecitabine compared with bevacizumab plus capecitabine in patients with previously treated metastatic breast cancer. J Clin Oncol 2005; 23: 792–9.
48. Brufsky A, Bondarenko IN, Smirnov V, et al. RIBBON-2: a randomized, double-blind, placebo-controlled, phase III trial evaluating the efficacy and safety of bevacizumab in combination with chemotherapy for second-line treatment of HER2-negative metastatic breast cancer. Cancer Res 2009; 69(Suppl): 495s (Abstract 42).
49. Miller K, Wang M, Gralow J, et al. Paclitaxel plus bevacizumab versus paclitaxel alone for metastatic breast cancer. N Engl J Med 2007; 357: 2666–76.
50. Miles DW, Chan A, Dirix LY, et al. Phase III study of bevacizumab plus docetaxel compared with placebo plus docetaxel for the first-line treatment of human epidermal growth factor receptor 2-negative metastatic breast cancer. J Clin Oncol 2010; 28: 3239–47.
51. Robert NJ, Diéras V, Glaspy J, et al. RIBBON-1: Randomized, double-blind, placebo-controlled, phase III trial of chemotherapy with or without bevacizumab for first-line treatment of human epidermal growth factor receptor 2-negative, locally recurrent or metastatic breast cancer. J Clin Oncol 2011; 29: 1252–60.

52. Gray R, Bhattacharya S, Bowden C, et al. Independent review of E2100: a phase III trial of bevacizumab plus paclitaxel versus paclitaxel in women with metastatic breast cancer. J Clin Oncol 2009; 27: 4966–72.

53. Smith IE, Pierga JY, Biganzoli L, et al. First-line bevacizumab plus taxane-based chemotherapy for locally recurrent or metastatic breast cancer: safety and efficacy in an open-label study in 2,251 patients. Ann Oncol 2011; 22: 595–602.

54. Biganzoli L, Di Vincenzo E, Jiang Z, et al. First-line bevacizumab-containing therapy for breast cancer: results in patients aged ≥70 years treated in the ATHENA study. Ann Oncol 2011 Mar 28. [Epub ahead of print.]

55. Robert NJ, Saleh MN, Paul D, et al. Sunitinib plus paclitaxel versus bevacizumab plus paclitaxel for first-line treatment of patients with advanced breast cancer: a phase III, randomized, open-label trial. Clin Breast Cancer 2011; 11: 82–92.

56. Bergh J, Greil R, Voytko N, et al. Sunitinib (SU) in combination with docetaxel (D) versus D alone for the first-line treatment of advanced breast cancer (ABC). J Clin Oncol 2010; 28(18S): LBA1010 (Abstract).

57. Crown J, Dieras V, Staroslawska E, et al. Phase III trial of sunitinib (SU) in combination with capecitabine (C) versus C in previously treated advanced breast cancer (ABC). J Clin Oncol 2010; 28(18S): LBA1011 (Abstract).

58. Barrios CH, Liu M-C, Lee SC, et al. Phase III randomized trial of sunitinib versus capecitabine in patients with previously treated HER2-negative advanced breast cancer. Breast Cancer Res Treat 2010; 121: 121–31.

59. Gradishar WJ, Kaklamani V, Prasad Sahoo T, et al. A double-blind, randomized, placebo-controlled, phase 2b study evaluating the efficacy and safety of sorafenib in combination with paclitaxel as a first-line therapy in patients with locally recurrent or metastatic breast cancer. Cancer Res 2009; 69(Suppl): 496s (Abstract 44).

60. Baselga J, Roché H, Costa F, et al. SOLTI-0701: a multinational double-blind randomized phase 2b study evaluating the efficacy and safety of sorafenib compared to placebo when administered in combination with capecitabine in patients with locally advanced or metastatic breast cancer (BC). Cancer Res 2009; 69(Suppl): 497s (Abstract 45).

61. Hudis C, Tauer KW, Hermann RC, et al. Sorafenib (SOR) plus chemotherapy (CRx) for patients (pts) with advanced (adv) breast cancer (BC) previously treated with bevacizumab (BEV). J Clin Oncol 2011; 29(15S): 1009 (Abstract).

62. Martin M, Roche H, Pinter T, et al. Motesanib, or open-label bevacizumab, in combination with paclitaxel, as first-line treatment for HER2-negative locally recurrent or metastatic breast cancer: a phase 2, randomised, double-blind, placebo-controlled study. Lancet Oncol 2011; 12: 369–76.

63. Rugo HS, Stopeck AT, Joy AA, et al. Randomized, placebo-controlled, double-blind, phase II study of axitinib plus docetaxel versus docetaxel plus placebo in patients with metastatic breast cancer. J Clin Oncol 2011; 29: 2459–65.

64. Boér K, Láng I, Llombart-Cussac A, et al. Vandetanib with docetaxel as second-line treatment for advanced breast cancer: a double-blind, placebo-controlled, randomized phase II study. Invest New Drugs 2010 Sep 10. [Epub ahead of print.]

65. Dieras V, Jassem J, Dirix LY, et al. A randomized, placebo-controlled phase II study of AMG 386 plus bevacizumab (Bev) and paclitaxel (P) or AMG 386 plus P as first-line therapy in patients (pts) with HER2-negative, locally recurrent or metastatic breast cancer (LR/MBC). J Clin Oncol 2011; 29(15S): 544 (Abstract).

66. Wildiers H, Fontaine C, Vuylsteke P, et al. Multicenter phase II randomized trial evaluating antiangiogenic therapy with sunitinib as consolidation after objective response to taxane chemotherapy in women with HER2-negative metastatic breast cancer. Breast Cancer Res Treat 2010; 123: 463–9.

67. Hu-Lowe DD, Zou HY, Grazzini ML, et al. Nonclinical antiangiogenesis and antitumor activities of axitinib (AG-013736), an oral, potent, and selective inhibitor of vascular endothelial growth factor receptor tyrosine kinases 1, 2, 3. Clin Cancer Res 2008; 14: 7272–83.

68. Taylor SK, Chia S, Dent S, et al. A phase II study of pazopanib in patients with recurrent or metastatic invasive breast carcinoma: a trial of the Princess Margaret Hospital phase II consortium. Oncologist 2010; 15: 810–8.

69. Moulder SL, Rivera E, Ensor J, et al. Phase I trial of escalating doses of weekly everolimus (RAD001) in combination with docetaxel for the treatment of metastatic breast cancer (MBC). J Clin Oncol 2009; 27(15S): 1066 (Abstract).

70. Chow LWC, Sun Y, Jassem J, et al. Phase 3 study of temsirolimus with letrozole or letrozole alone in postmenopausal women with locally advanced or metastatic breast cancer. Breast Cancer Res Treat 2006; 100(Suppl 1): S286 (Abstract 6091).

71. Bocci G, Nicolaou KC, Kerbel RS. Protracted low-dose effects on human endothelial cell proliferation and survival in vitro reveal a selective antiangiogenic window for various chemotherapeutic drugs. Cancer Res 2002; 62: 6938–43.

72. Colleoni M, Rocca A, Sandri MT, et al. Low-dose oral methotrexate and cyclophosphamide in metastatic breast cancer: Antitumor activity and correlation with vascular endothelial growth factor levels. Ann Oncol 2002; 13: 73–80

73. Belotti D, Vergani V, Drudis T, et al. The microtubule-affecting drug paclitaxel has antiangiogenic activity. Clin Cancer Res 1996; 2: 1843–9.

74. Laquente B, Viñals F, Germà JR. Metronomic chemotherapy: an antiangiogenic scheduling. Clin Transl Oncol 2007; 9: 93–8.

75. Dellapasqua S, Bertolini F, Bagnardi V, et al. Metronomic cyclophosphamide and capecitabine combined with bevacizumab in advanced breast cancer. J Clin Oncol 2008; 26: 4899–905.

76. Bagri A, Berry L, Gunter B, et al. Effects of anti-VEGF treatment duration on tumor growth, tumor regrowth, and treatment efficacy. Clin Cancer Res 2010; 16: 3887–900.

77. Miles D, Harbeck N, Escudier B, et al. Disease course patterns after discontinuation of bevacizumab: pooled analysis of randomized phase III trials. J Clin Oncol 2011; 29: 83–8.

78. Saad ED, Katz A, Buyse M. Overall survival and post-progression survival in advanced breast cancer: a review of recent randomized clinical trials. J Clin Oncol 2010; 28: 1958–62.

79. Broglio KR, Berry DA. Detecting an overall survival benefit that is derived from progression-free survival. J Natl Cancer Inst 2009; 101: 1642–9.

80. Miles DW, Romieu G, Dieras V, et al. Meta-analysis of patients (pts) previously treated with taxanes from three randomized trials of bevacizumab (BV) and first-line chemotherapy as treatment for metastatic breast cancer (MBC). Ann Oncol 2010; 21(Suppl 8): viii97 (Abstract 279PD).

81. O'Shaughnessy J, Romieu G, Dieras V, et al. Meta-analysis of patients with triple-negative breast cancer (TNBC) from three randomized trials of first-line bevacizumab (BV) and chemotherapy treatment for metastatic breast cancer (MBC). Cancer Res 2010; 70(24 Suppl): 452s (Abstract P6-12-03).

82. Brufsky A, Valero V, Tiangco B, et al. Impact of bevacizumab (BEV) on efficacy of second-line chemotherapy (CT) for triple-negative breast cancer (TNBC): analysis of RIBBON-2. J Clin Oncol 2011; 29(15S): 101 (Abstract).

83. O'Shaughnessy JA, Miles D, Gray RJ, et al. A meta-analysis of overall survival data from three randomized trials of bevacizumab (BV) and first-line chemotherapy as treatment for patients with metastatic breast cancer (MBC). J Clin Oncol 2010; 28(15S): 1005 (Abstract).

84. Schneider BP, Wang M, Radovich M, et al. Association of vascular endothelial growth factor and vascular endothelial growth factor receptor-2 genetic polymorphisms with outcome in a trial of paclitaxel compared with paclitaxel plus bevacizumab in advanced breast cancer: ECOG 2100. J Clin Oncol 2008; 26: 4672–8.

85. Miles DW, de Haas SL, Dirix L, et al. Plasma biomarker analyses in the AVADO phase III randomized study of first-line bevacizumab + docetaxel in patients with human epidermal growth factor receptor (HER) 2-negative metastatic breast cancer. Cancer Res 2010; 70(24 Suppl): 235s (Abstract P2-16-04).

86. Wen XF, Yang G, Mao W, et al. HER2 signaling modulates the equilibrium between pro- and antiangiogenic factors via distinct pathways: implications for HER2-targeted antibody therapy. Oncogene 2006; 25: 6986–96.

87. Hurvitz SA, Pegram MD, Lin L-S, et al. Final results of a phase II trial evaluating trastuzumab and bevacizumab as first line treatment of HER2-amplified advanced breast cancer. Cancer Res 2009; 69(Suppl): 854s (Abstract 6094).

9

Imaging in the management of metastatic breast cancer

David MacVicar

INTRODUCTION

Over the past 50 years there have been major shifts in practice regarding the diagnosis and treatment of breast cancer, with trends away from radical surgical procedures to breast conserving treatment. The national screening programme in the United Kingdom has been active for almost 20 years, targeted at patients between the age of 50 and 64, but available to patients outside this age range under certain circumstances. It has planned to extend the screening age group up to age 73, which raises capacity and resource issues for screening centres. Mammography, ultrasound (US), and fine needle aspiration cytology (FNAC) have facilitated the diagnosis of small tumours, and US, FNAC, and sentinel node imaging can detect the nodal disease prior to or at the time of primary surgery. Imaging assessment and clinical examination now guide the decision to treat with neoadjuvant chemotherapy which has been shown to reduce the need for mastectomy (1). The role of imaging is crucial and well defined in the diagnosis of locoregional disease and nodal metastasis, but how it should be deployed in the staging of breast cancer and search for metastatic disease at the time of diagnosis has been less clear-cut. In particular, screening programmes tend to discover early-stage tumours and a balance must be struck to find an appropriate level of imaging investigation.

STAGING OF BREAST CANCER AT DIAGNOSIS

The questions to be asked in this clinical setting are as follows:-

1. Which patients are likely to have distant metastatic disease at the time of diagnosis?
2. Is it justified to use imaging investigations to diagnose asymptomatic metastases?

Schneider et al. (2) described the cases of 488 consecutive patients with primary operable breast cancer who underwent surgery and a work-up for distant metastases including chest radiograph, called chest x-ray (CXR), liver US, and an isotope bone scan. Distant metastases were found in 3.9% (19 patients). Bone metastases were detected in 2.7%, liver metastases in 1%, and pulmonary metastases in 0.4%. Among patients with breast tumours less than 1 cm at pathological examination, none had metastatic deposits. In patients with pathological T4 tumours (e.g., extension to chest wall, skin oedema, and satellite nodules, and inflammatory carcinomas), the incidence of metastasis was 18%. This reflects other contributions to the literature which found that patients with T1 and T2 tumours (lesions up to 5 cm in diameter) had positive isotope bone scans in only 2% (3). The message here is unsurprising that locally advanced tumours are more likely to have metastasised at the time of diagnosis, and Schneider et al. conclude that the imaging work-up can be omitted in patients with small breast tumours presenting with symptoms of local disease only (2).

The question of whether it is worthwhile detecting metastatic disease which is asymptomatic at presentation was addressed by two multi-centre randomised trials conducted in Italy (4,5). Rosselli del Turco et al. (4) randomised a group of 1243 consecutive patients with no symptoms of metastases at the time of diagnosis of breast cancer into two groups. One group had physical examination and mammography at

6-monthly intervals whereas patients in the "intensive follow-up" group had, in addition, CXR and bone scan every 6 months. Vital status at 5 years was the main outcome measure. At the fifth year, 393 recurrences (104 local and 289 distant) were observed. Increased detection of isolated lung and bone deposits was evident in the intensive follow-up group compared with the clinical follow-up group. No difference in incidence was observed for metastasis at other sites or for local or regional recurrences. There was no difference in 5-year overall mortality, but the relapse-free survival rate was significantly higher in the group subjected to clinical follow-up only, with patients in the intensive follow-up group showing earlier detection of recurrence. This group followed up with 10-year statistics and, once again no difference in survival was detectable (6). In a similar study, the GIVIO investigators (5) randomised 1320 women into two groups, one group being assessed with clinical examination and an annual mammogram, the other being assessed with isotope bone scan and liver US at yearly intervals, CXR twice yearly, and laboratory blood tests every 3 months. Median follow-up was 71 months, and there was no overall difference in survival. They also measured health-related quality of life including quality of life perception, emotional well-being, body image, social functioning, satisfaction with care, and symptoms. No difference was found, so symptom relief cannot be used as a justification for attempts to detect metastatic disease early. Both trials came to the firm conclusion that the routine use of imaging investigations for patients with no symptoms of metastasis should be discouraged.

The faculty of Clinical Oncology of the Royal College of Radiologists (RCR) issued a document entitled *Imaging for Oncologists* (7) (2004) which recommended that CXR should be performed on women undergoing conservation surgery for T1 and T2 breast carcinomas, and CXR, isotope bone scan, and cross-sectional imaging of the liver should be performed on women undergoing mastectomy. This provoked a brisk response from diagnostic radiologists involved in the care of breast cancer patients (8). It was pointed out that it is illogical to use the type of surgery proposed as a prognostic indicator, as a patient with a small low-grade invasive tumour with extensive surrounding ductal carcinoma *in situ* (DCIS) needs a mastectomy, but is at low risk of developing metastases. However, a patient undergoing conservation surgery for a small high-grade invasive cancer may well have micrometastases which declare in future years. It was reiterated that there is no survival benefit in early detection of metastases, and attention was drawn to the likelihood of false-positive results generating anxiety and consuming resources unnecessarily. The decision to administer adjuvant therapy to patients with a poor prognosis is based on adverse pathological features. The Royal College of Radiologists subsequently amended the advice to the effect that prior to mastectomy, if there is any suspicion that patients may have metastatic disease, an isotope bone scan and a cross-sectional imaging of the liver should be employed. In the response (9) attention was drawn to the problem faced by oncologists treating patients that there is no reliable way of identifying patients with early metastasis, and therefore it is difficult to assess the effect of expensive modern cytotoxic drugs, bisphosphonates and emerging novel biological agents such as trastuzumab on the natural history of metastatic disease. It may be that there is a survival advantage for certain groups of patients who have a low-volume asymptomatic metastatic disease demonstrated by complex imaging techniques who are subsequently treated with systemic agents at an earlier point in the natural history of their disease. However, it is becoming clear that breast cancer is an example of a tumour with a wide range of molecular, biological, and clinical profiles. The studies of the 1990s (5,6) used relatively primitive imaging investigations. There may be a place for a reassessment of intensive use of imaging within a clinical trial. In practice what has happened is there has been a gradual drift towards imaging asymptomatic patients on an ad hoc basis. It is noticeable that in cash-driven sectors of health economies, the use of imaging seems to be more widespread.

Since a diagnosis of metastatic disease renders a patient "incurable", the diagnosis should be made with due circumspection and only when it is unequivocal. Modern imaging techniques are capable of throwing up a multitude of false-positive findings. Even in a patient with an established diagnosis of cancer the majority of radiological "abnormalities" will prove to be benign entities such as lung granulomas and liver cysts. Caution should be exercised by physicians requesting imaging studies with the intention of reassuring the patient, as they will frequently do the opposite. However, imaging studies come to the fore when symptoms develop which need investigation and for which systemic or local treatment may be beneficial.

IMAGING INVESTIGATIONS FOR SYMPTOMATIC METASTATIC DISEASE

Autopsy studies demonstrate that breast cancer is capable of metastasising to any organ. Lungs, bone, liver, and lymph nodes are the most frequent sites of metastatic disease. Lee (10) summarised the results of seven autopsy studies conducted between 1950 and 1982, and the more frequent sites of metastatic disease are as listed in Table 1. There are some surprising statistics, notably that CNS metastases seem under-represented by today's standards. It does seem that the pattern of metastatic disease is somewhat different in younger patients under the age of 50 years and in patients who have received prolonged cytotoxic chemotherapy in that these patients tend to have more sites of metastatic disease discovered at autopsy (11,12). Given that multiple sites of metastatic disease are frequently found, once metastatic disease has been diagnosed it is a reasonable proposition to trawl through various organs using cross-sectional imaging. The most versatile and readily available investigation is computed tomography (CT) but magnetic resonance imaging (MRI), US, isotope bone scanning, and positron emission tomography with 18-fluoro deoxyglucose (^{18}FDG-PET) may also be used. Such imaging techniques may be helpful in guiding the decision to change or abandon systemic treatment, and tumour assessment including volume measurement forms a part of many clinical trials. In the first instance, however, a symptom must be investigated with the intention of diagnosing and palliating metastatic disease, and each set of symptoms will require a tailored approach to investigations. A careful clinical history and physical examination are of inestimable value in providing clinical details which will guide appropriate investigation and enable the radiologist to interpret imaging findings. Incomplete information causes discrepancies of radiological interpretation which are detrimental to the patient.

TABLE 1   Breast Cancer: Sites of Metastasis at Autopsy

Site of metastasis	Percentage of patients affected
Lungs	71
Bone	71
Nodes	67
Liver	62
Pleura	51
Adrenal	41
Brain	26
Peritoneum	21
Ovaries	20
Dura	18
Leptomeninges	16
Pituitary	9
Spinal cord	8

Source: Adapted from Ref. 10.

Nodal Metastatic Disease

In the current (2009) version of the TNM staging system, metastatic disease in the supraclavicular fossa nodes is categorised as N3, although it has previously been staged as M1. Cervical nodal disease is considered metastatic. Most nodal metastases to the neck and axilla can be diagnosed by clinical examination, but CT and US (Fig. 1) may be used for confirmation in clinically equivocal cases and CT is useful for demonstrating mediastinal or retroperitoneal nodal metastasis.

Intrathoracic Metastatic Disease

Dyspnoea is the commonest symptom which raises the suspicion of pulmonary metastatic disease. This should be initially investigated by CXR. A baseline CXR is frequently

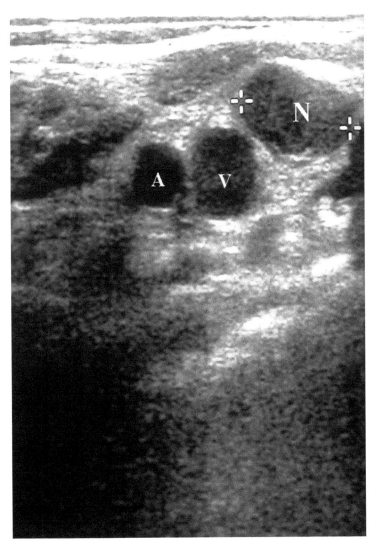

FIGURE 1   Ultrasound examination of the right infra-clavicular region showing a solid lymph node (N) in close proximity to the subclavian artery (A) and vein (V). There is no fat in the hilum of the node and it is of rounded rather than ovoid shape. It was also of increased vascularity on Doppler studies, and the size and characteristics were typical of a tumour-involved node, which was not clinically palpable.

available, although regular follow-up is not indicated (13) and any change in the appearance is relevant. CT may be helpful in discriminating metastases from other pathology such as intercurrent infection, but more often CXR is the only investigation necessary. Metastatic disease to the lungs typically takes the form of nodules which are usually slightly irregular and of different sizes throughout the lungs (Fig. 2).

Lymphangitis carcinomatosa is a common manifestation of metastatic breast cancer which presents with marked dyspnoea which is disproportionate to the often minimal radiographical changes. The classic appearance on CXR is of basal septal lines and peripheral reticulo-nodular shadowing, sometimes associated with small pleural effusions in the presence of a normal sized heart (Fig. 3). When CXR is normal or borderline abnormal, a high resolution CT can demonstrate limited degrees of lymphangitis.

Pulmonary involvement is frequently associated with intrathoracic nodal metastasis. This is best demonstrated by CT, and involved nodes may be discrete soft tissue masses, or as an infiltrative poorly defined process distorting the anatomy of the mediastinum (Fig. 4). This form of the disease is sometimes associated with venous obstruction and symptoms of vague chest pain and dysphagia.

Pleural disease is common and a majority present with pleural effusion which can be diagnosed by clinical examination and CXR, occasionally US is helpful if there is difficulty discriminating consolidation from effusion. US is increasingly being used to guide palliative pleural fluid aspiration (Fig. 5) (14).

Bone Metastases

In oncological practice, the clinical context of musculoskeletal pain is of paramount importance. Back pain in a patient with a previous diagnosis of breast cancer is a good example of how the clinical background fundamentally influences the selection of imaging tests and their subsequent interpretation. For example, a patient who had a 1-cm, grade 1 carcinoma of the breast for 15 years, with no nodes involved and reaches the age of 70 only to complain of low back pain while gardening, is likely to have degenerative disc disease. The chances of metastatic breast cancer being the

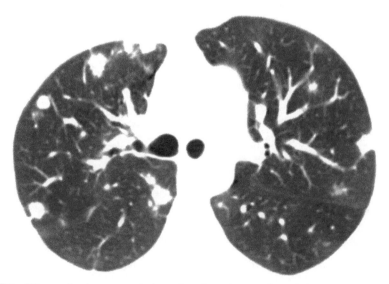

FIGURE 2 CT scan of pulmonary metastases from breast cancer. Irregularity of outline and variation in size are typical features.

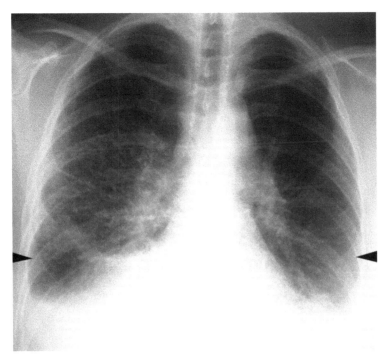

FIGURE 3   CXR showing lymphangitis carcinomatosa associated with breast cancer. Bilateral pleural effusions are present. Above these, horizontal septal lines are present (arrows) and the pulmonary interstitium is diffusely thickened giving a reticular pattern in the mid-zones of the lungs.

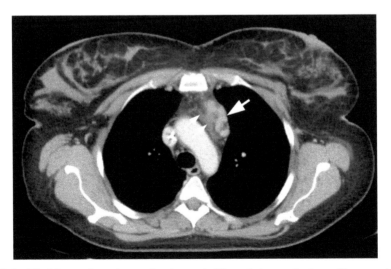

FIGURE 4   CT of thorax shows tumour involvement of the anterior mediastinum. There are irregular soft tissue masses anterior to the aortic arch which represent abnormal lymph nodes in the internal mammary and pre-vascular nodal groups (large arrow). There is also streaking of the mediastinal fat (small arrows) indicating infiltration beyond the discrete nodes, and this pattern is frequently observed in association with breast cancer metastatic to the mediastinum.

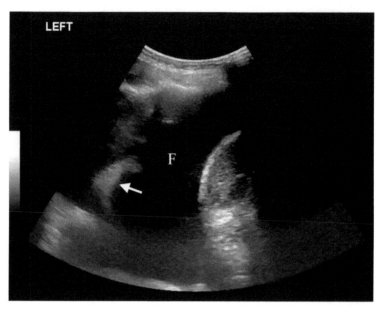

FIGURE 5 Ultrasound (US) of the left hemi-thorax. Pleural fluid (F) is present. This is a fairly large volume pleural effusion, with skin and a pleural thickness of approximately 2 cm and several-centimetre depth of fluid. The collapsed left lower lobe is seen as a beak-like structure dipping down into the fluid (arrow). Inferiorly, the curvi-linear structure is the left hemi-diaphragm. US is being increasingly used to guide appropriate points of insertion for therapeutic drainage of pleural effusion.

cause of these symptoms is low and a period of observation with no imaging tests would be appropriate. A plain radiograph of the lumbar spine may confirm degenerative change. An entirely different approach would be in order for a patient aged 40 years presenting with back pain 3 years after resection of a 5-cm grade 3 carcinoma with multiple involved nodes. In such a patient the likelihood of bony metastases is sufficiently high that plain film imaging, with its inherent lack of sensitivity, is scarcely worthwhile. An isotope bone scan would be an appropriate initial study and able to identify multiple sites of disease, thus confirming metastases. Full clinical details afford the investigating radiologist a far greater chance of interpreting the imaging findings appropriately. There is a small but important false-negative rate attached to isotope bone scanning, which is probably attributable to deposits which are confined to the bone marrow or which fail to excite any osteoblastic activity. If the clinical background is highly suggestive of metastatic disease, MRI is a suitable method of further evaluation of painful areas. T1-weighted spin-echo sequences yield good contrast between metastatic deposits and normal fatty bone marrow (Fig. 6A&B). Further sequences such as T2-weighted spin-echo and gradient-echo techniques and short tau inversion recovery (STIR) may be used at the discretion of the investigating radiologist. Approximately 7% of patients who have a normal isotope bone scan can be demonstrated to have spinal metastases using MRI (15,16).

In patients with a high risk of metastatic disease, a whole-body technique is appropriate. However, many patients will fall into a grey area where clinical suspicion is intermediate. Under these circumstances, it is appropriate to image the symptomatic area with plain radiography. Where typical features are observed, a diagnosis of metastatic disease may be made (Fig. 7). Bearing in mind the relative insensitivity of plain radiography, follow-up imaging may be necessary to confirm the diagnosis of metastatic disease.

(A)   (B)

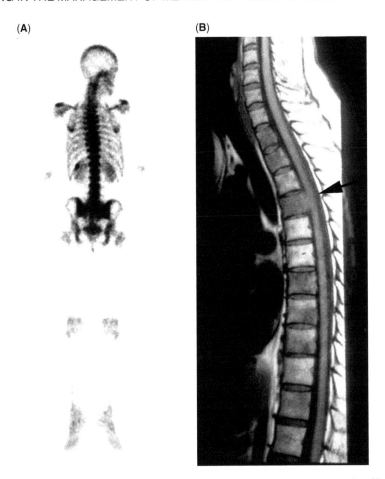

FIGURE 6 (**A**) Isotope bone scan of the whole body shows no focal increased uptake of isotope in the spine. (**B**) Owing to high clinical suspicion of metastatic breast cancer, an MRI was performed. Sagittal T1-weighted sequence shows high signal (white) return in normal marrow cavities. However, many vertebral bodies return lower (darker) signal, and these are tumour involved. An upper thoracic vertebra is threatening mechanical cord compression (arrow). The MRI study was performed 4 days after the isotope bone scan.

The American College of Radiology (ACR) has published "Appropriateness Criteria" for imaging investigations of metastatic bone disease. These describe a number of clinical scenarios which have been assessed by an expert panel using a modified Delphi technique. Recommendations are made for appropriate investigative pathways, depending on clinical presentation. It is of interest to note that for an asymptomatic patient with early breast cancer, any investigation for bony metastatic disease is deemed "least appropriate". This is in keeping with the RCR guidelines, "Making Best Use of a Radiology Department", which is now in its seventh edition. For patients with more advanced breast cancer and pain in back and hip, the ACR Appropriateness Criteria recommend isotope bone scan and symptom-directed plain radiographs; if this is negative, a whole-body FDG-PET can be used. Although far from comprehensive, the Appropriateness Criteria and RCR guidelines provide sound clinical advice aimed at a variety of users including general practitioners and non-specialists involved in breast cancer management (17,18).

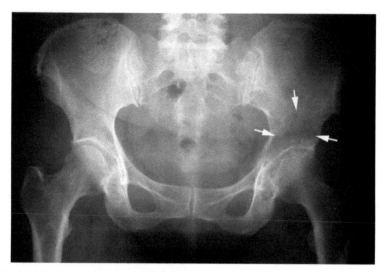

FIGURE 7 Pelvic radiograph in a patient with a past history of breast cancer complaining of left hip pain. There is a diffuse lytic lesion (arrows) in the iliac bone extending to the roof of the acetabulum. Typical features such as the loss of bony trabeculae and the wide zone of transition between normal and abnormal bone allow a confident diagnosis of a metastatic deposit to be made.

Despite the consensus view of the ACR, Costelloe et al. state "skeletal scintigraphy is very sensitive in the detection of osseous metastases and is recommended as the first imaging study in patients who are asymptomatic" (19). Clearly there is some inhomogeneity of practice and opinion. Perhaps the most polarised view comes from Yeh et al. who describe routine isotope bone scanning in patients with T1 and T2 breast carcinoma as a waste of money (20).

Liver Deposits
Statistically, liver deposits are slightly less common than bone and pulmonary deposits. Abdominal pain, hepatomegaly, and disturbance of liver biochemistry are the usual precipitants of a radiological search for liver metastases. It remains a moot point whether deranged liver function tests constitute a symptom. Initially investigation with US will usually make the diagnosis; breast deposits are typically hypoechoic and sometimes demonstrate a "target" lesion appearance (Fig. 8). Portal venous phase hepatic CT demonstrates focal breast metastases most frequently as rim-enhancing low attenuation lesions which are poorly defined but occasionally show a discrete well-circumscribed edge (Fig. 9). Small metastases may become confluent and diffuse, resulting in an imaging appearance similar to cirrhosis (Fig. 10A&B) (21,22). MRI is not routinely used in the evaluation of hepatic metastatic disease, but it has a useful problem-solving role, particularly in the evaluation of indeterminate focal lesions.

NEUROLOGICAL PRESENTATIONS IN PATIENTS WITH BREAST CANCER
In Lee's review of autopsy findings between 1950 and 1982, CNS metastases were found in 26% of patients (10). If a large number of autopsy studies were performed on patients with breast cancer today, it is difficult to imagine that the incidence would be as low as this figure. With modern chemotherapy, it seems that the CNS acts as a sanctuary site, possibly as a result of incomplete penetration of systemic chemotherapy beyond the blood–brain barrier, or alternatively because the natural history of the disease is altered in other ways. Intra-axial brain deposits are common, but there are

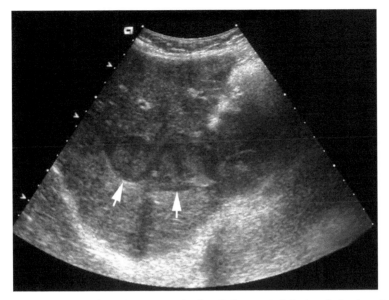

FIGURE 8 Liver ultrasound showing two predominantly hypo-echoic lesions in the hepatic paren-chyma (arrows). The diagnosis of hepatic metastatic disease is sometimes less straightforward than in this example.

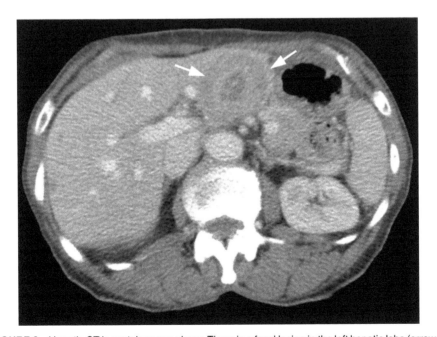

FIGURE 9 Hepatic CT in portal venous phase. There is a focal lesion in the left hepatic lobe (arrows). This is predominantly low attenuation with some enhancement at the rim. The outline of the metasta-sis is fairly well circumscribed. Metastases from breast cancer to the liver are frequently less well defined than this. Centrally, the area of lowest attenuation may represent necrosis within a rapidly growing deposit, and this appearance is sometimes referred to as a target lesion.

(A)   (B)

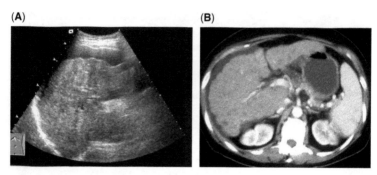

FIGURE 10   (**A**) Ultrasound of the liver shows ascites and diffuse abnormality of the echo texture. (**B**) The liver is not enlarged and shows diffuse mixed attenuation. A small volume of ascites is observed. Note that the spleen is of normal size, but there are dilated vascular channels around the greater curve of the stomach. This appearance of metastatic breast cancer (biopsy proven) is sometimes termed "pseudocirrhosis" and can cause diagnostic confusion. The appearance should be interpreted in the light of full clinical history.

several important ways in which metastatic breast cancer can affect the nervous system. Imaging with CT or MRI is employed to confirm suspected diagnoses. Neurological presentations can be complex, and it is extremely important to ensure that careful clinical assessment is undertaken. For example, a symptom such as inability to walk can result from a parafalcine brain deposit, cord compression, steroid myopathy, or general debility. It is unreasonable to image the entire neuraxis and carry out electrophysiological studies when a patient may simply need some rehydration, and the referring physician must try to localise the lesion clinically, even if only to place it above or below the foramen magnum.

Spinal Cord Compression

Epidural spinal cord compression (SCC) is a not-infrequent complication in patients with bony metastatic disease to the spine. The investigation of choice is MRI of the whole spine. It should be noted that pain is an almost invariable feature of true spinal cord compression, and loss of motor power is the most reliable physical sign. Sphincter disturbance, abnormalities of muscle tone, extensor plantar reflexes, and sensory signs are subjective and often unreliable.

In the presence of a convincing clinical picture, epidural cord compression may be diagnosed without a major degree of mechanical compression. The vascular supply of the cord is predominantly via the anterior spinal artery which forms an anastomotic chain running the length of the cord from T12 to C1. It is supplied by anterior radicular arteries which originate from the aorta, the proximal posterior intercostal artery, or vertebral arteries. Interruption of this blood supply can have a catastrophic clinical effect, as penetrating branches from the anterior spinal artery run into the anterior parts of the cord which carry the major descending motor pathways and the anterior horn cells. Infarction of the cord leads to power loss which is unlikely to recover, rendering the patient paraplegic. Metastases in the vertebral body, especially if associated with a soft tissue mass can put the blood supply of the cord at risk (Fig. 11).

On some occasions compression of the spinal cord may result from the expansion of the posterior elements of the vertebral body, particularly the pedicles. Pain will be the predominant clinical symptom, and power loss may be less marked than compression from deposits in the vertebral body. The imaging findings can be subtle, but trained radiographic staff will be able to perform

(A)   (B)

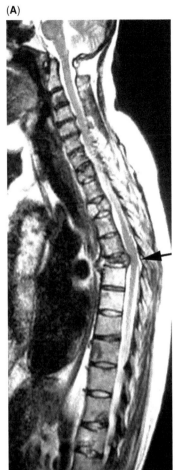
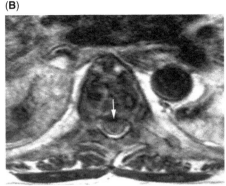

FIGURE 11   (**A**) Sagittal T2-weighted MRI showing metastatic disease at several levels with verte-bral collapse at D6 causing cord compression (arrow). Although the degree of mechanical compres-sion is less than what is sometimes seen, the patient was paraplegic. (**B**) Axial T2-weighted image which shows retropulsion of the metastasis in the vertebral body extending towards the site of the anterior spinal artery (arrow). Infarction of the cord at this level may be responsible for the clinical syndrome of cord compression.

supplementary sequences to confirm the diagnosis (Fig. 12). When investigating SCC, the entire spine should be imaged. Compression occurs frequently at multi-ple levels of the cord (Fig. 13A&B). In early SCC, the sensory level is usually sev-eral segments below the true level of compression, and as the syndrome develops the sensory level rises cranially.

When MRI is contraindicated, myelography and CT myelography may be per-formed, but they involve lumbar puncture which carries an increased risk to the patient as some cord compression syndromes worsen as a result of the procedure.

Spinal Meningeal Metastases
In a patient with metastatic breast cancer and definite neurological abnormality, men-ingeal metastatic disease should be considered. Poorly defined vague back pain and headache are usually present, and the neurological symptoms and signs cannot be

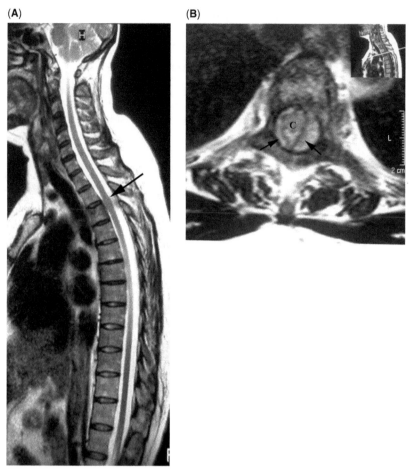

FIGURE 12 (**A**) T2-weighted sagittal section of the spine. Bony metastatic disease is present although not well demonstrated on this sequence. However, the apparent slight expansion of the cord (arrow) is a sinister sign. Axial T2-weighted images (**B**) are indicated and demonstrate soft tissue tumour (arrows) within the spinal canal compressing the cord (C) from a lateral direction predominantly. The blood supply of the cord may be preserved and the full clinical syndrome of cord compression may not be present, but some form of local treatment may be considered if clinically indicated.

correlated to a single anatomical site as should be the case with SCC. If clinical suspicion is high, MRI remains the investigation of choice but the technique will include gadolinium-enhanced T1-weighted imaging. The presence of meningeal metastatic disease gives typical nodular enhancement of the leptomeninges (Fig. 14). MRI is relatively insensitive in the detection of meningeal metastatic disease, so if clinical suspicion remains high, lumbar puncture and CSF cytology may be positive for tumour cells in the presence of a normal MRI study (23,24). Meningeal disease as the first manifestation of metastatic disease is extremely rare. Metastases to the spinal meninges may be a result of haematogenous spread, usually against a background of widely disseminated disease, but are also seen following radiation therapy for brain metastases. Intra-axial spinal cord deposits are present with similar clinical findings to meningeal metastases. They are usually associated with brain deposits and have a tendency to affect the conus (Fig. 15).

(A)   (B)

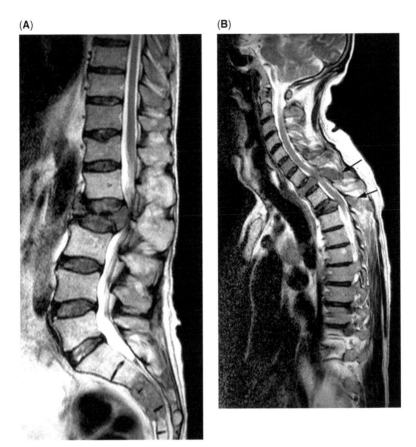

FIGURE 13 (**A**) T2-weighted sagittal MRI showing multiple levels of compression. At L2, there is a vertebral collapse and compression of the cauda equina. There is also a sacral deposit. The clinical presentation was of power loss with loss of muscle tone and hyporeflexia. Compression of the cauda equina may interrupt the reflex arc and obscure signs of upper motor neuron weakness as a result of compression of the cord at a more cranial level. MR of the entire spine should be undertaken when investigating suspected cord compression. (**B**) On this occasion, imaging of the cervical and thoracic region revealed two further compressive lesions at T1 and T3. Note the involvement of the posterior elements (spinous processes) of both of these vertebrae (arrows). The presence of an abnormal signal in the posterior elements of the vertebral body is a discriminator between malignant and osteoporotic vertebral collapse.

Brain Metastases

Brain metastases in breast cancer most frequently present with headache or convulsions. Localising signs such as hemiplegia or ataxia may be found. MRI is the most sensitive method of detecting small metastases, but CT is often adequate for diagnostic purposes. Breast metastases to the brain tend to be peripheral (Fig. 16), and an association between primary breast cancer and development of meningioma has been described. If a solitary cerebral deposit is identified it is tempting to suggest a diagnosis of meningioma. However, in the author's experience, a solitary brain deposit is much more frequent than an incidental meningioma and a pragmatic approach favours early follow-up investigation rather than immediate craniotomy. As with neurological presentations below the foramen magnum, leptomeningeal metastatic disease may result in a syndrome of diverse clinical signs, often affecting

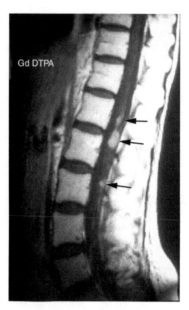

FIGURE 14 Gadolinium-enhanced T1-weighted images of lumbar spine show enhancing nodules (arrows), typical of meningeal metastases from breast cancer.

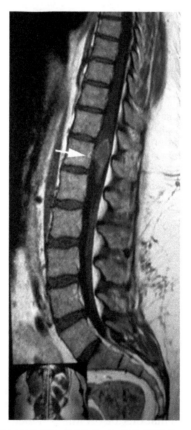

FIGURE 15 Gadolinium-enhanced T1-weighted sagittal MRI images showing an enhancing metastasis in the conus (arrow).

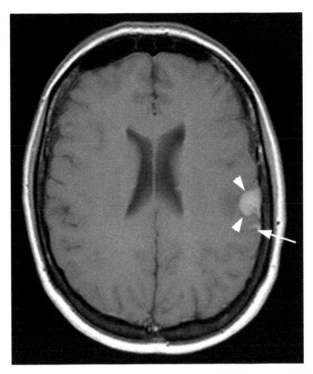

FIGURE 16 T1-weighted gadolinium-enhanced MRI of brain. A brain metastasis from breast cancer is shown in a typical location lying peripherally within the brain (arrowheads). There is some surrounding low-signal oedema. There is a broad base of contact with the meninges, a feature which emits meningioma. There is some faint leptomeningeal enhancement posterior to the lesion (curved arrow). Against a clinical background of metastatic breast cancer, an expectant approach is justified. If the lesion is truly solitary, some form of local treatment may be appropriate, but frequently further lesions will become apparent in due course.

cranial nerves. Contrast enhancement is routinely performed for MRI investigation of brain metastases, but different imaging planes may be used if cranial nerve palsies are observed, either as a result of meningeal metastatic disease or skull base deposits (Figs. 17 & 18). Dural metastatic disease has a different growth pattern and radiological appearance to leptomeningeal disease, and may be seen in association with adjacent bony metastases (Fig. 19).

Breast cancer also has a predilection for metastasising to the orbit. Solid deposits may be found on the ocular muscles, on the choroid or sclera, and it may also infiltrate the retro-orbital fat. Once again, clinical examination should direct the MR technique so that the orbits are studied in more detail. A tailored approach to demonstration of neuroanatomy on MRI can give exquisite detail, and the technique is at its best when used to answer specific questions (Figs. 20 & 21).

Brachial Plexopathy

Following treatment for breast cancer symptoms of pain down the arm raise the possibility of brachial plexopathy as a result of metastatic disease. True brachial plexopathy is characterised by power loss as well as sensory symptoms. The brachial plexus originates with the nerve roots of C5–T1, which exit the neural foramen and run between the anterior and middle scalene muscles. Upper, middle, and lower trunks are formed which give anterior and posterior divisions to re-form as the cords

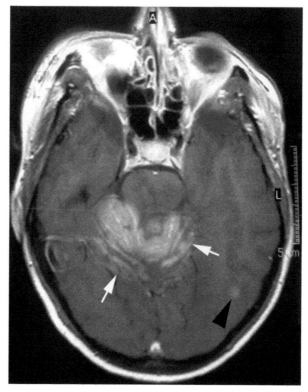

FIGURE 17   Meningeal metastatic disease. T1-weighted axial MRI study of brain with gadolinium enhancement. High signal over the tentorium (arrows) represents enhancement of meningeal metastatic disease. There is also an enhancing nodule (arrowhead) in the left temporo-parietal region which also represents leptomeningeal metastatic disease.

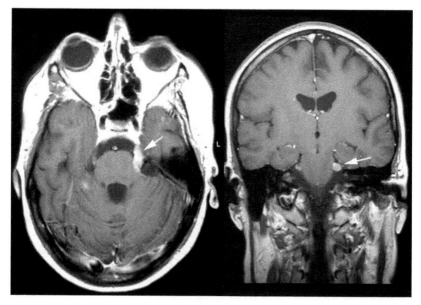

FIGURE 18   T1-weighted gadolinium-enhanced images in a patient with disseminated breast cancer and cranial nerve signs demonstrate enlargement and enhancement of the left 5th cranial nerve (arrows). Further meningeal metastases were present elsewhere in the cranial cavity.

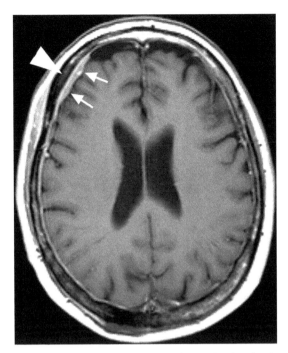

FIGURE 19 T1-weighted gadolinium-enhanced MRI of brain showing dural metastatic disease in association with adjacent bony disease. An irregular plaque of enhancing dura is seen over the right frontal lobe (arrows). Low signal within the marrow (arrowhead) indicates the presence of bony metastatic disease. Throughout the skull vault, inhomogeneity of marrow signal can be seen. The high-signal (white) areas are normal fatty marrow within the skull vault.

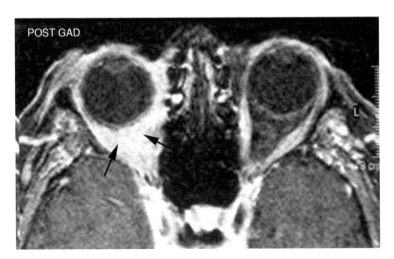

FIGURE 20 Fat-suppressed gadolinium-enhanced MRI of the orbits shows a diffuse high-signal mass lesion infiltrating the retro-orbital fat on the right (arrows). Using this sequence, the retro-orbital fat on the normal left side returns low signal. This type of MRI sequence is not routinely used unless orbital pathology is suspected.

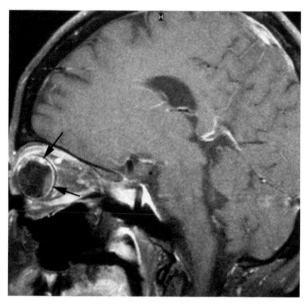

FIGURE 21 Fat-suppressed gadolinium-enhanced parasagittal T1-weighted images through the orbit demonstrating choroidal and retinal deposits (arrows).

of the brachial plexus which lie posterior to the subclavian vessels in the infra-clavicular or retro-clavicular region. Metastatic breast cancer can involve the brachial plexus at spinal level, cervical nodes may involve the plexus at the lateral border of the scalene muscles, but most frequently the point of involvement is where the cords lie behind the subclavian vessels. A detailed investigation of the symptoms should include the spine, and MRI has been demonstrated to be highly accurate in the diagnosis of tumour recurrence (25). As with nodal disease in the mediastinum, recurrence can take the form of infiltrative plaques rather than discrete lumps. However, a mass or plaque of tumour tissue around the brachial plexus is usually sufficient to confirm the diagnosis. In equivocal cases, US may be useful, as FNA cytology can be performed for disease confirmation (Fig. 22A&B). The main clinical differential diagnosis is with radiation plexopathy. This results in thickening in the elements of the brachial plexus within the radiation field. PET-CT is likely to be useful in this clinical context when there is no obvious mass lesion demonstrable by MRI, although there is little documented evidence in the literature as yet. There are also a number of recent technical advances in MRI which will refine the anatomical demonstration of the brachial plexus, for example MR neurography (26).

Intra-Abdominal Metastases
CT is an established and available method for investigating the abdomen in a patient with metastatic breast cancer. CT experience reflects the autopsy studies in that virtually any organ may be involved, including adrenals, spleen, pancreas, and ovaries. The serosa and mucosa of the gut may be involved, but peritoneal metastatic disease is notoriously difficult to diagnose on imaging. Infiltration of the retroperitoneum by small volume nodes is also an occasional manifestation of breast cancer metastases, and the disease can miss out the thoracic cavity completely and show up first in the

(A)

(B)

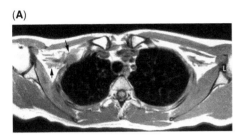
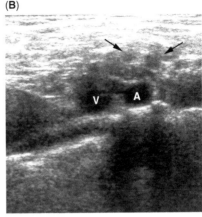

FIGURE 22 (A) T1-weighted axial images through the upper chest show diffuse thickening and a possible mass lesion in the region of the right brachial plexus (arrows). The likeliest diagnosis is of breast cancer recurrence, but this can be confirmed by ultrasound. (B) Ultrasound demonstrates poorly defined confluent small volume lymph nodes (arrows). These lie anterior to the subclavian artery (A) and vein (V). These nodes were subjected to FNAC which showed metastatic carcinoma.

abdomen. Peritoneal deposits in the abdomen are from lobular carcinoma in a disproportionate number of patients (27,28).

WHOLE-BODY IMAGING TECHNIQUES

Once a diagnosis of metastatic breast cancer has been made, there is some justification in imaging the whole body, as follow-up studies will be required to assess response to various lines of systemic treatment. CT is the most versatile technique, capable of demonstrating metastases to lymph nodes, lungs, liver, pleura, peritoneum, intra-abdominal organs, and bone. Assessment of the lesion size is the mainstay of response assessment, but in this approach there are many pitfalls. Bony deposits may become sclerotic and appear larger, but this may be a result of a healing response. Some assessments are beyond certain techniques, for example, CT cannot assess the meninges, and PET, owing to the high uptake of glucose in the brain, is unreliable in the detection of brain metastases. Whole-body MRI using the STIR sequence has been advocated for identifying metastases in all organs (29). However, the bony extremities, skull, and brain are not well imaged in this technique and MRI undoubtedly works better when targeted to a clinical problem. For the time being, diagnosis of symptoms is best achieved with a tailored approach using the single most appropriate imaging technique. In the assessment of response, CT will carry out most of the donkeywork at the present time owing to speed and availability of the technology.

CONCLUSION

With increasing complexity of available technological investigations, the fundamental message remains that to get the best out of these requires careful history taking and clinical examination. A sound knowledge of patterns of metastatic spread of breast cancer will allow appropriate use of imaging investigations, and a discussion of management at multidisciplinary team meetings involving imaging consultants will enhance patient care.

REFERENCES

1. Powles TJ, Hickish T, Makris A, et al. Randomized trial of chemoendocrine therapy started before or after surgery for treatment of primary breast cancer. J Clin Oncol 1995; 13: 547–52.
2. Schneider C, Fehr MK, Steiner RA, et al. Frequency and distribution pattern of distant metastases in breast cancer patients at the time of primary presentation. Arc Gynaecol Obstet 2003; 269: 9–12.
3. Khansur T, Haick A, Patel B. Evaluation of bone scan as a screening work-up in primary and local-regional recurrence of breast cancer. Am J Clin Oncol 1987; 10: 167–70.
4. Rosselli del Turco M, Palli D, Cariddi A, et al. Intensive diagnostic follow-up after treatment of primary breast cancer. A randomised trial. National Research Council project on Breast Cancer follow-up. JAMA 1994; 271: 1593–97.
5. GIVIO Investigators. Impact of follow-up testing on survival and health-related quality of life in breast cancer patients. A multicenter randomized controlled trial. JAMA 1994; 271: 1587–92.
6. Palli D, Russo A, Saieva C, et al. Intensive vs clinical follow-up after treatment of primary breast cancer: 10-year update of a randomised trial. National Research Council project on Breast Cancer follow-up. JAMA 1999; 281: 1586.
7. Board of the Faculty of Clinical Oncology, The Royal College of Radiologists. Imaging for Oncology. Collaboration between Clinical Radiologists and Clinical Oncologists in Diagnosis, Staging and Radiotherapy Planning. London: Royal College of Radiologists, 2004.
8. Evans AJ, Wilson R, Britton P, et al. Staging imaging in women with primary operable breast cancer. Clin Radiol 2005; 60: 520.
9. Hunter R. Staging imaging in women with primary operable breast cancer - response. Clin Radiol 2005; 60: 520–1.
10. Lee YT. Breast carcinoma: pattern of metastasis at autopsy. J Surg Oncol 1983; 23: 175–80.
11. Amer MH. Chemotherapy and pattern of metastases in breast cancer patients. J Surg Oncol 1982; 19: 101–5.
12. Viadana E, Cotter R, Pickren JW, et al. An autopsy study of metastatic sites of breast cancer. Cancer Res 1973; 33: 179–81.
13. Moskovic E, Parsons C, Baum M. Chest radiography in the management of breast cancer. Br J Radiol 1992; 65: 30–2.
14. Havelock T, Teoh R, Laws D, Gleeson F. Pleural procedures and thoracic ultrasound: British Thoracic Society pleural disease guideline 2010. Thorax 2010; 65: i61–76.
15. Jones AL, Williams MP, Powles TJ, et al. Magnetic resonance imaging in the detection of skeletal metastases in patients with breast cancer. Br J Cancer 1990; 62: 296–8.
16. Altehoefer C, Ghanem N, Hogerle S, et al. Comparative detectability of bone marrow metastases and impact on therapy of magnetic resonance imaging and bone scintigraphy in patients with breast cancer. Eur J Radiol 2001; 40: 16–23.
17. Roberts CC, Daffner RH, Weissman BN, et al. ACR Appropriateness Criteria ® metastatic bone disease. [online publication]. Reston (VA): American College of Radiology (ACR), 2009: 11p.
18. Board of the Faculty of Clinical Radiology, The Royal College of Radiologists. Making the best use of clinical radiology services (MBUR), 7th edn. London: Royal College of Radiologists, 2010; In press.
19. Costelloe CM, Rohren EM, Madewell JE, et al. Imaging bone metastases in breast cancer: techniques and recommendations for diagnosis. Lancet Oncol 2009; 10: 606–14.
20. Yeh KA, Fortunato L, Ridge JA, et al. Routine bone scanning in patients with T1 and T2 breast cancer: a waste of money. Ann Surg Oncol 1995; 2: 319–24.
21. Young ST, Paulson EK, Washington K, et al. CT of the liver in patients with metastatic breast carcinoma treated by chemotherapy: findings simulating cirrhosis. AJR Am J Roentgenol 1994; 163: 1385–8.
22. Brookes M, MacVicar D, Husband J. Metastatic carcinoma of the breast: the appearances of metastatic spread to the abdomen and pelvis as demonstrated by CT. Br J Radiol 2007; 80: 284–92.
23. Yousem DM, Patrone PM, Grossman RI. Leptomeningeal metastases: MR evaluation. J Comput Assist Tomogr 1990; 14: 255–61.

24. Collie DA, Brush JP, Lammie GA, et al. Imaging features of leptomeningeal metastases. Clin Radiol 1999; 54: 765–71.
25. Qayyum A, MacVicar AD, Padhani AR, et al. Symptomatic brachial plexopathy following treatment for breast cancer: utility of MR imaging with surface-coil techniques. Radiology 2000; 214: 837–42.
26. Takahara T, Hendrikse J, Yamashita T, et al. Diffusion-weighted MR neurography of the brachial plexus: feasibility study. Radiology 2008; 249: 653–60.
27. Lamovec J, Bracko M. Metastatic pattern of infiltrating lobular carcinoma of the breast: an autopsy study. J Surg Oncol 1991; 48: 28–33.
28. Ferlicot S, Vincent-Salomon A, Medioni J, et al. Wide metastatic spreading in infiltrating lobular carcinoma of breast. Eur J Cancer 2004; 40: 336–41.
29. Walker R, Kessar P, Blanchard R, et al. Turbo STIR magnetic resonance imaging as a whole-body screening tool for metastases in patients with breast carcinoma: Preliminary clinical experience. J Magn Reson Imaging 2000; 11: 343–50.

10

PET/CT in breast cancer

Asim Afaq and Bhupinder Sharma

INTRODUCTION

The morbidity and mortality related to metastatic breast cancer remains high, a fact which necessitates the optimisation of the role of imaging in breast cancer management. Functional imaging approaches are now being increasingly used in oncological management, the principal advantage relative to anatomical imaging being that sites of active disease are accurately assessed. A particularly exciting development in recent years has been that of the advent of positron emission tomography/computed tomography (PET/CT) scanners, providing functional information regarding disease status (defining sites of active/inactive disease) combined with the anatomical definition of CT.

The principal tracer used in clinical PET to date is 2-(fluorine-18) fluoro-2-deoxy-D-glucose (^{18}F-FDG). The extent of ^{18}F-FDG uptake in tumours is directly related to the number of viable tumour cells. In addition the number of viable tumour cells expressing the cell surface glucose transporter 1 (GLUT-1) best correlates with the extent of ^{18}F-FDG uptake in a given tumour; GLUT-1 being overexpressed in breast cancer (1). Once taken up by the cell ^{18}F-FDG undergoes a single phosphorylation step in the glycolytic pathway and is then retained.

This section will outline the role of PET/CT in breast cancer patients. The assessment of primary/axillary nodal disease will briefly be reviewed followed by the role of PET/CT in defining metastatic disease, treatment response assessment, and disease recurrence. Likely future applications of PET in breast cancer will also be briefly addressed.

PRIMARY STAGING

The evaluation of primary or axillary breast cancer disease status is not an "indication" for PET imaging. When PET studies are performed on patients with breast cancer, a significant proportion of primary breast cancers can be detected, including multifocal, bilateral, and occult disease. Likewise, a significant proportion of "involved axillae" will also be detected. PET often elegantly demonstrates axillary level I, II, and III disease, including occult disease in a significant proportion of patients as well as small volume nodal chain involvement (2).

For staging primary breast cancer, a number of studies have demonstrated that PET is not sufficiently accurate compared with the conventional breast work-up which includes triple assessment, including mammography, ultrasound, cyto/histology, and magnetic resonance imaging (MRI) where indicated. Therefore PET is not recommended for routine staging. Avril et al. (3) demonstrated a sensitivity range of 64–80% and specificity range of 94–75% for detection of breast malignancy by ^{18}F-FDG PET in 144 patients with known or suspected malignant breast masses, depending on whether conventional image reading (CIR) or sensitive image reading (SIR) respectively were used. For CIR only focal areas of markedly increased ^{18}F-FDG uptake were considered to represent malignancy, for SIR diffuse or focal areas of moderately increased tracer accumulation were also interpreted as representing malignancy. The same authors also demonstrated that the accuracy of whole-body ^{18}F-FDG PET in the detection of primary breast cancer depends on the lesion size; 0/4 stage pT1a tumours (0.5 cm or smaller) and 1/8 pT1b tumours were detected by PET;

81–92% (CIR and SIR respectively) of pT2 tumours (2–5 cm) were also demonstrated (Fig. 1).

False-negative findings are also observed with slow growing or well-differentiated tumours, non-invasive, tubular, ductal carcinoma *in situ* , and lobular tumours (a histological subtype which can often be [18]FDG PET "negative"/low grade, although they can be FDG avid in a small proportion of patients) (4).

It should also be recognised that ^{18}F-FDG is a glucose ligand, therefore, not truly a tumour-specific agent. False-positive uptake is therefore observed with inflammatory or infectious lesions and for a short interval after biopsy or surgery.

While there is some interest in the potential use of ^{18}F-FDG PET for axillary nodal staging, current whole-body PET/CT scanners are not quite of sufficient accuracy to replace the current "gold standard" of sentinel lymph node biopsy (SNLB) in routine clinical practice. Wahl et al. (5) conducted a prospective multicentre trial in 360 women with newly diagnosed invasive breast cancer, assessing 308 axillae with a gold standard of nodal pathology. With three highly experienced independent readers a sensitivity range of 54–67%, specificity of 79–81%, positive predictive value (PPV) of 62%, and negative predictive value (NPV) of 79% were observed. Although PET/CT cannot replace sentinel node biopsy or axillary clearance in first line clinical practice, there may be an adjunctive role. PPV for axillary nodal detection is more useful than the NPV (5). PET will demonstrate axillary level I , II, and III disease, and is particularly useful in the detection of level II and III involvement where disease is invariably occult, enabling appropriate surgical and radiotherapy treatment planning pre-operatively. It is now an accepted practice for breast surgeons to perform axillary dissections, without SNLB, where a PET is considered confidently positive for axillary nodal involvement, based on semi-quantitative standard uptake value (SUV). Conversely, because a "PET negative axilla" may reflect a "false negative" finding, an SNLB should be performed.

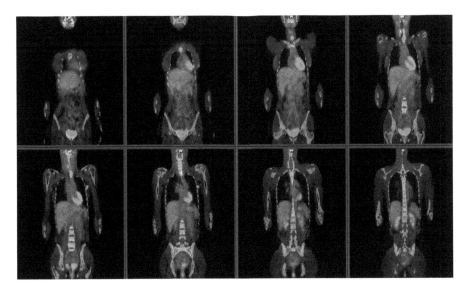

FIGURE 1 Primary disease. PET/CT performed to assess? recurrent laryngeal carcinoma (recurrence shown as "golden glow" of ^{18}F-FDG in laryngeal bed on coronal half body fused PET/CT images 3–5). An occult left breast primary tumour and involved left axillary adenopathy were also detected however, shown as focal tracer uptake in lower outer quadrant of the breast (2&3 upper row images) and nodal axillary uptake (5&6 lower row images); proved on ultrasound and biopsy subsequent to PET/CT findings (2-cm primary breast tumour).

Precise anatomical information can be given on extra-axillary sites including internal mammary chain and supraclavicular disease. Unlike CT alone, PET is able to detect occult small volume nodal disease in these distributions and also enables treatment planning such as radiotherapy.

There is also some evidence for greater FDG uptake in triple-negative cancers, raising the possibility for future PET use in staging specific tumour subtypes (6).

Currently, although moderately sensitive, PET is not routinely used for primary disease or axillary workup. Very useful clinical information can be provided in a significant number of cases when a PET study is performed in patients with breast cancer including the evaluation of local and distant disease.

DISTANT METASTATIC DISEASE

Converse to the assessment of primary disease, a large number of world-wide studies clearly demonstrate that PET/CT is the "single" most accurate imaging modality now available to stage metastatic disease, this technique providing both soft tissue and bony staging, often revealing unsuspected metastases in up to 30% of patients, with resultant management change (7).

The strengths of PET/CT are the fact that it is a whole-body scanning modality, accurately assessing the soft tissues, viscera, and skeleton with "one" test and with the ability to define the sites of active tumour (Fig. 2).

The technique is particularly effective in demonstrating small (sub 5–10 mm) metastatic nodal sites of involvement and bony disease. With anatomical CT imaging

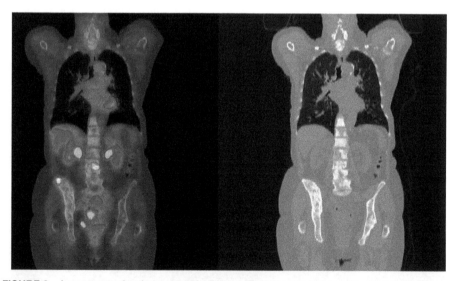

FIGURE 2   Assessment of active metastatic disease. Patient with a history of metastatic breast cancer treated with chemotherapy and hormone therapy. The PET/CT image (fused coronal colour scale image) (*left*) shows intense FDG uptake by (active) tumour involving L3, the right ilium (upper half) with a few small foci of active disease in the right acetabulum (not all shown on this single coronal image). Note the CT bony window component of the PET/CT however (*right*) showing very extensive sclerotic and lytic metastatic disease throughout much of the axial skeleton (throughout the length of the spine in particular). This case illustrates the value of PET in defining active as opposed to inactive sites of disease; although active disease is shown, in this study a key observation also being that the vast majority of the extensive bony metastatic disease (shown on the CT component) is PET negative indicating that there, in fact, has been a very good metabolic response to therapy.

the significance of small (sub 1 cm) sites of change (adenopathy) is difficult to assess (e.g., in axillary levels II and III, the internal mammary and mediastinal stations); PET can indicate pathology in small nodes, in patients otherwise thought to be "disease free". As mentioned above, the lack of a tumour-specific PET tracer raises the risk of false-positive studies. For example, entities such as sarcoidosis will cause increased FDG accumulation, with mediastinal and bilateral hila nodal uptake (8).

Therefore, it is important to always interpret scan findings in the clinical context and use all the imaging findings in order to provide an accurate diagnosis. A useful rule in daily clinical practice is that "a 'positive' [18]FDG PET does not always imply malignancy and a 'negative' [18]FDG PET does not always imply that malignancy is absent".

Technetium-99m methylene diphosphonate (99mTc MDP) bone scintigraphy is conventionally used to assess the skeleton but is not a specific technique as an osteoblastic response is imaged. False-positive uptake is seen with a degenerative change, trauma, inflammation, and infection. In addition, bone scan is not sensitive in the context of lytic metastatic disease when a significant osteoblastic response may not occur, and areas of resulting photopaenia can be difficult to identify (9).

CT bony window assessment is insufficiently sensitive for staging. MRI, although a sensitive technique, is targeted to certain parts of the skeleton, not currently being a whole-body-scan modality in clinical practice. Diffusion-weighted MRI is an interesting new technique, with protocols being developed in relation to whole-body imaging. However this technique remains of research interest and has not been sufficiently developed at present for routine clinical practice (10).

^{18}F-FDG PET is a more specific modality than bone scan as it demonstrates sites of viable tumour cells in the skeleton. The other significant benefit of PET over bone scan is the improved accuracy in the detection of lytic metastatic disease. Cook et al. (11) assessed 23 patients with known bony metastatic disease using ^{18}F-FDG PET and 99mTc MDP bone scintigraphy. Overall, PET detected more sites of disease than bone scan (mean 14.1 vs. 7.8 lesions respectively). The difference was greatest with osteolytic disease. As lytic disease is associated with a more aggressive breast cancer and a worse prognosis, an earlier and more accurate detection by FDG PET is of particular importance. The current sensitivity of bone scan is considered to be 75%, whereas FDG PET has a sensitivity of 85% for lytic bone disease. A large retrospective study from the Royal Marsden Hospital, evaluating 233 PET/CT studies over a 4-year period found that PET/CT was particularly useful in evaluating lytic disease (12).

The entity of the bone scan-negative PET-positive patient with bony metastatic disease is now clearly recognised; these patients virtually always have lytic lesions (Fig. 3). If a "negative bone scan" is observed in a patient, where the clinical index for suspicion of bony disease is high, in the context of bone pain or a raised alkaline phosphatase, an [18]FDG PET scan should be considered.

PET/CT can lack sensitivity to sclerotic (osteoblastic) bone metastases in small numbers of patients, and a combined approach, where the underlying CT bone window aspect of PET/CT that is also evaluated in detail, may be useful to avoid false negatives (13).

A recent study of 163 women found a high concordance between PET/CT and bone scan results (81%). Of those discordant cases, approximately 1/3 had pathologically confirmed bone metastases, most of which were detected by PET/CT (14).

Comparing whole-body diffusion weighted imaging (DWI) with PET/CT for the detection of bony metastases in patients with breast cancer, Heusner et al. found DWI to be a sensitive but unspecific modality for the detection of locoregional or metastatic disease. In the 11 patients evaluated, PET/CT had higher sensitivity and specificity (94% and 99% compared with 91% and 72%) (15).

(A)   (B)

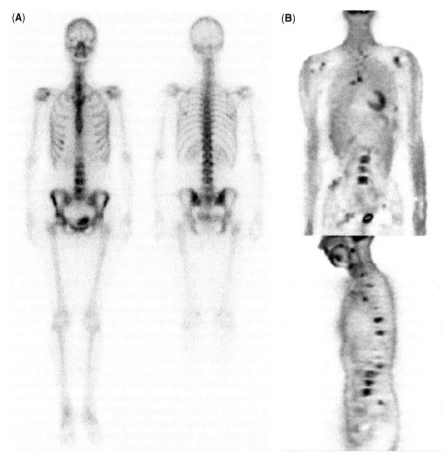

FIGURE 3   Assessment of metastatic disease. Patient with a history of breast cancer presenting with bony aches and pains. Negative 99mTc-MDP whole-body bone scan (**A**). A PET study performed within 1 month of bone scintigram shows a number of scattered bony metastases (sites of increased uptake on coronal and sagittal inverse gray scale FDG-PET images, (**B**)).

Grankvist et al. found MRI, including DWI, to be comparable to PET/CT in the detection of bone metastases. In 13 patients, MRI was able to identify 59 of the 60 lesions described on PET/CT (16).

[18]FDG PET is also extremely useful for liver disease evaluation. The concept of the indeterminate liver lesion is well known on ultrasound, CT, and liver MRI, which sometimes requires biopsy. However this can constitute risk to the patient if the lesion is in a challenging anatomical location or is hypervascular. The key advantage of PET over MRI in the evaluation of liver lesions is that benign vascular liver lesions such as haemangiomas, focal nodular hyperplasia, and adenomas, with "atypical appearances" on CT and MRI are FDG negative. Conversely, liver metastases from breast cancer, including small liver metastatic lesions, are PET positive (17).

Limitations

Limitations of PET/CT include the lack of ability to effectively evaluate the neuroaxis. Metastatic lesions in the brain parenchyma and leptomeningeal disease are difficult to identify on PET due to physiological FDG brain uptake (18).

Although PET will detect moderate or larger volume intracranial metastases and we have found PET to detect leptomeningeal disease in a small number of patients, gadolinium-enhanced MRI of the craniospinal axis is the gold standard modality for CNS evaluation. However, an area where PET is increasingly useful is with gamma knife intracranial surgery. This technique is being used in a proportion of patients with breast cancer depending on the number of intracranial deposits, thereby avoiding whole-brain radiotherapy (WBRT). Post gamma knife, active or recurrent disease can be very difficult to differentiate from radionecrosis on MRI imaging. Correlation and fusion of post-gamma knife PET cranial studies with MRI is useful in this context as radionecrosis is PET negative and active/recurrent disease is [18]FDG avid (19).

PET also has difficulties in fluid compartment assessment. Due to the tumour cell density being low in fluid, [18]FDG PET will not differentiate benign from malignant fluid. Hence, the technique will not differentiate benign from metastatic pleural or pericardial effusions or ascites. In a study of ascites of undetermined origin, the sensitivity, specificity, and accuracy of PET/CT in detecting the primary cause of ascites were 63.3%, 70.0%, and 65.0%, respectively (20).

It is critical to always evaluate these anatomical compartments on the underlying CT aspect of PET/CT when analysing PET data. Likewise, although a PET signal will usually be seen in the context of omental/peritoneal disease infiltration, a significant PET signal may not be seen with fine peritoneal stranding/infiltration. This highlights the importance of reviewing the peritoneal spaces on the anatomical CT fusion component of PET.

Despite the few limitations, clinicians need to recognise that in a proportion of patients, disease will be detected by this new, more sensitive imaging modality at an earlier stage and smaller anatomical volume than with "CT or bone scan".

Given that PET/CT is the most sensitive current imaging modality to define metastatic disease there is clearly an argument that it should be used as the first-line investigation in patients with metastatic breast cancer. This would reduce the need for serial investigations which may include plain films, bone scintigraphy, CT, MRI, and biopsy prior to a PET/CT scan. As PET/CT accurately defines the disease status early in the patient's workup, the management pathway can become more efficient and cost effective.

ASSESSING RESPONSE TO TREATMENT

^{18}F-FDG PET is useful in assessing response to a number of different types of treatment, particularly hormone/endocrine therapy, chemotherapy, radiotherapy, and surgery. It is also now being used with radiofrequency (RF)/laser ablation and post cyberknife therapy (21,22).

The large Royal Marsden Hospital PET/Breast Cancer series (12) showed that PET/CT studies over a 4-year period at this institution were useful in the management of patients, with up to one-third of all studies performed for response evaluation.

Because PET will give a very useful indication of the overall "active" disease burden, it provides clinicians with important information regarding the timing and use of non-toxic treatment/maintenance strategies, such as hormone treatment for example, where "metabolic low volume" active disease, or "metabolic low intensity (low SUVmax), disease remains and the need for/use of more toxic systemic single/combination chemotherapy treatment strategies (where metabolically large volume and/or intensely FDG-avid disease is present).

Early Treatment Response Assessment

The early assessment of treatment response is a particularly exciting use of functional imaging, as metabolic changes in tumours occur before morphological (anatomical) changes occur. The early differentiation of responding from non-responding patients would allow for alteration/discontinuation of ineffective treatment, improving patient morbidity and mortality, and also leading to public health care savings.

Data indicate that PET may be of clinical value in predicting response to chemotherapy in patients with metastatic breast cancer earlier than any other method used (23,24). Gennari et al. (23) evaluated the treatment response to an epirubicin/paclitaxel chemotherapy regimen in 13 patients with metastatic breast cancer. Response was evaluated in a conventional manner, clinically and radiographically after every two cycles. This was compared with baseline PET (within a week before treatment initiation), day 8 PET (after the first chemotherapy course), and end of chemotherapy PET studies being performed. Qualitative (visual) and semi-quantitative (SUV) analysis of the PET data were performed. In six patients who achieved a response to treatment (by clinical and conventional imaging criteria) ^{18}FDG uptake diminished substantially (median SUV at baseline 7.65 (range 3.4–12.3); 5.7 (range 2.8–7.6) at day 8; and 1.2 (range 0.99–1.3) at the end of the planned six cycles of chemotherapy. Three patients who achieved stable disease as best response had no significant qualitative or semi-quantitative reduction in FDG uptake, while non-responding patients also had no significant modification at day 8 from baseline FDG levels. Kumar et al. showed that PET/CT was able to identify 16 responders and 7 non-responders in 23 patients two cycles after neoadjuvant chemotherapy. Differentiation of responders from non-responders had a sensitivity of 93%, specificity of 75%, and accuracy of 87% (4). Straver et al. studied 38 patients with PET/CT and found the modality to effectively monitor axillary response in triple-negative tumours (25).

These studies indicate that FDG PET scanning of metastatic breast cancer has the ability to detect rapid and significant reduction in glucose metabolism in responding patients, whereas no significant reduction is seen in non-responding patients. Although the optimum time for the investigation of treatment response has not yet been established, the response/ non-response differentiation is possible as early as day 8 after the first cycle of chemotherapy. The use of SUVs for serial response evaluation is part of our routine daily clinical practice, baseline marker SUVmax (standard uptake value maximum) levels being documented with marker levels at different body sites of involvement, such as primary breast, nodal, lung, liver, and bone marker measurements. This allows a serial semi-quantitative PET analysis, as well as visual scan analysis, on subsequent studies as demonstrated in the large clinical series audit of Royal Marsden Hospital (12). The role of MRI is also under active investigation in treatment response in the neoadjuvant setting (26).

RF Ablation/Laser Therapy

Early assessment of complete tumour destruction following RF ablation (RFA) and a subsequent follow-up of RFA sites is difficult with conventional imaging. Ultrasound, CT, and MRI all have limitations with regard to sensitivity and specificity. PET is a modality which is particularly useful in this regard, enabling both early assessment of complete/incomplete tumour destruction and also being a sensitive and an accurate modality in subsequent follow-up (27–29).

Carditello et al. (28) assessed treatment response of liver metastases from a number of different primaries (including breast); a larger series being that of Donckier et al. (29) (colorectal hepatic metastases being assessed). In this series 28 lesions were assessed in 17 patients, CT and FDG PET being preoperatively, at 1 week, 1 month, and 3 months post RFA. In 24/28 lesions PET and CT were negative post RFA, none of these patients subsequently developing local recurrence. In four patients PET at 1 week and 1 month showed recurrence, CT being negative. Recurrence was confirmed in three out of these four patients by biopsy, recurrence in the fourth being confirmed by follow up. A key point is that PET is a useful modality for the early detection of efficacy of complete ablation/incomplete tumour destruction, which can be very difficult to difficult to distinguish with anatomical CT and MRI imaging.

Bone Response Assessment

Response assessment of bony metastatic disease is a difficult area with conventional imaging. While assessment of disease progression with CT, MRI, or bone scan for example is often "straightforward", determination of response and evaluation of the presence of active disease (as opposed to inactive disease) is problematic. This is because once a lesion is present on CT (bony windows) or MRI the bony texture/destruction will often remain relatively abnormal, even after treatment. Increasing dense sclerosis (with reducing lytic change) on both CT bone windows and MRI are a feature of response to treatment; however, a time-point is often reached in patients where diffuse dense sclerotic infiltration appears static on CT and MRI. 99m Tc MDP bone scintigraphy is also relatively non-sensitive as visualisation of lesions depends on an osteoblastic response, this often lagging behind changes in the tumour component itself. Lesions can remain "positive" or increasingly "positive" on 99Tc MDP bone scan therefore, despite the fact that the patient is responding (the persistent or increasing bone scan activity in some cases reflecting osteoblastic bone healing and repair and not disease progression) (30).

FDG PET is an excellent modality to assess bony response (31) (Fig. 4). Viable tumour cells only show a significant FDG uptake (^{18}FDG PET not "relying" on an

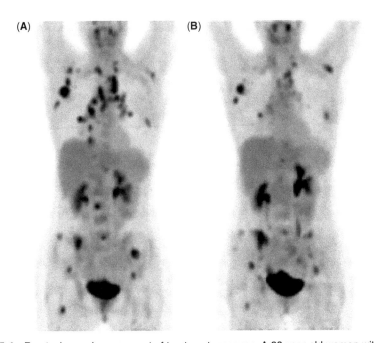

FIGURE 4 Re-staging and assessment of treatment response. A 38-year-old woman with a 4-year history of treatment for metastatic breast cancer. Presentation with right arm pain associated with progressive weakness and numbness. MRI brachial plexus negative. (**A**) The image (inverse gray scale PET image) shows numerous intensely FDG avid metastases involving the axial skeleton and proximal appendicular skeleton together with involved neck, axillary, and mediastinal nodal disease. Right axillary nodal disease was responsible for the right upper limb symptoms. (**B**) The coronal PET image shows a good partial response to weekly Taxol chemotherapy, there being a clear reduction in the extent of metabolically active disease. (*Continued*)

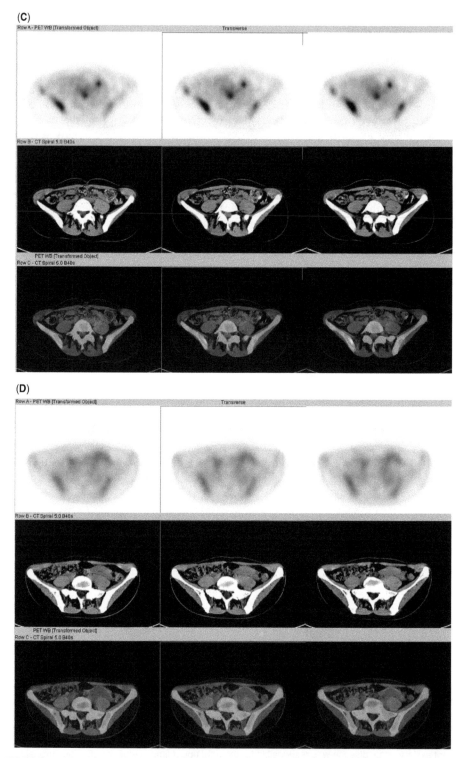

FIGURE 4 (*Continued*) This is also illustrated in (**C, D**) (axial inverse grey scale PET, CT, and fused PET/CT images) of the bony disease in the pelvis (before and after Taxol chemotherapy; note that response would be difficult to define on CT bony windows alone.

indirect signal such as osteoblastic activity, which is the case with MDP bone scan) and therefore response assessment of bony lesions can be performed early and accurately; bone windows of the CT correlate (of the PET/CT) demonstrating the underlying anatomical bony change (lysis, sclerosis, cortical expansion/ disruption, vertebral body compression, soft tissue change, or pathological fracture).

In addition to visual PET analysis, the semi-quantitative SUVmax measurement is also very useful in providing a semi-objective measurement regarding bone disease status. Our standard practice is to document a series of SUVmax baseline marker measurements when reporting clinical and research protocol PET studies with further "marker" measurements on subsequent scans allowing a comparison and more accurate judgment regarding metabolic complete response (CR), partial response (PR), stable disease (SD), or disease progression (PD).

Although PET/CT can be used "early" for response evaluation and has been usefully performed within 1 week of chemotherapy in certain tumour types, a practical issue is the presence of physiological bone marrow reactivation due to chemotherapy, which will cause a generalised increased marrow activity on ^{18}FDG PET studies (32).

This is not an "issue" when looking at soft tissue (liver, nodal, lung) response, but can limit interpretation when evaluating bone response. In general it is better to delay the "Early Response Evaluation" PET study, in the context of assessing bone response, for as long as possible; for example, if the patient is on a weekly chemotherapy regimen, to perform the PET at day 6 or day 5 (i.e., circa 1 or 2 days before the next treatment cycle is due), thus reducing the extent of marrow reactivation effects. If detailed care is taken comparatively analysing the data, sometimes PET bone response can still be interpreted despite marrow reactivation, because the exact anatomical bone sites which were involved on baseline PET will show diminished activity, that is, a reduced SUVmax measurement or metabolic photopaenia, whereas the rest of the marrow will have reactivated elsewhere (i.e., marrow at the site of metastatic bone/bone marrow involvement not showing "physiological" reactivation). This principle also applies to previous radiotherapy fields— metabolic photopaenia being shown on PET at treated and responding radiotherapy field sites (a few months and onwards after radiotherapy). This is also very useful for defining disease recurrence/tumour activity within previous radiotherapy beds, disease recurrence showing an increased PET signal, recurrence often being difficult to objectively define on CT or MRI, with clinical problems of patient pain and changing tumour markers often also being an issue in this clinical scenario.

Liver Response

Liver ultrasound and CT (MRI when required) are useful modalities for liver metastatic disease evaluation. However, in a proportion of patients, objective or convincing subjective response evaluation can be difficult with these modalities, particularly with the "workhorse modality" of CT in the situation where widespread liver abnormality is often present. It can be very difficult to evaluate whether liver disease is progressing, active, responding, or showing a mixed response. Dual (arterial and venous phase) liver imaging can be helpful and is the preferred CT protocol wherever possible. However, technical differences in timing of scans can cause differences in the appearances of angiogenic enhancement and/or conspicuity of lesions. The other principal clinical problem faced in breast practice is the situation of "hepatic pseudo-cirrhosis of malignancy". The liver developing a contracted irregular fibrotic appearance, with scattered fibrotic residua within/variable enhancement. This is an appearance observed after treatment response of extensive liver disease involvement. However, it is often impossible to define whether clinically significant active liver disease is present in this situation, or to reliably detect changes in liver disease status at an "early stage".

Akin to the situation of PET providing a signal in the context of widespread bone infiltration, PET is very useful for defining the control of liver disease or disease reactivation. We find PET particularly useful in the context of liver residual changes and "liver pseudocirrhosis of malignancy" (12), the PET simply being "negative" in the context of a controlled "fibrotic" liver, whereas the metabolic volume and metabolic intensity (SUVmax) of liver disease activity/reactivation can be clearly visualised and documented on PET (Fig. 5). This is important, as extensive liver

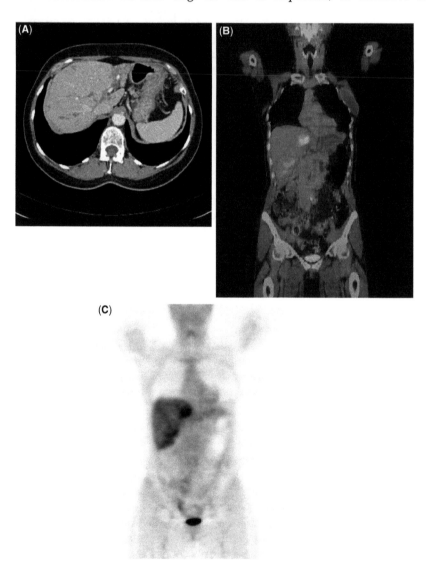

FIGURE 5   PET and liver pseudocirrhosis/liver response evaluation. A 36-year-old woman with metastatic breast cancer (liver) and multiple previous treatment lines. (A) Contrast-enhanced CT shows a "typical" fibrotic pseudocirrhotic appearance of malignancy. CT stable compared with previous, difficult to accurately define disease activity or control. (B,C) Coronal fused PET/CT colour and inverse grey scale data confirm disease has reactivated far into left lateral liver and inferior right liver segments ("yellow colour" on fused colour scale image; "black" appearance on inverse grey scale PET data). (*Continued*)

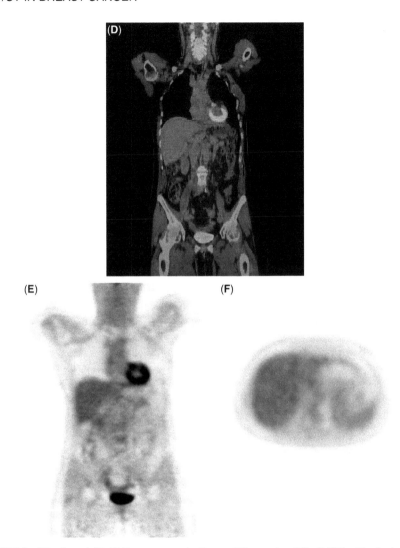

FIGURE 5 (*Continued*) (**D–F**) Response evaluation on CT was also difficult (CT subjectively similar). PET confirms an excellent response to chemotherapy however, with a complete metabolic remission being shown on PET imaging (the PET signal being useful to accurately and confidently assess disease activity and response therefore, judgements are very difficult in this type of situation with cross-sectional CT or MRI alone).

involvement/active disease is a life threatening situation in breast cancer, the PET providing information regarding liver disease status and therefore enabling appropriate treatment.

Response to Radiotherapy, Surgery, and Cyberknife

The evaluation of residual/active metastatic disease following radiotherapy and surgery is difficult with conventional imaging (CT and MRI) in a proportion of patients; this is particularly the case in the spine, for example.

PET/CT is very useful as an imaging tool in this scenario. For example, a widespread diffuse marrow and bony disease infiltration, throughout the axial and proximal appendicular skeleton, with a widespread sclerotic/lytic infiltration, and previous multilevel spinal surgical stabilisation and radiotherapy, with patient pain/changing tumour markers, is not an uncommon clinical problem. The cause for the patient's symptomatology (e.g., low back or pelvic pain) is often very difficult or impossible to define on CT and MRI imaging, in the presence of such a widespread anatomical abnormality and multiple pre-treatments. PET is extremely useful in this clinical situation, highlighting sites of tumour activity/sites of control, thus enabling further targeted (radiotherapy) or systemic treatments as clinically appropriate (12). Clinical Oncology colleagues find the PET/CT data extremely useful in this situation, planning patient radiotherapy treatment fields based on the PET/CT fused data.

PET/CT can be useful in this regard but there are some limitations with this modality. Some FDG uptake will be observed at the radiotherapy site for a short term (of the order of a few weeks at least) after treatment due to (benign) granulation tissue uptake and macrophage activity. Fortunately however, immediate post-radio-therapy imaging at a recently radiotherapy treated site is usually not clinically required—the PET being performed to evaluate disease status elsewhere (33).

Cyberknife is a relatively new treatment technique used in certain patient situations. Experience of PET with cyberknife is limited at present. As with radiotherapy, PET is very useful in defining sites/volumes suitable for cyberknife treatment, aiding cyberknife planning (19).

Post cyberknife, FDG PET shows increased activity in the "treatment bed" for a longer time period than with radiotherapy, more of an intense macrophage inflammatory reaction being incited with this highly targeted "radiotherapy technique". At present we do not know the period of time that this PET inflammatory appearance is likely to persist for (with moderate or intense SUVmax), although I would predict that the reaction is likely to persist for more than 3 months, possibly several months. This is a subject of our analysis at this time.

Limitations and Caveats

Small (sub 7 mm in particular) lung nodules can be beyond the resolution of current PET scanners, therefore, it is important to always scrutinise the underlying CT anatomical lung window component of PET/CT. As discussed above, fluid compartment assessment is also limited.

Krukenberg deposits can also be misinterpreted in pre-menopausal women. This is because cyclical physiological ovarian activity can be seen as a normal appearance on [18]FDG PET imaging. Whilst in a post-menopausal woman, adnexal [18]FDG increased activity is considered to usually reflect disease involvement, in a pre-menopausal woman again due consideration needs to be given to the CT appearance in the adnexum, occasionally a trans-vaginal ultrasound or pelvic MRI being needed for further clarification (34).

Pleurodesis is a situation where care is needed regarding the interpretation of PET data/response evaluation. Pleurodesis incites an intense inflammatory reaction, with activated macrophages and granulation tissue; these cells will of course take up the FDG radiotracer (which is a glucose analogue). When PET imaging is performed post pleurodesis, one invariably sees an intense PET activity encasing a hemithorax. Furthermore, serial SUVmax measurements are not helpful in this situation, as the degree of pleurodesis metabolic activity can "wax and wane" for a number of months and years following the procedure (12). On a very detailed analysis, the sites of increased pleurodesis-related PET activity usually correspond to "typical high-attenuation CT sites of pleurodesis change" on the underlying CT aspect of PET, however. Pleural disease recurrence/progression is usually shown by an increase in pleurally based soft tissue change on review of the underlying CT aspect of PET (as well as associated PET changes) and/or re-accumulation/a significant increase in pleural fluid volume.

PET is very useful for bone response evaluation, including post surgery and post radiotherapy, as described earlier. A potential pitfall when reporting PET studies is in the context of vertebroplasty procedures, however (35).

This is because "high attenuation" vertebroplasty cement (shown on the CT aspect) causes an "attenuation correction artefact" on PET studies, implying a "PET positive" appearance (reminiscent of active disease). Again, as always for appropriate patient data interpretation/reporting it is very important to analyse the underlying CT soft tissue and bone window appearances of PET/CT and not to just assess PET data in "isolation". If a high-attenuation typical "cement" appearance is seen on CT, then evaluation of the source "non-attenuation" corrected PET data on the workstation is appropriate. An "attenuation correction artefact signal" will not be seen on the source data. These steps will avoid the possibility of calling "false positive" sites of disease.

THE CONCEPT OF "OLIGOMETASTATIC" DISEASE

PET is critical for the appropriate selection of patients with metastatic breast cancer for novel treatment strategies such as surgery for "oligometastatic disease" (e.g., sternal disease resection and chest wall reconstruction) or planning potential liver RFA. PET is able to define the disease extent and is crucial for the detection of clinically important occult disease.

The use of novel techniques such as RFA has lead to improved patient quality of life, prolonged survival, reduced requirements for toxic systemic chemotherapy treatments, and improved overall outcomes (36).

Although metastatic breast cancer is by definition considered to be an "incurable" systemic condition, approaches such as RFA and surgery can be very effective in a small cohort of patients with metastatic breast cancer, sometimes rendering the patient in a radiological "Complete Remission" status for a number of months or years.

Patient pre-selection prior to these approaches is critical, however. If the patient is considered to have one site (or a couple of much localised sites) of metastatic disease, demonstrating stability over a period of time (or response), these novel procedures may be of therapeutic benefit. PET/CT is indicated prior to embarking upon potential surgical or RFA procedures in metastatic breast cancer patients, as PET is the most accurate modality which we currently have for defining the disease and occult disease extent, and therefore deciding whether these approaches (which have associated morbidity, affect patient expectations and hopes, and health and economic costs) are appropriate for any given patient. Our standard paradigm is therefore to perform a PET study prior to significant procedures such as chest wall/sternal surgical resection and reconstruction for what is considered to be "stable isolated sternal recurrence" for example; PET should also be used prior to liver RFA procedures. Unfortunately, we have seen a large number of patients referred from various centres where liver RFA was performed without PET as part of the patient work-up. This led to the underestimation of the disease, which was not visualised on single-phase CT or MRI. Follow-up imaging often revealed widespread metastatic disease with PET, which may have been present pre-procedure, but not detected with other modalities.

PET AND PROGNOSTICATION

In breast cancer PET will provide prognostic information on treatment responsiveness and whether the particular regimen can be used again in future for example, also highlighting when treatment resistance has developed.

PET can show treatment response to hormone and systemic chemotherapy. This provides very useful clinical information. For example, if a patient has a substantial "PET metabolic volume" and "PET metabolic intensity" (SUVmax) and early response to agents such as capecitabine, or vinorelbine/herceptin, or avastin, this provides useful treatment prognostic information. It implies that continued treatment with this regimen is reasonable and may be used again in future, in the event of patient relapse. Serial PET studies may be performed, to confirm ongoing treatment responsiveness, until PET shows that treatment resistance to a particular regimen has developed. "Resistance" to the particular regime can eventually develop after it has been used two to three times in a treatment pathway. In other cases the PET may show that the SUVmax levels do not change substantially, for example, the SUVmax may change from 10 to 9, in which case the patient is not particularly responsive to the particular regimen in question, and a different regimen may be considered.

Unfortunately, unlike the situation of PET in some other tumour types such as Hodgkin's lymphoma, PET will not provide prognostic information regarding "durability" of treatment response in breast cancer (37).

A patient may show a complete metabolic "switch off" of disease activity on PET imaging, for example (metabolic complete response/remission CR). The NPV of PET CR in Hodgkin's lymphoma is 82–90%. This does not apply for PET and breast cancer. A PET CR in breast cancer does not provide any prognostic information regarding the durability of response. Despite a PET CR, the patient's breast cancer can reactivate at any future time (Fig. 6). The key consideration after achieving PET CR in breast cancer is treatment consolidation and maintaining a non-toxic treatment strategy.

There is evidence to suggest that some prognostic information regarding durability of response can be obtained. Tateishi et al. retrospectively evaluated 102 patients with metastatic breast cancer with PET/CT before and after treatment. This study

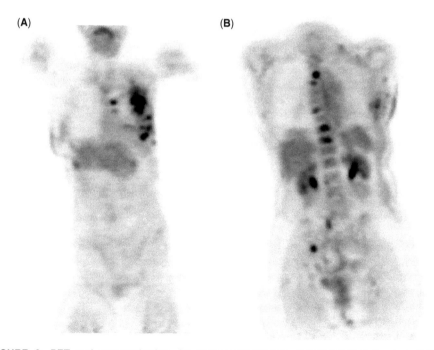

FIGURE 6 PET and prognostication. An 81-year-old woman, recent mastectomy and ALND, completely excised grade III IDC with associated DCIS, 2/16 nodes ER, PR, HER2⁺. (**A**, **B**) PET inverse grey scale coronal images, 5 months post op, unfortunately shows florid mastectomy bed and left anterolateral chest wall recurrence (SUVmax up to 10.7, a high intensity level), with scattered bony metastases, spine and pelvis (note physiological renal FDG excretion in addition). (*Continued*)

(C)   (D)

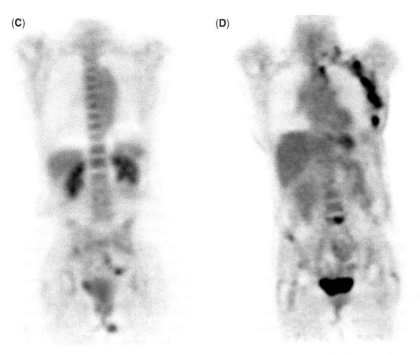

FIGURE 6 (*Continued*) (**C**) Inverse grey scale early response evaluation PET, 2 months post op. Capecitabine shows a dramatic complete metabolic response that is, confirming *prognostic exquisite chemo-responsiveness* to this treatment regimen. (**D**) PET unfortunately does not provide *prognostic information regarding durability* of response; follow-up PET 6 months later showed an extensive disease reactivation in the left anterolateral chest wall. Previous PET imaging had shown excellent responsiveness to capecitabine however; therefore, the patient was usefully rechallenged with capecitabine.

found a decrease in SUV after treatment was an independent predictor of response duration in patients with metastatic breast cancer who had bone metastases (38). However, in general terms, although PET will provide prognostic information as to whether a treatment regimen works, and when resistance is developing, it does not provide prognostic predictive information regarding the duration of response.

RECURRENT DISEASE
PET/CT is an extremely useful modality in defining and re-staging disease recurrence.

If equivocal conventional imaging findings are obtained, as opposed to repeating bone scan, ultrasound, CT, and MRI at an interval (e.g., 3–6 months), a PET/CT will very often provide a categorical answer regarding the disease status. PET is a very useful "diagnostic problem solving tool" in the context of indeterminate imaging findings/ indeterminate patient clinical status.

PET is not highly accurate in defining local recurrence in the breast due to the limitations as described for primary breast cancer, low grade tumours, and false-positive uptake. PET is currently the most accurate modality available to define metastatic disease recurrence and to re-stage metastatic disease extent, enabling evaluation of the soft tissue and bony sites with one test. PET/CT is particularly effective relative to other modalities in the context of defining bony disease recurrence, difficult to image sites (e.g., the brachial plexus, chest wall), post-surgery and post-radiotherapy (39–42) (Fig. 7).

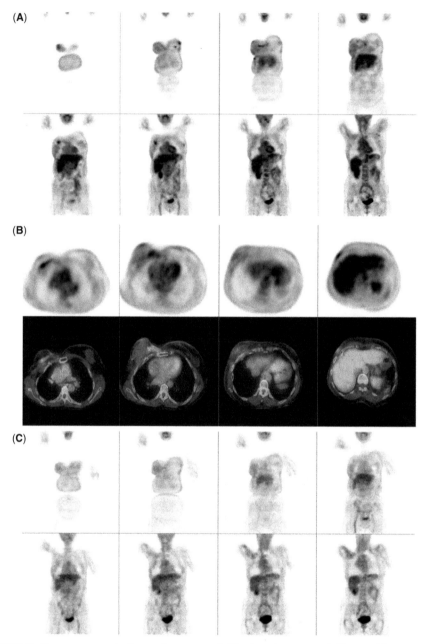

FIGURE 7 Recurrence, re-staging, and assessment of treatment response. A 69-year-old woman with known (biopsy proven) anterior chest wall recurrence of breast cancer. Re-staging PET/CT shows of the order of 12 focal sites of FDG uptake in the anterior chest wall (cutaneous/subcutaneous and related to chest wall musculature) together with FDG uptake in left axillary adenopathy; indicative of sites of disease recurrence. No visceral (pulmonary, hepatic) or bony sites of recurrence are defined however (1st and 2nd images). A subsequent follow-up PET/CT performed after Letrozole therapy (ER+ tumour) shows an excellent metabolic response, no metabolically active disease being defined on this study (confirming a very good clinical response). This study also demonstrates the utility of PET in "difficult to image sites", contrast-enhanced breast MRI being the only other imaging test which would reliably depict disease at this site; breast MRI not staging the remainder of the body and treatment response also being categorically shown on PET, "complete response" being a more difficult judgement on MRI.

PET is not highly accurate in the context of lobular disease (lobular histology disease often being "false negative" or low grade on [18]FDG PET imaging), but it is accurate with other breast cancer histological subtypes. Although PET is useful for detecting chest wall sites of disease (parasternal, subcutaneous, and intramuscular deposits), it is not accurate for cutaneous chest wall infiltration (where clinical visual inspection and punch biopsy are more accurate than [18]FDG PET).

In a systematic review involving 808 patients, Isasi et al. found PET to effectively detect recurrent disease, with a sensitivity of 90% and specificity of 87% (42).

In the "Recommendations on the use of FDG PET in Oncology" from the American Society of Clinical Oncology, the panel found its main benefit was avoiding futile surgery. Moderate evidence was found that PET improved health-care outcomes and to support the routine addition of PET to the work-up of detecting recurrent breast cancer (43).

Although MRI is clearly an accurate modality in the assessment of bony disease, PET has the advantage of being a whole-body technique, and is effective in the evaluation of indeterminate bony lesions. This also applies to soft tissue sites such as the brachial plexus. The differentiation of disease recurrence as opposed to radiation damage causing unilateral upper limb oedema is a not an uncommon clinical problem in the follow-up of patients with breast cancer. Although MRI will usually accurately define recurrent disease in this setting, it is well recognised that a small number of MRIs will be indeterminate (in these cases diffuse altered signal change usually being observed in the brachial plexus, e.g., diffuse high signal on the STIR sequence, as opposed to discrete "measurable" masses which would indicate disease recurrence). Hathaway et al. (44) assessed 10 patients with suspected locoregional disease involving the supraclavicular fossa/brachial plexus with MRI and PET. MRI was diagnostic for recurrence in five patients and indeterminate in four patients. PET positively identified tumour in all nine patients, being particularly helpful just outside the region of the axilla and in the chest wall (1 patient out of the 10 having concordant benign findings on both MRI and PET). In the situation of an equivocal/ "negative" MRI with a high index of clinical suspicion, PET is virtually always a useful problem solving test for the brachial plexus, accurately defining as to whether recurrent disease is present or not (radiation-induced fibrosis being "PET negative", whereas disease recurrence causing lymphoedema is "PET positive" (Fig. 8).

RISING/DISCORDANT TUMOUR MARKERS: UNCERTAIN SIGNIFICANCE
PET/CT is a useful technique for detecting recurrent disease in patients with elevated tumour marker levels of unknown cause. It is also of clinical use in the context of discordant tumour marker fluctuations and has an important clinical impact on the management of these patients.

PET/CT is indicated in the evaluation of patients with a tumour of unknown primary and for patients with the paraneoplastic syndrome. It is also useful in breast cancer in the context of patients with elevated CA 15-3, CA 19-9, CA 125, and/or CEA tumour marker levels in otherwise apparent remission/of uncertain significance (45–47).

Suarez et al. (45) performed PET in 45 women in apparent clinical and imaging remission from histologically proven breast cancer, in whom CA 15-3 and/ or CEA were elevated. PET results were validated by histological sampling wherever possible, otherwise by other imaging techniques (x-ray, ultrasound, CT, MRI) and/or by clinical follow-up of at least 12 months. Fifty-four sites of focal intense FDG uptake were shown in 27 patients (19 skeleton, 18 lymph node sites, 5 liver, 5 pelvic, 1 lung, 1 pericardium, 1 pleura, 1 contralateral breast, 2 peritoneum, and 1 thyroid bed), with 48 of these lesions subsequently being proved to be metastases. In 11 further patients

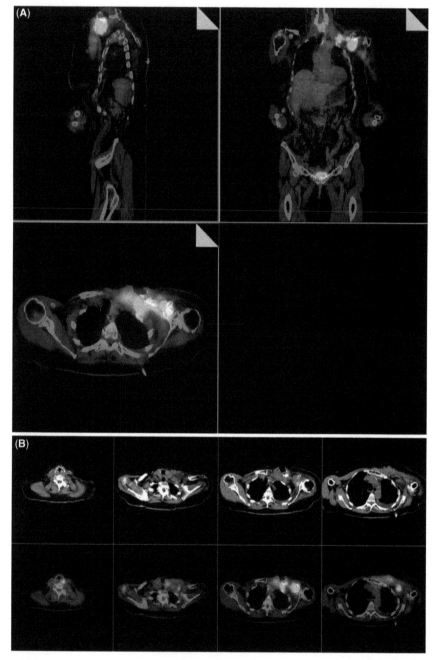

FIGURE 8 Disease recurrence. A patient with a 19-year "disease-free interval" after treatment (including radiotherapy) for a left-sided lobular breast cancer. Increasing left upper limb lymphoedema. Clinical evaluation, ultrasound, CT, MRI brachial plexus, and percutaneous biopsy negative/equivocal; ? recurrent breast cancer. PET/CT shows focal sites of intense FDG uptake in the left axilla/neck, indicative of sites of active tumour. Note the superficial (anterior) skin breakdown and ulceration shown in the left superior chest wall in addition (on the CT component of the PET/CT). The question of "disease recurrence or treatment/radiotherapy-related lymphoedema" usually occurs of the order of years after radiotherapy, PET therefore being an effective modality (some radiotherapy-related FDG uptake being observed for at least a few weeks after radiotherapy, however intense (benign) uptake certainly not usually being observed more than 6 months after radiotherapy).

9 true negative and 2 false-negative results were obtained. The sensitivity in this series was 92%, specificity 75%, PPV 89%, NPV 82%, and accuracy 87%. Liu et al. (46) retrospectively evaluated 30 patients in a similar series finding a sensitivity of 96% and accuracy of 90%.

In a study of 89 women with breast cancer and rising tumour markers, with negative clinical examination and conventional imaging, Grassetto et al. used PET/CT to identify active disease in 40 patients. Occult locations of disease were found in the chest wall, internal mammary nodes, lungs, liver, and bony skeleton (48).

PET is also useful in the context of discordant tumour marker levels, when certain tumour markers increase and others decrease. This can theoretically reflect discordant changes in bone and soft tissue disease status. For example, when bone disease status worsens/improves, while soft tissue disease status conversely improves/worsens. PET can be very useful in this situation, particularly given that patients may have been extensively pre-treated and there may be extensive liver and bone residual changes. The PET uptake can differentiate areas of metabolic progression from response and metabolic control.

CURRENT AND FUTURE PRACTICE

Given the current resource limitations of PET/CT, conventional work-up/assessment, bone scan and CT, currently remain the "workhorse" modalities to define metastatic/recurrent disease and assess treatment response. Clearly, CT is a suitable modality in a vast majority of patients (>99%) in this regard. We currently recommend that PET/CT should be performed in the following:

1. a small percentage of patients where there is true clinical/imaging equivocation/uncertainty regarding recurrent/metastatic disease status (and where clinical management will be influenced by the result), as PET is very useful in this regard as a diagnostic problem-solving tool;
2. where treatment response cannot be reliably assessed by other means, PET provides a useful signal for response evaluation.

A further important development is the development of more tumour-specific radiotracers suitable for clinical practice. Exciting ligands, which are currently under research development, include radiolabelled antibodies targeting the HER2/neu receptor and markers of apoptosis such as annexin V have also been tested in preclinical studies (49).

FLT, a marker of cell proliferation has been tested in clinical studies and may have a role in detecting early treatment response. FES, a radioligand of oestrogen receptors has also been tested in clinical studies and may have a role in distinguishing hormone-sensitive tumours from hormone-resistant ones (50,51). The advent of tumour-specific radiotracers will imply that PET/CT imaging will be more powerful again, enabling receptor-specific targeting, with receptor-targeted drug delivery.

As PET/CT becomes more widely available, patient management pathways will change, and PET/CT is likely to be used early and extensively in the management of patients with metastatic breast cancer. Functional imaging will have an increasing role to play in patient management in years to come.

CONCLUSION

PET/CT is fundamental for the appropriate and optimal management of breast cancer patients. With current clinical radiotracers and technology it is not accurate enough to be used in routine clinical practice in the context of primary breast disease/axillary nodal assessment, conventional work-up remaining the gold standard (although PET when performed in a breast cancer patient will provide useful primary breast and axillary staging information in a significant number of patients). However, the converse is true regarding defining recurrent disease, re-staging metastatic disease extent, and for treatment response assessment; PET proves to be a very useful diagnostic imaging problem solving tool in the context of imaging or clinical uncertainty. PET/CT is currently the most accurate imaging modality available for defining recurrent/metastatic disease, a key advantage being a whole-body assessment (soft tissue, nodal, visceral, and bony sites) with one test. Despite the fact that current ^{18}F-FDG PET/CT cannot rule out microscopic disease, it does provide a reliable assessment of the true extent of macroscopic metabolically active disease. It is also a highly effective and useful test to define treatment response, key strengths being early response assessment and the differentiation of active from inactive disease sites. Bony response assessment is a particularly exciting area—this being difficult with other imaging approaches. As PET/CT resource becomes more widely available in the coming years, it is likely that patient management pathways will change, with PET/CT being increasingly widely used early in the breast cancer disease course.

REFERENCES

1. Brown RS, Wahl RL. Over expression of Glut-1 glucose transporter in human breast cancer: an immunohistochemical study. Cancer 1993; 72: 2979–85.
2. Stadnik TW, Everaert H, Makkat S, et al. Breast imaging. Preoperative breast cancer staging: comparison of USPIO-enhanced MR imaging and 18F-fluorodeoxyglucose (FDC) positron emission tomography (PET) imaging for axillary lymph node staging–initial findings. Eur Radiol 2006; 16: 2153–60.
3. Avril N, Rose CA, Schelling M, et al. Breast imaging with positron emission tomography and fluorine –18 fluorodeoxyglucose: use and limitations. J Clin Oncol 2000; 18: 3495–502.
4. Kumar R, Chauhan A, Zhuang H, et al. Clinicopathologic factors associated with false negative FDG-PET in primary breast cancer. Breast Cancer Res Treat 2006; 98: 267–74.
5. Wahl RL, et al. Prospective multicentre study of axillary nodal staging by positron emission tomography in breast cancer: a report of the staging breast cancer by PET Study Group. J Clin Oncol 2004; 22: 277–85.
6. Basu S, Chen W, Tchou J, et al. Comparison of triple-negative and estrogen receptor-positive/progesterone receptor-positive/ HER2-negative breast carcinoma using quantitative fluorine-18 fluorodeoxyglucose/positron emission tomography imaging parameters: a potentially useful method for disease characterization. Cancer 2008; 112: 995–1000.
7. Groheux D, Giacchetti S, Rubello D, et al. The evolving role of PET/CT in breast cancer. Nucl Med Commun 2010; 31: 271–3.
8. Basu S, Saboury B, Werner T, et al. Clinical utility of FDG-PET and PET/CT in non-malignant thoracic disorders. Mol Imaging Biol 2010. [Epub ahead of print].
9. Love C, Din AS, Tomas MB, et al. Radionuclide bone imaging: an illustrative review. Radiographics 2003; 23: 341–58.
10. Kwee TC, Takahara T, Ochiai R, et al. Whole-body diffusion-weighted magnetic resonance imaging. Eur J Radiol 2009; 70: 409–17.
11. Cook GJ, Houston S, Rubens R, et al. Detection of bone metastases in breast cancer by 18FDG PET: differing metabolic activity in osteoblastic and osteolytic lesions. J Clin Oncol 1998; 16: 3375–9.
12. Constantinidou A, Martin A, Sharma B, et al. Positron emission tomography/computed tomography in the management of recurrent/metastatic breast cancer: a large retrospective study from the Royal Marsden Hospital. Ann Oncol 2010. [Epub ahead of print].
13. Nakai T, Okuyama C, Kubota T, et al. Pitfalls of FDG-PET for the diagnosis of osteoblastic bone metastases in patients with breast cancer. Eur J Nucl Med Mol Imaging 2005; 32: 1253–8.
14. Morris PG, Lynch C, Feeney JN, et al. Integrated positron emission tomography/computed tomography may render bone scintgraphy unnecessary to investigate suspected metastatic breast cancer. J Clin Oncol 2010; 28: 3154–9.

15. Heusner TA, Kuemmel S, Koeninger A, et al. Diagnostic value of diffusion weighted magnetic resonance imaging (DWI) compared to FDG PET/CT for whole-body breast cancer staging. Eur J Nucl Med Mol Imaging 2010; 37: 1077–86.
16. Grankvist J, Fisker R, Iyer V, et al. MRI and PET/CT of patients with bone metastases from breast carcinoma. Eur J Radiol 2011. [Epub ahead of print]
17. Shimada K, Nakamoto Y, Isoda H, et al. FDG PET for giant cavernous hemangioma: important clue to differentiate from a malignant vascular tumor in the liver. Clin Nucl Med 2010; 35: 924–6.
18. Kitajima K, Nakamoto Y, Okizuka H, et al. Accuracy of whole-body FDG-PET/CT for detecting brain metastases from non-central nervous system tumors. Ann Nucl Med 2008; 22: 595–602.
19. Lartigau E, Mirabel X, Prevost B, et al. Extracranial stereotactic radiotherapy: preliminary results with the CyberKnife. Onkologie 2009; 32: 209–15.
20. Zhang M, Jiang X, Zhang M, et al. The role of 18F-FDG PET/CT in the evaluation of Ascites of Undetermined Origin. J Nucl Med 2009; 50: 506–12.
21. Rajagopalan MS, Heron DE. Role of PET/CT imaging in stereotactic body radiotherapy. Future Oncol 2010; 6: 305–17.
22. Heron DE, Andrade RS, Beriwal S, Smith RP. PET-CT in radiation oncology: the impact on diagnosis, treatment planning, and assessment of treatment response. Am J Clin Oncol 2008; 31: 352–62.
23. Dose Schwarz J, Bader M, Jenicke L, et al. Early prediction of response to chemotherapy in metastatic breast cancer using sequential 18F-FDG PET. J Nucl Med 2005; 46: 1144–50.
24. Gennari A, Donati S, Salvadori B, et al. Role of 2-(18F)-fluorodeoxyglucose (FDG) positron emission tomography (PET) in the early assessment of response. Clin Breast Cancer 2000; 1: 156–61.
25. Straver ME, Aukema TS, Olmos RA, et al. Feasibility of FDG PET/CT to monitor the response of axillary lymph node metastases to neoadjuvant chemotherapy in breast cancer patients. Eur J Nucl Mol Imaging 2010; 37: 1069–76.
26. Choi JH, Lim HI, Lee SK, et al. The role of PET CT to evaluate the response to neoadjuvant chemotherapy in advanced breast cancer: comparison with ultrasonography and magnetic resonance imaging. J Surg Oncol 2009; doi:10.1002/jso.21424.
27. Nair N, Ali A, Dowlatshahi K, et al. Positron emission tomography with fluorine-18 fluorodeoxyglucose to evaluate response of early breast carcinoma treated with stereotaxic interstitial laser therapy. Clin Nucl Med 2000; 25: 505–7.
28. Carditello A, Scisca C, David A, et al. Radiofrequency ablation in primary and secondary liver tumours. Chir Hal 2002; 54: 83–6.
29. Donkier V, Van Laethem JL, Goldman S, et al. (F-18) fluorodeoxyglucose positron emission tomography as a tool for early recognition of incomplete tumour destruction after radiofrequency ablation for liver metastases. J Surg Oncol 2003; 84: 215–23.
30. Cook GJ. PET and PET/CT imaging of skeletal metastases. Cancer Imaging 2010; 10: 1–8.
31. Stafford SE, Gralow JR, Schubert EK, et al. Use of serial FDG-PET to measure the response of bone-dominant breast cancer to therapy. Acad Radiol 2002; 9: 913–21.
32. Chua S, Gnanasegaran G, Cook GJ. Miscellaneous cancers (lung, thyroid, renal cancer, myeloma, and neuroendocrine tumors): role of SPECT and PET in imaging bone metastases. Semin Nucl Med 2009; 39: 416–30.
33. Bussink J, Kaanders JH, van der Graaf WT, et al. PET-CT for radiotherapy treatment planning and response monitoring in solid tumors. Nat Rev Clin Oncol 2011. [Epub ahead of print].
34. Grigsby PW. Role of PET in gynecologic malignancy [review]. Curr Opin Oncol 2009; 21: 420–4.
35. Kuo PH, Cheng DW. Artifactual spinal metastases imaged by PET/CT: a case report. J Nucl Med Technol 2005; 33: 230–1.
36. Purandare NC, Rangarajan V, Shah SA, et al. Therapeutic response to radiofrequency ablation of neoplastic lesions: FDG PET/CT findings. Radiographics 2011; 31: 201–13.
37. Dunleavy K, Mikhaeel G, Sehn LH, et al. The value of positron emission tomography in prognosis and response assessment in non-Hodgkin lymphoma. Leuk Lymphoma 2010; 51(Suppl 1): 28–33.

38. Tateishi U, Gamez C, Dawood S, et al. Bone metastases in patients with metastatic breast cancer: morphologic and metabolic monitoring of response to systemic therapy with integrated PET/CT. Radiology 2008; 247: 189–96.
39. Lonneux M, Borbath I, Berliere M, et al. The place of whole-body PET FDG for the diagnosis of distant recurrence of breast cancer. Clin Positron Imaging 2000; 3: 45–9.
40. Gallowititsch HJ, Kresnik E, Gasser J, et al. F-18 fluorodeoxyglucose positron-emission tomography in the diagnosis of tumour recurrence and metastases in the follow-up of patients with breast carcinoma; a comparison to conventional imaging. Invest Radiol 2003; 38: 250–6.
41. Eubank WB, Mankoff D, Bhattacharya M, et al. Impact of FDG PET on defining the extent of disease and on the treatment of patients with recurrent or metastatic breast cancer. AJR 2004; 183: 479–85.
42. Isasi CR, Moadel RM, Blaofox MD. A meta-analysis of FDG-PET for the evaluation of breast cancer recurrence and metastases. Breast Cancer Res Treat 2005; 90: 105–12.
43. Fletcher JW, Djulbegovic B, Soares HP, et al. Recommendations on the use of 18F-FDG PET in oncology. J Nucl Med 2008; 49: 480–508.
44. Hathaway PB, Mankoff DA, Maravilla KR, et al. Value of combined FDG PET and MR imaging in the evaluation of suspected recurrent local-regional breast cancer: preliminary experience. Radiology 1999; 210: 807–14.
45. Suarez M, Perez-Castejon MJ, Jimenez A, et al. Early diagnosis of recurrent breast cancer with FDG-PET in patients with progressive elevation of serum tumour markers. Q J Nucl Med 2002; 46: 113–21.
46. Liu CS, Shen YY, Lin CC, et al. Clinical impact of (18)F FDG-PET in patients with suspected recurrent breast cancer based on asymptomatically elevated tumour marker serum levels: a preliminary report. Jpn J Clin Oncol 2002; 32: 244–7.
47. Siggelkow W, Rath W, Buell U, et al. FDG PET and tumour markers in the diagnosis of recurrent and metastatic breast cancer. Eur J Nucl Med Mol Imaging 2004; 31(Suppl 1): S118–24.
48. Grassetton G, Fornasiero A, Otello D, et al. (18)F-FDG-PET/CT in patients with breast cancer and rising Ca 15-3 with negative conventional imaging: a multicentre study. Eur J Radiol 2010; doi:10.1016/j.ejrad.2010.04.029.
49. Yagle KJ, Eary JF, Tait JF, et al. Evaluation of 18F-annexin V as a PET imaging agent in an animal model of apoptosis. J Nucl Med 2005; 46: 658–66.
50. Kenny L, Coombes RC, Vigushin DM, et al. Imaging early changes in proliferation at 1 week post chemotherapy: a pilot study in breast cancer patients with 30-deoxy-30-[18F] fluorothymidine positron emission tomography. Eur J Nucl Med Mol Imaging 2007; 34: 1339–47.
51. Peterson LM, Mankoff DA, Lawton T, et al. Quantitative imaging of estrogen receptor expression in breast cancer with PET and 18F-fluoroestradiol. J Nucl Med 2008; 49: 367–74.

Novel biomarker approaches for improving therapeutic strategies in metastatic breast cancer

Roberta Ferraldeschi and Gerhardt Attard

INTRODUCTION

Breast cancer is a heterogeneous disease that encompasses several distinct entities with different biological characteristics and clinical behaviors. Currently, treatment decisions for metastatic breast cancer patients are made based on a small number of well-established molecular biomarkers, including the oestrogen receptor (ER), progesterone receptor (PR), and the human epidermal growth receptor 2 (HER2), as well as clinicopathological features. The biological importance of these established biomarkers has been reinforced over the last decade with the identification of discrete genetic subtypes of breast cancer with distinct prognoses (section "Established Biomarkers" and chap 4) (1,2). Advances in high throughput technologies including proteomics, expression array technologies, copy number measurements, and most recently next generation sequencing, will significantly increase the potential to identify a variety of biomarkers and assign single tumours to specific molecular subgroups, even when small amounts of tumour tissue are available (3). Furthermore, the study of circulating biomarkers (section "Circulating Biomarkers") offers the promise of analysing tumours comprehensively at the molecular level in "real-time" without subjecting patients to multiple clinical interventions to obtain tissue. This chapter will focus on recent advances in biomarker research, especially the use of circulating biomarkers, and will give some examples as to how these could impact the management of breast cancer patients.

TYPES OF BIOMARKERS AND THEIR APPLICATION

A biomarker is a characteristic that is objectively measured as an indicator of normal biological or pathogenic processes, or pharmacological responses to a therapeutic intervention. Prior to the routine use of a biomarker in clinical practice, a biomarker requires analytical and clinical validation. Analytical validation establishes the performance characteristics and the range of conditions under which an assay gives reproducible and accurate data; certification by an accredited authority is usually required. Clinical validation refers to the process of linking a biomarker with biological processes or clinical endpoints in the context of the intended use. In the clinic, biomarkers could be used for patient selection for treatment based upon an estimation of the natural history of the disease (prognostic biomarkers) or an estimation of probability of response to a specific agent (predictive biomarkers) (Table 1). In practice, many biomarkers have both predictive and prognostic impact as, for example ER and HER2. Predictive biomarkers are potentially the most useful for clinical decision-making, providing an estimate of probability of response to therapy or risk of unacceptable toxicity. Therefore, such biomarkers may reduce late-stage drug attrition in clinical trials and help control health economic costs. In the early clinical drug development process, biomarkers can also be used to measure pharmacokinetic parameters of drug exposure or pharmacodynamic endpoints of drug effect that can be used to guide dose selection (4). In later stages of drug development, biomarkers can be used as surrogate endpoints to identify treatment efficacy and clinical benefit at an earlier time point than would be required to attain the traditional clinical endpoints

TABLE 1 Application of Biomarkers in the Clinical Management of Cancer Patients

Prognostic biomarkers	Indicate the probability of a specific clinical outcome, such as recurrence, progression, or survival independent from treatment
Predictive biomarkers/classifiers	Identify the chance of response to a specific therapy and allow enrichment with patient sub-groups more likely to have disease sensitive to a therapy
Response indicators	Monitor response and could assist in "stop vs. continue" treatment decisions
Pharmacokinetic biomarkers	Measure pharmacokinetic parameters of drug exposure
Pharmacodynamic biomarkers	Measure endpoints of drug effect on target, pathway, and downstream biological processes
Intermediate endpoint biomarkers	Reflect treatment efficacy and clinical benefit at an earlier time point than would be required to attain the traditional clinical endpoints

(i.e., intermediate/surrogate endpoint biomarkers). The use of surrogates is aimed at accelerating trial completion and minimising cost, patient numbers, and risk of failure and is routinely used in several fields outside cancer. Finally, biomarker studies may also identify the development or cause of treatment resistance in patients receiving a therapy, such as loss of expression of the target or secondary site mutations, thus allowing treatment discontinuation or combination with a second therapy.

TUMOUR TISSUE–BASED BIOMARKERS
Established Biomarkers
ER status has been used since the mid-1970s in the clinical management of breast cancer patients and undoubtedly remains the most important prognostic factor and predictive marker for response to endocrine therapy (chap 3). ER status therefore forms part of the U.K. minimum dataset for histopathology reporting of invasive breast cancer (5). ER is routinely determined on all invasive breast cancers and reported using a standardised technique. However, up to 40% of ER-positive metastatic breast cancers respond to endocrine therapy (6), and additional predictive biomarkers are required. The expression of PR is strongly dependent on the presence of ER and in fact ER-negative PR-positive tumours, which represent up to 5% of patients, should undergo re-testing of their ER status to eliminate false ER negativity (7). Although some studies have reported ER-positive tumours weakly expressing PR respond poorly to tamoxifen, the predictive value of PR status for response to aromatase inhibitors remains unclear (7,8). Some have argued for discontinuation of routine PR testing but this is controversial, especially given that PR-positive ER-negative patients could benefit from hormone therapy (7,9). Another well-established predictive biomarker is HER2. The observation that overexpression of HER2 was present in approximately one quarter of breast cancers and was associated with worse prognosis (10) led to the biomarker-driven use of trastuzumab in patients with tumour overexpression or amplification of HER2 (11). Analytically validated protocols for immunohistochemistry and *in situ* hybridisation techniques for defining HER2 status as a predictive biomarker for anti-HER2 therapy (chap 4) are well established (12).

Emerging Biomarkers
An emerging example of a biomarker-driven therapeutic strategy is the selection of patients with a BRCA1 or BRCA2 mutant tumour for treatment with a

poly(ADP-ribose) polymerase (PARP) inhibitor (chap 5). PARP is involved in the repair of single-strand DNA breaks, and inhibition of the enzyme results in an impairment of DNA repair and an augmentation in the number of double-strand DNA breaks. Both BRCA1- and BRCA2-mutated tumours have a defect in homologous DNA repair and pre-clinical models demonstrated PARP inhibition was especially detrimental to cells with no intact BRCA1 or BRCA2 function (so-called synthetic lethality) (13). Phase I and II studies confirmed these pre-clinical observations (14,15) and phase III trials of PARP inhibitors in BRCA-mutant cancers are anticipated. Several groups are also now evaluating biomarkers of sensitivity to PARPi and other synthetic lethal approaches in sporadic cancers (16).

It is unlikely that a single biomarker will be sufficiently sensitive to effectively predict response, especially in the presence of complex redundant signalling networks that can rapidly cause resistance. For example, approximately one-third of HER2-positive tumours respond to trastuzumab monotherapy (17) and the majority of patients with HER2-positive metastatic breast cancer who initially respond to trastuzumab or lapatinib will eventually develop disease progression. Efforts are therefore ongoing to develop panels of biomarkers that include both predictors of response and resistance. A number of candidate biomarkers that associate with resistance have been identified, for example aberrant activation of the PI3K/AKT pathway downstream of HER2 secondary to activating mutations of PI3K or loss of function of PTEN (18). However, it is probable that a comprehensive evaluation of resistance mechanisms will be required as evaluation of solely one biomarker, for example PTEN loss, is unlikely to identify all tumours resistant to HER2-targeting therapies (19). Also, biomarker panels could be increasingly drug specific, as for example, truncated forms of the HER2 receptor known as p95HER2 that lack the trastuzumab-binding domain but retain tyrosine kinase activity and are detected in 20–40% of HER2-positive tumours cause resistance to trastuzumab but not to lapatinib (20,21).

Proliferation is a key hallmark of cancer and can be evaluated by the immunohistochemical assessment of the nuclear antigen Ki-67. Several studies have investigated the use of Ki-67 as a prognostic and predictive biomarker in early and locally advanced breast cancer (22). Studies in the neoadjuvant setting suggest that a change in Ki67 could predict benefit from treatment and on-treatment Ki-67 measurements could be superior predictors of long-term outcome than pre-treatment levels (23). The peri-operative endocrine treatment for individualising care (POETIC) trial is evaluating whether the measurement of Ki-67 after 2 weeks of pre-surgical treatment with an aromatase inhibitor is sufficiently predictive of outcome to warrant its introduction into routine clinical practice.

Multigene Signatures

The underlying genetic basis for the clinical and biological heterogeneity of breast cancer has been confirmed by pioneer studies with gene expression profiling from patient tumour samples. These studies have demonstrated that breast cancer can be divided into at least five distinct molecular subtypes (so-called intrinsic subtypes): hormone receptor (HR)-positive luminal A and B, HER2-positive, basal-like, and normal-like breast cancer (1) (chap 2). These subtypes have different histopathological, molecular, and clinical features and require different therapeutic approaches (Table 2). However, although whole-genome expression profiling is a powerful tool in population-based studies, assignment of a single tumour to a specific molecular sub-type based on currently used methodologies is largely inaccurate and more stringent definitions are required to allow incorporation into routine clinical practice and treatment decision-making (2). Also, the differences between luminal A and B are very subtle and controversy surrounds the true definition of "normal-like" breast

TABLE 2   General Characteristics of Breast Cancer Subtypes

Luminal A	ER$^+$ and/or PR$^+$, HER2$^-$, low Ki-67
Luminal B	ER$^+$ and/or PR$^+$, HER2$^+$ (or HER2$^-$ with high Ki67)
HER2	ER$^-$, PR$^-$, HER2$^+$
Basal like	ER$^-$, PR$^-$, HER2$^-$, cytokeratin 5/6$^+$ and/or EGFR$^+$

Abbreviations: EGFR, epidermal growth factor receptor; ER, oestrogen receptor; HER2, human epidermal growth factor receptor; PR, progesterone receptor.

TABLE 3   Selected Prognostic Multigene Signatures in Breast Cancer

Signature	Platform	Number of genes	Type of tissue samples
MammaPrint	Microarray	70	Fresh frozen
Rotterdam Signature	Microarray	76	Fresh frozen
Genomic grade index	Microarray	97	Fresh frozen
Mammostrat	IHC	5	FFPE
Oncotype DX	qRT-PCR	21	FFPE

Abbreviations: FFPE, formalin-fixed paraffin embedded; IHC, immunohistochemistry; qRT-PCR, quantitative reverse transcriptase-polymerase chain reaction.

cancer that may be an artefact of tumour contaminated by high normal cell content (2). Moreover, gene expression profile analysis is technically challenging and costly, especially when only small amounts of poor-quality tumour tissue are available. A number of multigene classifiers and outcome predictors have been introduced to date, but none has become universally accepted, although several have been analytically and clinically validated and commercialised (Table 3). The multigene assays, 21-gene recurrence score Oncotype DX® (Genomic Health, CA, USA) and 70-gene signature MammaPrint® (Agendia BV, The Netherlands; and Agendia, Inc., CA, USA) are the most widely used.

In February 2007, Agendia's MammaPrint became the first *in vitro* diagnostic multivariate index assay to receive clearance from the FDA. Specifically, the 70-gene microarray-based test was originally developed as a general prognostic test in untreated patients with lymph node-negative disease and validated retrospectively on a set of 295 patients including both lymph node-positive and -negative disease (24). It gauges the risk of breast recurrence within 5 years following surgery, and stratifies patients into either low risk or high risk of distant recurrence. The real-time PCR-based Oncotype DX was designed to improve prediction of the risk of distant recurrence in patients with ER-positive, node-negative cancers treated with tamoxifen. It assesses the expression of 21 genes and yields a recurrence score (RS) between 0 and 100, which correlates with metastatic disease within 10 years. A high RS was also found to predict the benefit from adjuvant chemotherapy in ER-positive, tamoxifen-treated patients (25,26). Oncotype DX is similar to MammaPrint in that both tests place their highest weight on gene expression in three major pathways: proliferation, ER, and HER2. However, Oncotype DX has the advantages of ease of use on formalin-fixed paraffin-embedded tissues and the ability to serve as both a prognostic test and predictive test for certain chemotherapeutic agents. Two large, prospective trials are ongoing that aim to evaluate the clinical usefulness of both tools in comparison with the existing clinical prognostic tools: the Microarray in Node-Negative Disease May Avoid Chemotherapy (MINDACT) trial for MammaPrint, and the Trial Assigning Individualized Options for Treatment (TAILORx) trial for Oncotype DX.

CIRCULATING BIOMARKERS
Circulating Tumour Cells

For metastases to develop, it is probable that tumour cell dissemination occurs prior to primary therapy. A number of studies conducted through the 1980s and 1990s identified a significant association between the presence of bone marrow micrometastases in breast cancer patients with no radiological evidence of local disease or distant metastases and disease-free survival (DFS) and overall survival (OS) (27). However interestingly, not all patients with bone marrow micrometastases died from their breast cancer. Moreover, the invasive nature of serial bone marrow aspirates limits their clinical utility. It can be hypothesised that for blood-borne metastases to develop, cells must circulate through blood, introducing the possibility that circulating tumour cells (CTC) could be identified in and extracted from a blood sample. This has led to vast research investment in the field of CTC studies in the past decade, with an exponential increase in the number of papers published and clinical studies conducted (28). The mechanisms that underlie the existence of cancer cells in blood are poorly understood but most sources agree on estimates that when present, the concentration is in the order of one in a billion normal cells (29). The technological challenge of isolating such rare events is obvious. Ideally, a platform for capturing CTC should be highly sensitive (detects every single circulating cancer cell), very specific (does not define events as CTC when they are not: this can be initially evaluated by studies in healthy volunteers when detection of any event is assumed to be a false positive) and reproducible (with minimal intra- and inter-operator variability). Furthermore, although the presence of CTC may give prognostic information, the impact on clinical practice could be greater if this is combined with molecular characterisation studies. To allow these analyses, a CTC isolation platform will ideally isolate a highly pure CTC-containing sample with no or minimal contaminating normal cells (e.g., leukocytes) and preserve CTC viability, morphology, protein, and nucleic acids. Finally, for widespread use a CTC isolation platform needs to be well priced, allowing low-cost, high-throughput processing of samples with minimal operator time requirements.

Aiming to achieve these requirements, CTC isolation technology platforms have attempted to exploit characteristics specific to CTC. CTC enrichment strategies can be broadly divided into positive (capture of cells with characteristics specific to CTC) or negative selection (capture of cells with features not shared by CTC, for example the capture and depletion of CD45-positive cells). The first platform to achieve robust clinical and analytical validation is CellSearch™, developed by Immunicon and now owned and distributed by Veridex (NJ, U.S.A.). As the first and to date the only CTC isolation platform to achieve FDA clearance for the prognostic evaluation of breast, colorectal, and prostate cancer patients, CellSearch has set the standard for CTC isolation and enumeration. CellSearch uses EpCAM-bound ferrofluids to capture all EpCAM-expressing events in a magnetic field. This has the potential advantage of utilising all EpCAM antigens on the three-dimensional surface of a CTC and has shown successful capture of cells within a wide range of expression of cell-surface EpCAM antigens (30). A second "CTC identification" step is required that uses permeabilisation and immunofluorescence with a nuclear stain [4',2- diamidino-2-phenylindole, dihydrochloride (DAPI)], an antibody staining CK 8, 18, and 19 and an antibody to CD45. The images of all captured events are then displayed to operators centrally trained by the distributing company (Veridex) who identify and count all cells that meet a definition for a CTC that was established during the development of this platform. This definition involves enumerating only CTCs that are positive for CK 8, 18, or 19, negative for CD45, at least $4 \times 4\ \mu m^2$ in size and have an intra-cellular DAPI-staining nucleus. Using this definition, <0.3% of healthy volunteers have two or more CTCs in 7.5 mL blood (Fig. 1) (31).

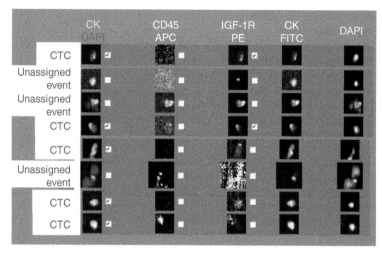

FIGURE 1 EpCAM-positive events captured by CellSearch and as presented to operators in the browser window. Examples of CTC are shown that stain positive for cytokeratin, negative for CD45, have an intracellular DAPI-staining nucleus and are at least 4 μm in size. Events that do not meet these criteria are termed "unassigned events". IGF-1R immunofluorescence has also been utilised to identify IGF-1R-positive (marked boxes) and IGF-1R-negative CTC. *Source*: Adapted from Ref. 50.

Circulating Tumour Cell Enumeration

The first prospective, multicentre study to be conducted using CellSearch was in 177 advanced breast cancer patients with progressive, measurable metastatic disease and due to commence a new systemic therapy (32). This study was industry-sponsored by Immunicon but subsequent academic studies have reported similar findings. Using a training set of 102 patients, the median progression-free survival (PFS) of patients with CTC counts above or below 1, 2, 3, 4, 5 and so on per 7.5 ml of blood prior to start of treatment, was calculated using a Cox proportional-hazards model. A plateau in Cox hazard ratio was reached at approximately ≥5 CTCs per 7.5 ml of blood, which was selected to identify two similarly-sized patient sub-groups with significantly different outcomes. The median OS of the favourable group (<5 CTC/7.5 mL) prior to start of treatment was 21.9 months and the median OS of the unfavourable group (≥5 CTC/7.5 mL) was 10.9 months that were significantly different (p < 0.0001) (Table 4) (33). Similarly the PFS was significantly different for the favourable and unfavourable groups, namely 2.1 versus 7 months (32). Moreover, using multivariate Cox regression analysis a CTC count ≥5 versus <5 both prior to start of treatment (HR = 4.26, p < 0.001) and after once cycle of treatment (HR = 6.49, p < 0.001) was the parameter most significantly associated with OS when a wide range of clinical variables were considered, including HER2 status, type of therapy, and performance status (PS). The clinical value of a prognostic tool for patients who require treatment for their metastatic disease is however limited as it does not usually change physicians' practice. Of greater interest is the evaluation of CTC count after one cycle of treatment. The median OS of patients whose CTC count remained <5 CTC/7.5 mL was 22.6 months and for patients with ≥5 CTC/7.5mL after one cycle of treatment the median OS was 4.1 months. Patients who had a decline in count from ≥5 to <5 had an improvement in their median OS to 19.8 months and similarly, the median OS of patients whose CTC count rose from <5 to ≥5 declined to 10.6 months (33) (Fig. 2). These observations introduce the interesting possibility that a change in CTC count after solely one cycle of treatment from an unfavourable to a favourable

TABLE 4 Median Overall Survival in Patients with Metastatic Breast Cancer Commencing a New Line of Therapy Split by Circulating Tumour Cell Count Enumerated Using CellSearch (32,33)

	Total number of patients	From blood draw prior to commencement of cytotoxic treatment		Difference between 2 groups	At 3 weeks after commencement of treatment			
		Favourable group (<5 CTC/7.5 mL)	Unfavourable group (≥5 CTC/7.5 mL)	Log rank P value	Remained favourable	Remained unfavourable	Favourable converted to unfavourable	Unfavourable converted to favourable
Median overall survival (months)	177	21.9	10.9	<0.0001	22.6	4.1	10.6	19.8

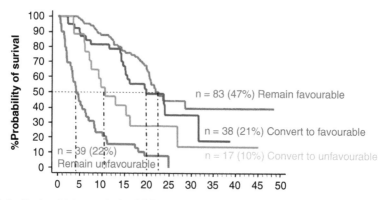

FIGURE 2 Kaplan–Meier analysis dividing patients with metastatic breast cancer, due to start a new treatment, into four groups based on CTC count. Remain Favourable: <5 CTC/7.5 mL remain <5 CTC/7.5 mL after one cycle of treatment. Convert to Favourable: ≥5 CTC/7.5 mL decline to <5 CTC/7.5 mL on treatment; Convert to Unfavourable: <5 CTC/7.5 mL increase to ≥5 CTC/7.5 mL; Remain Unfavourable: ≥5 CTC/7.5 mL remain ≥5 CTC/7.5 mL on treatment. *Source*: Courtesy of Professor Leon Terstappen, University of Twente, The Netherlands.

value is associated with treatment benefit, while conversion to, or persistence of an unfavourable CTC count suggests treatment failure. In addition to giving an earlier read-out, CTC enumeration is subject to significantly less inter-reader variability than imaging (34). Prospective studies in advanced breast cancer are currently evaluating whether an early change in treatment is indicated for patients whose CTC count rises (e.g., http://www.cancer.gov/clinicaltrials/SWOG-S0500).

Better risk-stratification of patients with early disease who are scheduled to receive or have received radical treatment to their primary tumour into those who will not relapse with haematogenous metastases (no detectable CTC) versus those with a high chance of relapsing could improve on current paradigms for selecting patients for adjuvant treatment. Predictably, CTCs are less prevalent in early breast cancer with ≥1 CTC/7.5 mL detected using CellSearch in up to 25% of patients and ≥5 CTC/7.5 mL detected in <5% of patients (35–37). There was no concordance between CTC count and clinicopathological variables except for HER2-positivity that is associated with a higher prevalence of CTC. Importantly, these early reports suggest a worse outcome for patients with detectable CTC after completing adjuvant chemotherapy. It is probable that additional molecular characterisation studies that specifically identify CTCs which have the potential to form metastases would further improve on the prognostic potential of unselected enumeration. Also, the detection rate in early disease could be improved by analysing larger volumes of blood, for example 30 mL. CTC evaluation in the (neo)adjuvant setting is currently under clinical evaluation in a number of multicentre studies.

The use of a dichotomous variable may miss important information: for example, a decline in CTC count from >200 to 6 would not result in conversion from an unfavourable to a favourable group but may signify treatment benefit. Attempts have therefore been made to evaluate the association between CTC count as a continuous variable and robust clinical endpoints (38). Although there is very high concordance of CTC counts between different operators at low CTC numbers, the inter- and intra-operator variability appears to increase with higher CTC counts (33). To this effect, algorithm-driven software is being developed that could allow automation of CTC enumeration that in addition to minimising operator time (and therefore cost) will eliminate high CTC count variability. Also interestingly, preliminary reports suggest that less stringent definitions for what constitutes a CTC, including for example CK-positive, CD45-negative "fragments" that lack a nucleus, are also significantly associated with OS despite the presence of significant, albeit lower numbers, of these events in healthy volunteers (39). A potential benefit of using a less stringent definition for CTC is the potential to identify significant numbers of events in more patients, especially in the adjuvant setting. In a prospective study of 91 early breast cancer patients receiving adjuvant therapy, patients who had a 10-fold rise in CK-positive, CD45-negative events had a significantly shorter time to relapse than patients who did not have a rise, while patients who had a 10-fold decrease were significantly less likely to relapse (40).

The inevitable limitation of the current CellSearch set-up is that only EpCAM-expressing CTCs are isolated. The presence and relevance of non-EpCAM expressing CTC is controversial but these could include biologically important events. For example, it has been suggested that normal-like breast cancer circulating cells do not express EpCAM (41). Also, "poorly-differentiated, stem-cell-like" cells or cells in epithelial–mesenchymal transition could be EpCAM-negative and although rare, could represent a biologically important sub-group (42). Combinations of antibodies could be used to capture different sub-populations of CTC but this strategy has not been extensively studied and preliminary reports in breast cancer patients suggest that there was no gain in sensitivity by targeting multiple cell surface receptors (30). An alternative strategy could utilise CTC capture by size that is not dependent on CTC surface expression. Platforms have been developed that exploit the observation that CTCs have a larger median diameter than normal cells. In these systems blood is filtered through pores (usually 8 μm in diameter) with the aim of trapping events larger than the maximum pore diameter (43–45). The success of this process is dependent on a number of factors that include blood flow rate, uniformity of pore size, and rigidity of the membrane. High flow rates can cause CTC to "squeeze" through pores and the membrane to warp. Very slow flow rates cause excess accumulation of leukocytes, clotting of blood and prolong the processing time. Cheaper materials and high-throughput coring of membranes keep costs down but compromise on the consistency of pore diameter and the uniformity of pores across the membrane (e.g., the pores in some types of membranes are random and can adjoin, thus resulting in larger openings). To improve capture rate, membranes could be coated with antibodies to CTC cell-surface markers. However, filtration will inevitably lose CTC equal in size or smaller than the pore diameter whilst capturing leukocytes and other debris that are larger: secondary identification of CTC amongst captured cells based on staining for CK, CD45, or other tumour markers; morphology; nuclear size etc. will remain necessary. Newer approaches utilise nano-technology to exploit the difference in CTC flow dynamics in blood filtered through nano-chambers with unique characteristics. The recently described microfluidic biochip uses thousands of pores coated with an antibody of interest (e.g., EpCAM) to increase the chance of exposure of EpCAM-positive events (including CTC) to EpCAM antibody-coated surfaces as blood flows through the chip (29,46).

Circulating Tumour Cell Molecular Characterisation

The greatest limitation of the CellSearch studies to impact clinical care was the failure to define an indication that would change treatment strategy. As patients with advanced cancer have a fatal disease that requires treatment, the key issue is not "who to treat?" but "what treatment to use?". Immunofluorescence or FISH identifying HER2 gain in CTC could improve patient selection for treatment with HER2 targeting treatments. Using CTC in addition to primary tissue could identify HER2-positive patients who were previously classified as HER2 negative based on their primary tumour (47). Similarly, evolution of a dominant HER2-negative clone following multiple treatments of a HER2-positive primary cancer could predict drug resistance. In fact, HER2 copy number in primary tumour often matches CTC except in patients treated with trastuzumab when in some cases, the majority of CTCs do not have HER2 gain by FISH (35,47,48). The DETECT study prospectively compared HER2 status of the baseline, primary tumour to that of CTC from patients on relapse of their disease evaluated by immunofluorescence and also reported a discordance in HER2 status: one-third of HER2-negative tumours had HER2-positive CTC and nearly half of patients with HER2-positive primary tumours had solely HER2-negative CTC at relapse (49). Similarly, discordance has been reported between the HER2 status of CTC and primary tissue in early breast cancer patients receiving (neo)adjuvant treatment (35). The implications of these results are significant as they identify a sub-group of patients who may benefit from HER2-targeting therapies that are currently not being offered treatment and a proportion of patients who currently would be administered treatment, but may be less likely to benefit. Similarly, evaluation of ER and PR status in CTC could distinguish hormone-sensitive metastatic disease from disease that is no longer hormone-receptor positive. However, due to CTC heterogeneity, large numbers of patients will be required to identify clinically relevant cut-offs for defining a patient's molecular status based on CTC. For example, should a patient with any HER2-positive CTC receive treatment or should one select patients with a minimum number or proportion of HER2-positive CTC? Furthermore, immunostaining on CTC may be more variable than for tissue and new, more stringent quantitation protocols may be required.

Characterisation of CTC acquired from patients on treatment could evaluate drug effect on target (pharmacodynamic studies), selective reduction of genetically distinct sub-populations of CTC (e.g., a reduction in IGF-1R expressing CTCs in patients treated with an IGF-1R targeting agent (Fig. 1)) (50) or the onset of changes associated with resistance. For example, CTC studies in non-small cell lung cancer patients receiving treatment with an EGFR small-molecule tyrosine kinase inhibitor have reported that the presence of the activating mutation prior to commencement of therapy was associated with response and the previously described T790M mutation was associated with resistance; sequential studies of CTC showed that frequently, analysis of CTC from responders who lacked the T790M mutation prior to treatment had developed this mutation at disease progression (51). Concerns remain that pharmacodynamic studies on CTC (even when these match the primary tumour or metastases) may yield different effects to the biological impact of therapeutics on solid lesions due to the different "milieu" of the two cell populations. For example, therapeutics that have an effect on CTC mobilisation could disproportionately affect CTC counts relative to the cytotoxic action of the drug.

Most CTC biomarker studies to date have been limited to the evaluation of stable proteins by immunofluorescence or immunohistochemistry, gene copy number or chromosomal aberrations by FISH, and sequencing of known gene mutations (47,48,51–53). Moreover, these commonly involve the analyses of up to two or three genes using one or two modalities. To date, global gene expression profiling studies have only been possible on those rare patients with large numbers of CTCs, which allowed differences in expression to be identified despite contamination with leukocyte RNA (54). As technological advances make single-cell whole genome, transcriptome, and proteome analyses more feasible and economical (28), the transfer of these technologies to the CTC arena could allow analysis of CTC with "multigene" biomarker assessments that are established in tissue.

Studies on CTC captured using CellSearch report that a significant number of cells are apoptotic and that the proportion of apoptotic cells increases with increasing CTC count (53,55). FISH analysis is not feasible on all CTCs captured using CellSearch, with cells appearing apoptotic [more likely to have granulated CK staining and to stain positive for M30 (55)) less likely to generate a FISH signal (FISH signals were seen in adjacent control leukocytes) (53). As apoptotic CTC are not amenable to molecular characterisation, platforms that cause *ex vivo* cell death will limit their potential utility for these studies. It is however not clear whether a significant proportion of *in vivo* CTCs are undergoing apoptosis, or whether cell death occurs after blood draw and could be reduced by CTC capture involving fewer steps. The developers of CellSearch released a product called the CellProfile™ kit that allows immunomagnetical enrichment of EpCAM-positive events followed by collection of the sample for molecular characterisation studies (with omission of the permeabilisation and immunofluorescence steps required for enumeration). However CTCs remain bound to ferrofluids that may interfere with molecular characterisation protocols. It is possible that the multiple processing steps used by CellSearch and the shearing pressures exerted by immunomagnetical separation may reduce cell viability when compared with processes based on the gentle flow of blood through a chamber, but formal comparisons have not yet been published (29).

Circulating Plasma Nucleic Acids

A molecular tool that could also complement or improve on CTC evaluation is the analysis of circulating tumour nucleic acids in plasma (Table 5). The existence of circulating tumour nucleic acids is a common and relatively early phenomenon in breast cancer patients and similarly to CTC, appears to be associated with blood-borne metastases. Emerging evidence suggests that tumours shed large amounts of nucleic acids into blood either as a free circulating molecule or possibly protected from degradation in exosomes; another explanation for the detection of circulating nucleic acids could be apoptosis of CTCs and release of their nuclear material (56). However, although circulating plasma nucleic acid concentrations are associated with CTC counts, circulating tumour-related DNA has been detected in the absence of CTC and may be more prevalent in early disease than CTC. Nonetheless, this could be a consequence of the sensitivity of detection of currently available CTC technologies. Importantly, tumour-associated aberrations can be detected in DNA extracted from plasma (57). Also, plasma DNA concentrations are higher in advanced cancer patients and associate with worse prognosis (58,59). These two observations introduce the possibility that the evaluation of circulating tumour nucleic acids could give predictive and prognostic information for guiding the treatment of breast cancer patients. Unlike CTC, no analytically or clinically validated assays are available and although several promising studies have been published, well-powered, prospective multicentre studies will not be feasible in the absence of an analytically validated platform. Most studies of circulating tumour nucleic acids to date have been restricted to the analyses of DNA; due to its less stable properties and the presence of circulating RNAses, extracting viable RNA has been challenging although technological improvements may make this possible.

Evaluation of cancer patients and healthy volunteers (ideally age-matched) could identify tumour-specific aberrations (e.g., hypermethylation) in circulating tumour nucleic acids that allow prognostic stratification of early or advanced breast cancer patients, possibly in combination with other biomarkers. For example, evaluation of methylation of PITX2 and RASSF1A in plasma from early breast cancer patients undergoing surgery was significantly associated with OS and DFS (60). Moreover, early reports describe changes in circulating DNA levels with treatment suggesting that the concentration of free tumour nucleic acids or the presence of cancer-specific aberrations in plasma could be used to monitor response to treatment similar to the monitoring of blood BCR-ABL transcripts in Philadelphia-positive myeloid leukemia patients receiving treatment with imatinib (61). The molecular characterisation of nucleic acids extracted from plasma could also be used to select

TABLE 5 Comparison of Circulating Plasma DNA as a Biomarker to Circulating Tumour Cell Detection—Current State of Research

	Circulating tumour DNA	Circulating tumour cells
Methodology	Extraction of DNA from plasma followed by quantitation and analyses using standard platforms	Relatively complex, multistep process that involves rare cell isolation followed by secondary staining and image capture on dedicated platforms
As a diagnostic tool	Promising but partly contradictory results (58,60)	High false-negative rate with current platforms
Prevalence in early breast cancer	Tumour-specific circulating nucleic aberrations detected in up to 50–70% of early breast cancer patients	Using CellSearch, ≥1 CTC/7.5 mL detected in ~25% of patients and ≥5 CTC/7.5 mL detected in <5% (35–37). Newer platforms report higher detection rates but further validation is required (29). Less stringent definitions for circulating tumour-associated events may be useful in adjuvant setting (40)
Prognostic relevance in adjuvant setting	Potentially yes; for example, persistent methylated serum RASSF1A is associated with shorter PFS and OS (60)	Multiple academic studies investigating CTC in early breast cancer are ongoing but early data suggest patients with ≥5 CTC on/after adjuvant treatment have a worse outcome (35–37)
Prevalence in advanced breast cancer	Early data suggest circulating tumour-specific DNA can be detected in >75%. Prevalence increased with more advanced disease	Using CellSearch, 50–75% have ≥5 CTC/7.5 mL. Associated with blood-borne metastases. Prevalence increased with more advanced disease
Prognostic relevance in advanced cancer	Multiple small studies report association between DNA levels and OS and PFS (58,59)	Industry-sponsored, multicentre, prospective study confirms association with OS and PFS (29)
Therapy monitoring in metastatic patients	No conclusive data available yet	Changes in CTC count associated with OS (Fig. 2). Studies evaluating a change in CTC count as a surrogate endpoint are ongoing
Analytically validated protocol	Protocol not yet analytically validated	One FDA cleared platform (CellSearch). Multiple other platforms in phase I development.
Molecular characterisation options	Identification of genomic mutations and hypermethylation	Immunostaining and *in situ* hybridisation studies can be performed on isolated CTC. Nucleic acids can also be extracted for analyses

Abbreviations: CTC, circulating tumour cell; OS, overall survival; PFS, progression-free survival.

patients for specific treatments. Similarly to CTC studies, these analyses could allow repeated, minimally-invasive testing of patients for selection for specific treatments and the detection of molecular changes that associate with the development of resistance. Both studies of circulating tumour somatic mutations and hyper-methylation of cancer-associated genes have been reported to date. Analyses of somatic mutations has been restricted to specific, known mutations and whole genome sequencing studies or new mutation discovery has to date not been feasible due to the quality of extracted nucleic acids and dilution by wild-type nucleic acids. A PCR-based system using Amplification Refractory Mutation System (ARMS) primers and Scorpion probes has been used to detect PIK3CA mutations in metastatic tumour biopsies and plasma from matched patients. PIK3CA mutations were detected in 28% of patients with a 95% concordance between plasma-derived and tumour DNA (59). A similar protocol was used to detect EGFR mutations in non-small cell lung cancer patients receiving treatment with EGFR small-molecule tyrosine kinase inhibitors (51). In this study, analyses of plasma DNA appeared to be less sensitive than DNA extracted from CTC but it is possible that the sensitivity of plasma DNA studies will increase with improved platforms and more experience. The Sequenom platform uses mass spectroscopy to screen for hundreds of known mutations in several known onco-genes and tumour suppressor genes (62). It is able to detect mutations at concentrations as low as 1–5% which is a significant advantage in the analysis of mutations in DNA from plasma which will be expected to be frequently diluted by wild-type loci from normal cells and non-mutated tumour cells. Preliminary reports suggest that the detection of multiple common mutations in plasma is feasible and shows a high concordance with patient-matched tumour samples. The analyses of circulating tumour-associated mutations may be most useful in advanced cancer patients as early cancer patients have significantly lower concentrations of circulating plasma nucleic acids and the majority will undergo a diagnostic biopsy or surgical resection.

HOST BIOMARKERS

Identifying germline, or inherited, genetic variants (e.g., single nucleotide polymorphisms, copy number variations) associated with treatment benefit and/or drug toxicity has the potential to provide crucially important data on selecting treatment and its dosing (63). Due to technological advances and large scale DNA sequencing projects, pharmacogenetics research has made tremendous progress in recent years, with the identification of numerous inherited variants that influence drug response. As a result, many drug labels have been updated with information about the relevance of pharmacogenetic biomarkers (http://www.fda.gov/Drugs/ScienceResearch/ResearchAreas/Pharmacogenetics/ucm083378). Germline DNA may be obtained from a diverse array of biological sources including leukocytes from blood, mucosal cells from sputum, and even adjacent normal tissue from the same organ as the cancer, rendering germline evaluation a practical and attractive field of research and one that can be easily translated into the clinical setting. Recently, increasing attention has been paid to the pharmacogenetics of tamoxifen. Tamoxifen is a pro-drug and its efficacy depends on the biotransformation, predominantly via the enzyme Cytochrome P450 2D6 (CYP2D6), to its active metabolite endoxifen (64). Among Caucasians, approximately 7–10% are deficient in CYP2D6 metabolism and these individuals convert tamoxifen to endoxifen poorly. Several studies addressing the interaction between CYP2D6 genotype and outcomes in women treated with tamoxifen in adjuvant and metastatic settings have been conducted and reported contradictory results (65). Recently, retrospective analyses from two large adjuvant randomised trials—ATAC and BIG 1-98, presented at the 33rd Annual San Antonio Breast Cancer Symposium (SABCS)—have found no association between the CYP2D6 genotype and the effectiveness of tamoxifen in preventing breast cancer recurrence, in contrast to several previous positive studies (66,67). The International Tamoxifen Pharmacogenetics Consortium has been established to collect the worldwide experience relating to genetic variation in CYP2D6 and the outcomes of women treated with adjuvant tamoxifen and results of these analyses are awaited with interest. Emerging data suggest that host factors may also predict inter-patient variability in response to aromatase inhibitors (68).

CONCLUSION

As an increased understanding of the molecular biology underlying cancer leads to a plethora of novel targeted agents entering clinical trials and routine patient treatment, there is an urgent, rapidly increasing demand for diagnostics that sub-classify patients based on molecular profiles and allow patient selection for specific targeted treatments. The sub-classification of patients based on their original primary tumour (as currently invariably practised) may be misleading due to (i) molecular changes that occur secondary to treatment pressures; (ii) intra-patient tumour heterogeneity resulting in missed unevaluated areas in the primary tumour containing the sub-clones that ultimately lead to drug-resistant disease (28). Ideally patients should therefore be classified based on the profile of their metastatic disease; this is however often not feasible. Collection of blood and isolation and evaluation of CTC or circulating nucleic acids could serve as a "liquid biopsy" allowing minimally invasive, real-time molecular characterisation of metastatic cancer to identify biomarkers that associate with specific sub-groups and detect biomarkers of resistance developing during the course of treatment. This is a novel, rapidly evolving field that holds great promise. However, the technological and practical limitations of identifying and studying circulating biomarkers in all patients remain a challenge. The interpretation of data from circulating biomarkers may therefore be most useful in combination with tissue-based biomarker analyses.

A number of challenges exist for biomarker development that include, but are not restricted to, the relatively high cost and significant operator time required, tumour heterogeneity (resulting in missing of a biomarker in tissue sections or CTC analyses etc.), and pharmaceutical industry politics that may fail to include potentially useful biomarkers for patient selection in appropriately designed prospective clinical studies. Nonetheless, an increasing number of clinical studies now incorporate biomarker-driven patient selection and treatment monitoring with the aim of drug approval for a specific treatment linked to a diagnostic test that has been prospectively clinically validated in parallel with or as an integral part of phase III therapeutic efficacy studies.

REFERENCES

1. Sørlie T, Perou CM, Tibshirani R, et al. Gene expression patterns of breast carcinomas distinguish tumor subclasses with clinical implications. Proc Natl Acad Sci USA 2001; 98: 10869–74.
2. Weigelt B, Mackay A, A'hern R, et al. Breast cancer molecular profiling with single sample predictors: a retrospective analysis. Lancet Oncol 2010; 11: 339–49.
3. Gonzalez-Angulo AM, Hennessy BT, Mills GB. Future of personalized medicine in oncology: a systems biology approach. J Clin Oncol 2010; 28: 2777–83.
4. Yap TA, Sandhu SK, Workman P, et al. Envisioning the future of early anticancer drug development. Nat Rev Cancer 2010; 10: 514–23.
5. Pathology reporting of breast disease. A joint document incorporating the third edition of the NHS breast screening programme's guidelines for pathology reporting in breast cancer screening and the second edition of The Royal College of Pathologists' minimum dataset for breast cancer histopathology. NHS BSP Publication 58.
6. Johnston SRD. New strategies in estrogen receptor-positive breast cancer. Clin Cancer Res 2010; 16: 1979–87.
7. Weigel MT, Dowsett M. Current and emerging biomarkers in breast cancer: prognosis and prediction. Endocr Relat Cancer 2010; 17: R245–62.
8. Hammond ME, Hayes DF, Dowsett M, et al. American Society of Clinical Oncology/College of American Pathologists guideline recommendations for immunohistochemical testing of estrogen and progesterone receptors in breast cancer (unabridged version). Arch Pathol Lab Med 2010; 134: e48–72.

9. Olivotto IA, Truong PT, Speers CH, et al. Time to stop progesterone receptor testing in breast cancer management. J Clin Oncol 2004; 22: 1769–70.
10. Slamon DJ, Clark GM, Wong SG, et al. Human-breast cancer-correlation of relapse and survival with amplification of the HER-neu oncogene. Science 1987; 235: 177–82.
11. Slamon DJ, Leyland-Jones B, Shak S, et al. Use of chemotherapy plus a monoclonal antibody against HER2 for metastatic breast cancer that overexpresses HER2. N Engl J Med 2001; 344: 783–92.
12. Wolff AC, Hammond ME, Schwartz JN, et al. American Society of Clinical Oncology/College of American Pathologists guideline recommendations for human epidermal growth factor receptor 2 testing in breast cancer. Arch Pathol Lab Med 2007; 131: 18–43.
13. Farmer H, McCabe N, Lord CJ, et al. Targeting the DNA repair defect in BRCA mutant cells as a therapeutic strategy. Nature 2005; 434: 917–21.
14. Tutt A, Robson M, Garber JE, et al. Oral poly(ADP-ribose) polymerase inhibitor olaparib in patients with BRCA1 or BRCA2 mutations and advanced breast cancer: a proof-of-concept trial. Lancet 2010; 376: 235–44.
15. Fong PC, Boss DS, Yap TA, et al. Inhibition of poly(ADP-Ribose) polymerase in tumors from BRCA mutation carriers. N Engl J Med 2009; 361: 123–34.
16. Turner NC, Ashworth A. Biomarkers of PARP inhibitor sensitivity. Breast Cancer Res Treat 2011; 127: 283–6.
17. Vogel CL, Cobleigh MA, Tripathy D, et al. Efficacy and safety of trastuzumab as a single agent in first-line treatment of HER2-overexpressing metastatic breast cancer. J Clin Oncol 2002; 20: 719–726.
18. Esteva FJ, Guo H, Zhang S, et al. PTEN, PIK3CA, p-AKT, and p-p70S6K status association with trastuzumab response and survival in patients with HER2-positive metastatic breast cancer. Am J Pathol 2010; 177: 1647–56.
19. Johnston S, Trudeau M, Kaufman B, et al. Phase II study of predictive biomarker profiles for response targeting human epidermal growth factor receptor 2 (HER-2) in advanced inflammatory breast cancer with lapatinib monotherapy. J Clin Oncol 2008; 26: 1066–72.
20. Scaltriti M, Rojo F, Ocaña A, et al. Expression of p95HER2, a truncated form of the HER2 receptor, and response to anti-HER2 therapies in breast cancer. J Natl Cancer Inst 2007; 99: 628–38.
21. Scaltriti M, Chandarlapaty S, Prudkin L, et al. Clinical benefit of lapatinib-based therapy in patients with human epidermal growth factor receptor 2-positive breast tumors coexpressing the truncated p95HER2 receptor. Clin Cancer Res 2010; 16: 2688–95.
22. Weigel MT, Dowsett M. Current and emerging biomarkers in breast cancer: prognosis and prediction. Endocr Relat Cancer 2010; 17: R245–62.
23. Dowsett M, Smith IE, Ebbs SR, et al. Prognostic value of Ki67 expression after short-term presurgical endocrine therapy for primary breast cancer. J Natl Cancer Institute 2007; 99: 167–70.
24. van't Veer LJ, Dai H, van de Vijver MJ, et al. Gene expression profiling predicts clinical outcome of breast cancer. Nature 2002; 415: 530–6.
25. Paik S, Tang G, Shak S, et al. Gene expression and benefit of chemotherapy in women with node-negative estrogen receptor-positive breast cancer. J Clin Oncol 2006; 24: 3726–34.
26. Albain KS, Barlow WE, Shak S, et al. Prognostic and predictive value of the 21-gene recurrence score assay in postmenopausal women with node-positive, oestrogen-receptor-positive breast cancer on chemotherapy: a retrospective analysis of a randomised trial. Lancet Oncol 2010; 11: 55–65.
27. Braun S, Vogl FD, Naume B, et al. A pooled analysis of bone marrow micrometastasis in breast cancer. N Engl J Med 2005; 353: 793–802.
28. Attard G, de Bono JS. Utilizing circulating tumor cells: challenges and pitfalls. Curr Opin Genet Dev 2011; 21: 50–8.
29. Nagrath S, Sequist LV, Maheswaran S, et al. Isolation of rare circulating tumour cells in cancer patients by microchip technology. Nature 2007; 450: 1235–9.
30. Connelly M, Wang Y, Doyle GV, et al. Re: Anti-epithelial cell adhesion molecule antibodies and the detection of circulating normal-like breast tumor cells. J Natl Cancer Inst 2009; 101: 895; author reply 896–7.
31. Allard WJ, Matera J, Miller MC, et al. Tumor cells circulate in the peripheral blood of all major carcinomas but not in healthy subjects or patients with nonmalignant diseases. Clin Cancer Res 2004; 10: 6897–904.

32. Cristofanilli M, Budd GT, Ellis MJ, et al. Circulating tumor cells, disease progression, and survival in metastatic breast cancer. N Engl J Med 2004; 351: 781–91.
33. Miller MC, Doyle GV, Terstappen LW. Significance of circulating tumor cells detected by the cellsearch system in patients with metastatic breast colorectal and prostate cancer. J Oncol 2010; 2010: 617421.
34. Budd GT, Cristofanilli M, Ellis MJ, et al. Circulating tumor cells versus imaging-predicting overall survival in metastatic breast cancer. Clin Cancer Res 2006; 12: 6403–9.
35. Riethdorf S, Müller V, Zhang L, et al. Detection and HER2 expression of circulating tumor cells: prospective monitoring in breast cancer patients treated in the neoadjuvant Gepar-Quattro trial. Clin Cancer Res 2010; 16: 2634–45.
36. Pierga JY, Bidard FC, Mathiot C, et al. Circulating tumor cell detection predicts early metastatic relapse after neoadjuvant chemotherapy in large operable and locally advanced breast cancer in a phase II randomized trial. Clin Cancer Res 2008; 14: 7004–10.
37. Lang JE, Mosalpuria K, Cristofanilli M, et al. HER2 status predicts the presence of circulating tumor cells in patients with.operable breast cancer. Breast Cancer Res Treat 2009; 113: 501–7.
38. Scher HI, Jia X, de Bono JS, et al. Circulating tumour cells as prognostic markers in progressive, castrationresistant prostate cancer: a reanalysis of IMMC38 trial data. Lancet Oncol 2009; 10: 233–9.
39. Coumans FA, Doggen CJ, Attard G, et al. All circulating EpCAM+CK+CD45-objects predict overall survival in castration-resistant prostate cancer. Ann Oncol 2010; 21: 1851–7.
40. Pachmann K, Camara O, Kavallaris A, et al. Monitoring the response of circulating epithelial tumor cells to adjuvant chemotherapy in breast cancer allows detection of patients at risk of early relapse. J Clin Oncol 2008; 26: 1208–15.
41. Sieuwerts AM, Kraan J, Bolt J, et al. Anti-epithelial cell adhesion molecule antibodies and the detection of circulating normal-like breast tumor cells. J Natl Cancer Inst 2009; 101: 61–6.
42. Mani SA, Guo W, Liao MJ, et al. The epithelial-mesenchymal transition generates cells with properties of stem cells. Cell 2008; 133: 704–15.
43. Ntouroupi TG, Ashraf SQ, McGregor SB, et al. Detection of circulating tumour cells in peripheral blood with an automated scanning fluorescence microscope. Br J Cancer 2008; 99: 789–95.
44. Vona G, Sabile A, Louha M, et al. Isolation by size of epithelial tumor cells: a new method for the immunomorphological and molecular characterization of circulating tumor cells. Am J Pathol 2000; 156: 57–63.
45. De Giorgi V, Pinzani P, Salvianti F, et al. Application of a filtration- and isolation-by-size technique for the detection of circulating tumor cells in cutaneous melanoma. J Invest Dermatol 2010; 130: 2440–7.
46. Racila E, Euhus D, Weiss AJ, et al. Detection and characterization of carcinoma cells in the blood. Proc Natl Acad Sci USA 1998; 95: 4589–94.
47. Meng S, Tripathy D, Shete S, et al. HER-2 gene amplification can be acquired as breast cancer progresses. Proc Natl Acad Sci USA 2004; 101: 9393–8.
48. Punnoose EA, Atwal SK, Spoerke JM, et al. Molecular biomarker analyses using circulating tumor cells. PLoS ONE 2010; 5: e12517.
49. Fehm T, Müller V, Aktas B, et al. HER2 status of circulating tumor cells in patients with metastatic breast cancer: a prospective, multicenter trial. Breast Cancer Res Treat 2010; 124: 403–12.
50. de Bono JS, Attard G, Adjei A, et al. Potential applications for circulating tumor cells expressing the insulinlike.growth factor-I receptor. Clin Cancer Res 2007; 13: 3611–16.
51. Maheswaran S, Sequist LV, Nagrath S, et al. Detection of mutations in EGFR in circulating lung-cancer cells. N Engl J Med 2008; 359: 366–77.
52. Shaffer DR, Leversha MA, Danila DC, et al. Circulating tumor cell analysis in patients with progressive castrationresistant prostate cancer. Clin Cancer Res 2007; 13: 2023–9.
53. Attard G, Swennenhuis JF, Olmos D, et al. Characterization of ERG, AR and PTEN gene status in circulating tumor cells from patients with castration-resistant prostate cancer. Cancer Res 2009; 69: 2912–18.
54. Smirnov DA, Zweitzig DR, Foulk BW, et al. Global gene expression profiling of circulating tumor cells. Cancer Res 2005; 65: 4993–7.

55. Swennenhuis JF, Tibbe AG, Levink R, et al. Characterization of circulating tumor cells by fluorescence in situ hybridization. Cytometry A 2009; 75: 520–7.
56. Fehm T, Banys M. Circulating free DNA: a new surrogate marker for minimal residual disease? Breast Cancer Res Treat 2011 Feb 15. [Epub ahead of print].
57. Chen X, Bonnefoi H, Diebold-Berger S, et al. Detecting tumor-related alterations in plasma or serum DNA of patients diagnosed with breast cancer. Clin Cancer Res 1999; 5: 2297–303.
58. Schwarzenbach H, Alix-Panabières C, Müller I, et al. Cell-free tumor DNA in blood plasma as a marker for circulating tumor cells in prostate cancer. Clin Cancer Res 2009; 15: 1032–8.
59. Board RE, Wardley AM, Dixon JM, et al. Detection of PIK3CA mutations in circulating free DNA in patients with breast cancer. Breast Cancer Res Treat 2010; 120: 461–7.
60. Göbel G, Auer D, Gaugg I, et al. Prognostic significance of methylated RASSF1A and PITX2 genes in blood and bone marrow plasma of breast cancer patients. Breast Cancer Res Treat 2011 Jan 8. [Epub ahead of print].
61. Druker BJ, Talpaz M, Resta DJ, et al. Efficacy and safety of a specific inhibitor of the BCR-ABL tyrosine kinase in chronic myeloid leukemia. N Engl J Med 2001; 344: 1031–7.
62. MacConaill LE, Campbell CD, Kehoe SM, et al. Profiling critical cancer gene mutations in clinical tumor samples. PLoS ONE 2009; 4: e7887.
63. Coate L, Cuffe S, Horgan A, et al. Germline genetic variation, cancer outcome, and pharmacogenetics. J Clin Oncol 2010; 28: 4029–37.
64. Johnson MD, et al. Pharmacological characterization of 4-hydroxy-N-desmethyl tamoxifen, a novel active metabolite of tamoxifen. Breast Cancer Res Treat 2004; 85: 151–9.
65. Ferraldeschi R, Newman WG. The impact of CYP2D6 genotyping on tamoxifen treatment. Pharmaceuticals 2010; 3: 1122–38.
66. Rae JM, Drury S, Hayes DF, et al. Lack of correlation between gene variants in tamoxifen metabolizing enymes with primary endpoints in the ATAC trial. San Antonio, Texas: December 8–12, 2010. Program and abstracts of the 33rd Annual San Antonio Breast Cancer Symposium [abstract S1-7].
67. Leyland-Jones B, Regan MM, Bouzyk M, et al. Outcome according to CYP2D6 genotype among postmenopausal women with endocrine-responsive early invasive breast cancer randomized in the BIG 1-98 trial. San Antonio, Texas: December 8–12, 2010. Program and abstracts of the 33rd Annual San Antonio Breast Cancer Symposium [abstract S1-8].
68. Ingle JN, Schaid DJ, Goss PE, et al. Genome-wide associations and functional genomic studies of musculoskeletal adverse events in women receiving aromatase inhibitors. J Clin Oncol 2010; 28: 4674–82.

12 Palliative radiotherapy in the management of metastatic breast cancer

Anthony Chalmers and Richard Simcock

INTRODUCTION

External beam radiotherapy (EBRT) is a cost-effective and reliable modality in the palliation of metastatic breast cancer. It is useful in the management of localisable lesions and contributes to symptom relief through local control but rarely to survival benefit. In this chapter, theoretical and practical issues surrounding the role of radiotherapy in the management of bone deposits, spinal cord compression, chest wall disease, and choroidal and cerebral metastases will be discussed.

FRACTIONATION

When considering radiation it is important to address the issue of dose fractionation. EBRT is delivered in a number of treatments (fractions) that make up the overall dose. The total radiation dose measured in Gray (abbreviated to Gy) will have a biological effect that is determined by the number of fractions, the dose per fraction, the total time taken to deliver the course of treatment, and the radiosensitivity of the tissues being irradiated. The biological effects of the treatment may be crudely separated into acute and late effects, which in turn are mediated by the rate of turnover in the relevant tissue. In radical treatments, a beneficial therapeutic ratio is obtained by delivering a dose that is unlikely to cause late effects while maximising acute effects within the tumour. This is usually achieved by delivering daily doses of approximately 2 Gy, five times per week over a period of 5–7 weeks. In the palliative setting, much larger doses per fraction may be delivered over shorter overall treatment times in order to achieve a rapid tumour kill. This approach is unlikely to eradicate tumour deposits at the treated site, but palliation is often achieved and the theoretical risk of late radiation effects on normal tissues is not usually clinically relevant in the patient's lifetime. With improved treatment for metastatic disease, stage shift through better imaging, and earlier treatment of oligometastatic disease it may be necessary in the modern era to be more mindful of possible late effects of hypofractionated radiotherapy.

Through a combination of radiobiological modelling and clinical experience the trend in palliative fractionation has been to give smaller numbers of treatments at higher doses per fraction (hypofractionation). There are clear advantages to the patient: clinical isoeffectiveness, a very low risk of complications, and a reduced number of visits for treatment. Most palliative treatments may therefore be delivered in 1–5 fractions, with the caveat that in those patients where survival may be measured in years a larger number of smaller doses may be appropriate.

BONE METASTASES

Bone is the most common site of metastatic disease in breast cancer and affects up to 70% of women with metastases. Disease is most often in the axial skeleton but all bones may be affected including the base of the skull and skull vault. The prevalence of bone metastases is twice the incidence (1), and the prevalence is likely to increase as systemic therapies for metastatic disease become more effective. Two-thirds of patients with bone metastases will experience skeletal-related events (fracture, orthopaedic intervention, spinal cord compression, or radiotherapy) (2).

Median survival after development of bone metastases is 19–25 months, falling to 12 months following a pathological fracture (3). There is a long tail on the survival curve, with a small number of very long term survivors. Good prognostic factors for survival are a low histological grade, positive oestrogen receptor status, bone disease at initial presentation, long disease-free interval, and increasing age. Bone-only disease has a better prognosis than disease associated with visceral involvement.

Whilst bone-dominant disease may be adequately controlled by endocrine therapies and bisphosphonates radiotherapy remains an important part of the treatment algorithm. Patients receiving radiotherapy for bone metastases form the largest group of patients receiving any form of palliative radiotherapy. It is of particular benefit for those patients with painful bone disease or spinal cord compression and as an adjuvant therapy to orthopaedic intervention and can be a useful treatment even in the face of a large burden of metastatic disease due to the high response rate and low toxicity.

Effect of Radiotherapy on Bone
Within bone affected by metastatic tumour there are conflicting processes of destruction and new bone formation. The majority of bone destruction is mediated by osteoclasts, which are in turn influenced by humoral factors released by a tumour. Malignant stimulation of the RANK signalling pathway increases the osteoclastic activity (4). New bone formation is predominantly reactive (as seen in healthy bone after fracture), but may be exuberant, generating new bone that often lacks the strength of normal lamellar bone. Although it is often not possible to determine histologically the balance of destruction and new bone formation, imaging studies will indicate whether the metastatic process is predominantly sclerotic, lytic, or mixed. Malignant bone pain has a statistically significant negative correlation with bone density (5).

Bone pain is the most common complication of metastatic bone disease. Pain may be either nociceptive (mediated by prostaglandins, substance P, and other cytokines) or neuropathic (as a result of bone destruction and increased resorption, peri-osteal irritation and nerve entrapment). The mechanism by which radiotherapy improves pain is not clearly understood. The fact that pain relief associated with radiotherapy treatment often occurs very rapidly makes it unlikely that the effect is mediated entirely through cytotoxic effects on the tumour. Despite some limited evidence of dose response with radiotherapy (6) useful palliative responses often occur without any reduction in the size of bone lesions. It is not known at what doses of radiation changes in the RANK pathway occur. A prompt reduction in peri-tumoural oedema may be responsible for the rapid relief of neuropathic pain. Pre-clinical studies also suggest that the shared action of radiotherapy and bisphosphonates on osteoclasts may provide an enabling synergy leading to osteoblastic bone remodelling (7,8).

Response to Treatment
Evaluation of bone radiotherapy has previously been made difficult by a literature which used a heterogeneous group of response assessments at differing time points and with varying awareness of the confounding effects of analgesia. The International Bone Metastasis Consensus working party has produced standardised definitions of response which allow comparisons of datasets (Table 1) (9). Using these definitions, an analysis of the existing data reveals that responses to radiotherapy are independent of the age of the patient (10) and the baseline pain level (11). Radiotherapy should therefore be offered early before pain becomes severe and should be used without hesitation in elderly patients in whom its low toxicity make it an attractive palliative option.

TABLE 1   Bone Metastasis Consensus Criteria for Response Assessment (9)

Patients score pain according to Brief Pain Inventory pre-treatment and one-month post treatment

Complete response

     Worst pain of 0 with no concomitant increase in analgesic uptake (stable or reducing analgesics in daily oral morphine equivalents)

Partial response

     Worst pain score reduction of 2 or more at the treated site without analgesic increase

     Opioid analgesic reduction of 25% or more from baseline without an increase in worst pain score

Progression

     Either an increase in worst pain score or 2 or more points above baseline at the treated site without reduction in analgesic use or an increase of 25% or more in daily oral morphine equivalent compared with baseline without a reduction in baseline worst pain score

---

A large study (n = 125) of urinary markers of bone resorption (pyridinoline and deoxypyridinoline), measured before and after radiotherapy for bone pain failed to show any association between response and markers of turnover (12). This is in contrast to earlier smaller studies and the literature on bisphosphonates. Bone marker levels cannot currently be used to predict which patients are likely to respond to therapy.

Fractionation in the Treatment of Localised Bone Metastases

For many years, fractionation has been a major focus of research in this area. The body of evidence addressing this question since 1982 amounts to at least 26 published trials, 5 published overviews, an overview of the overviews, and a Cochrane review. These trials have studied over 6500 patients. Despite these numbers, only a small fraction of the total number of patients treated over this time has entered clinical trials; the largest single randomised study—The Dutch Bone Metastasis Study (DBMS) (13)—randomised only 29% of eligible patients. All of the randomised studies included multiple different tumour types, but in all cases breast and/or prostate cancer formed the predominant patient groups. In the DBMS, 49.7% of the 1157 patients had breast cancer.

In the overviews (14,15) neither overall response rate nor complete response rate (by intention to treat) was significantly different in the multiple- or single-fraction arms of the study. A single fraction of 8 Gy delivered for palliation achieves a 60% response rate by intention-to-treat analysis. Approximately one-third of patients treated have a complete pain response. Overall, mean time to response is 3 weeks and mean duration of remission is 18 weeks, although in the Dutch study response rates in breast cancer patients were higher than average (78%) and responses more sustained (24 weeks) than for other tumour types.

The consistently repeated message from these studies and overviews is that multiple fractions of radiotherapy offer no advantage over a single fraction of treatment. Single fractions are clearly more convenient for the patient and increase treatment capacity for the radiotherapy centre. Delivering treatment as a single fraction further increases the cost efficiency of an already cost-effective treatment (16).

Despite this considerable body of evidence (which continues to grow), the discrepancy between published recommendations and clinical practice persists. In a survey of nearly a thousand radiation oncologists, 101 different radiotherapy schedules were described with a clear preference expressed for multiple fraction regimens (17). Persistent physician bias must also be at least partly responsible for the continuing geographical variation in prescribing habits. While single fractions are commonly employed in the United Kingdom and Canada, fractionated regimens such as 20 Gy in 5 fractions or 30 Gy in 10 fractions are the norm in the rest of the world (18).

Re-Treatment of Bone Deposits

Critics of single-fraction treatment have pointed to the higher levels of re-treatment required in the single-fraction arms of the randomised studies. Re-treatment after a single fraction is recorded for 21.5% of patients as compared with 7.4% of those receiving multiple fractions. However, pain relief levels are similar, and the higher re-treatment rates are likely to reflect a bias among treating physicians not to re-treat those patients who have previously received a higher dose through multiple fractions. This view is strongly supported by a reanalysis of the DBMS, controlling for the effect of re-treatment (19).

What Dose should be Given to a Previously Treated Area?

Re-treatment is worthwhile and produces good responses. Among breast cancer patients experiencing progressive pain who had previously responded to treatment, 89% derived benefit from re-treatment. Perhaps more importantly, 82% of those who had not previously responded experienced symptomatic relief from re-treatment.

Many physicians have taken the view that if the patient previously received a single fraction yet progressed or failed to achieve a complete response, re-treatment should be delivered to a higher fractionated dose. Neither retrospective studies (20) nor the final analysis of the re-treatment data from the Dutch bone study supports this view and a single fraction may be delivered for re-treatment as effectively as multiple fractions.

Cost effectiveness analysis of the most recent US trial [Radiation Therapy Oncology Group (RTOG) 97-14] of single versus multiple fraction radiotherapy demonstrates that a single fraction is significantly more cost effective, even when factoring in re-treatment costs, with an incremental cost of nearly US$7000 per quality-adjusted life year for multiple fraction treatments (21).

Neuropathic Bone Pain

Single-fraction treatment has also been tested against multiple fractions in the treatment of neuropathic bone pain, where it has been argued that multiple fractions are required to reduce tumour mass and relieve pressure on nerves. The Trans-Tasman group (22) randomised 272 patients with neuropathic bone pain between five 2-Gy fractions and a single 8-Gy fraction. The difference in overall response rates between the two arms (53% for single fraction and 61% for multiple fractions) was small and not statistically significant (P = 0.18). It therefore seems appropriate to conclude that whereas 20 Gy in 5 fractions may be a slightly better choice for patients with neuropathic pain, a single fraction is still entirely appropriate for patients with poor performance status, limited prognosis, or difficult access to radiotherapy facilities.

Spinal Cord Compression

Compression of the spinal cord or cauda equina by vertebral collapse or by direct spread of metastatic disease is a particularly important consequence of bone disease because in addition to the problems of neuropathic pain, the patient faces the prospect of neurological disability. Metastatic spinal cord compression (MSCC) therefore deserves special consideration, with ambulatory status an important outcome measure. Epidemiology and presentation are dealt with in the chapter entitled "Management of Neurological Complications in Metastatic Breast Cancer". The same chapter also indicates which patients should be considered for surgery.

U.K. guidelines suggest using a single fraction (8 Gy) for patients with poor prognosis and established neurological deficit but fractionated regimens for all others (23). This advice seems reasonable based on the results of the studies published thus far (24) although a U.K. trial of a single 8-Gy fraction versus 20 Gy in 5 fractions is ongoing (the SCORAD study). A randomised study of two "long course"

TABLE 2 Scoring System for Outcome after Diagnosis of Metastatic Spinal Cord Compression

Variable	Post RT ambulatory rate (%)	Score
Breast cancer diagnosis	81%	8
Interval from tumour diagnosis to MSCC		
≤15 months	58	6
> 15 months	78	8
Visceral metastases		
Yes	54	5
No	78	8
Motor function before RT		
Ambulatory without aid	98	10
Ambulatory with aid	89	9
Not ambulatory	28	3
Paraplegic	7	1
Time of developing motor deficit before RT		
1-7 days before	37	4
8-14 days before	69	7
>14 days before	88	9

Total score	Post ambulatory rate (%)	6 month survival (%)
≤28	6	6
29-31	44	31
32-34	70	42
35-37	86	61
≥38	99	98

Source: Adapted from Ref. 28.

regimens (30 Gy in 10 fractions or 40 Gy in 20 fractions) in 214 patients (28% breast cancers) showed no advantage to the longer regimen with over 40% of patients experiencing an improved motor function with either schedule (25). These two regimens have been grouped and compared to two "short course" regimens (20 Gy in 5 fractions or 8 Gy in a single fraction). This non-randomised prospective comparison showed no difference in improved motor function, but there was a statistically significant difference in in-field recurrence rates (9% for longer fractionations compared with 18% for short fractionations). In the longer fractionation group recurrences occurred on average 2.5 months later than in the other group (7.5 months, p = 0.001) (26). These data lend support for a longer fractionation in patients with a prognosis anticipated to exceed 6 months. Median survival in a review of over 300 breast cancer patients with MSCC was 20 months. Breast cancer often responds better to treatment than other solid organ malignancies, and the best outcomes are achieved in those patients with limited bone disease, no visceral involvement, good performance status and long interval between initial diagnosis and MSCC (27). Patients who report a very rapid reduction of motor function prior to treatment often do poorly with radiotherapy as tumour growth in these cases has most often caused spinal cord infarction which leads to irreversible disability.

The largest ever retrospective analysis in MSCC (over 2000 patients) by Rades has produced a useful scoring system to predict outcome (Table 2). A score of ≤28 predicts for poor prognosis in both survival and functional outcome and may therefore indicate those patients for whom short fractionation and/or best supportive care are appropriate (28).

If it is possible to offer surgical intervention as the first treatment for MSCC then radiotherapy should be offered afterwards. This statement is supported by a randomised study of 101 patients (12 with breast cancer) who were offered surgery and adjuvant radiotherapy or radiotherapy alone; 62% of patients in the surgery group retained the ability to walk compared with only 19% in the radiotherapy-alone group (29).

Re-Treatment in MSCC

The spinal cord lies within the high dose region of treatment and therefore the total dose becomes important in re-treatment because of the risk of exceeding the normal tissue tolerance of the spinal cord and causing disability through irreversible myelopathy. The same factors that predict response to the first treatment hold true for re-treatment although surprisingly neither the cumulative dose nor the interval to re-treatment has been shown to be significant with regard to outcome (30). In a study of 124 re-treated patients the cumulative biological effective dose (BED) was less than $120\,Gy$ ($\alpha/\beta=2$) in 92% and no myelopathy was observed. This is the equivalent of two separate courses of $20\,Gy$ in 5 fractions (assuming no normal tissue recovery between courses). In a separate study of a mixed group of 35 patients with radiation myelopathy, none had received a BED of less than $100\,Gy$ (31), which is equivalent to $20\,Gy$ in 5 fractions followed by a single fraction of $8\,Gy$. These data provide reassurance that re-treatment is effective and safe at conventional dose levels.

Stereotactic Body Radiosurgery and Volumetric Arc Therapy for Spinal Metastases

Because of concern with respect to spinal cord tolerance, stereotactic radiosurgery has been employed to deliver high radiation doses to spinal and para-spinal tumours while limiting the dose to the spinal cord. Stereotactic radiotherapy/surgery uses multiple small beams of radiotherapy targeted on a single small area to provide high dose with minimal toxicity to surrounding tissues. Gantry-based systems [using a Linear Accelerator (Linac)] have been used for many years with the limitation of beam entry points all needing to be in the same axial plane. Newer technologies put the beam on a robotic arm allowing beam entry points to be non-co-planar and more flexible (e.g., Cyberknife system). Proof of principle has been established in over a dozen studies comprising more than 700 treatments, often for primary spinal tumours (32,33). Similar results are now also demonstrated using volumetric arc therapy (a complex treatment planning algorithm based on a radiation gantry rotating around the patient delivering differing doses around a central point) (34).

However, these treatments are costly to provide and are resource intensive for personnel, equipment, and patient. So far, cost efficacy has not been demonstrated (35) but these innovative treatment approaches may have value for patients who have received more than one treatment with EBRT and who present with progressive MSCC and in-field recurrence, yet maintain good prognosis, as indicated by high scores on the Rades scale (see the previous section).

Radiotherapy for Bone Metastases: Techniques

Magnetic resonance imaging (MRI) of the whole spine is recommended prior to the treatment of spinal lesions, as this investigation reveals additional, often asymptomatic, lesions in a large number of cases (36) as well as allowing accurate calculation of treatment depth. For other sites, information from bone scans and plain radiographs is usually sufficient for treatment planning. In cases of MSCC the treatment should be delivered urgently.

The patient requires immobilisation before simulation and treatment. In the majority of patients cushioning will be adequate but vacuum bag fixation may be required to assure the comfort of some patients. Rigid fixation is almost never required. Computed tomography (CT) or fluoroscopic simulation should always be available and, with treatment possible from under the couch; it should not be necessary to place the patient in an uncomfortable and unstable prone position.

For most of the sites, treatment should be prescribed as an applied dose for single-incident fields and at mid-plane for opposed fields. The treatment volume should include at least one vertebral body above and below the painful vertebra(e) and at least a 2-cm margin on long bones (9). Because there is a high rate of re-treatment or subsequent treatment of adjacent areas, simulation and verification films are recommended to document target localisation along with permanent skin marking of the treatment fields. When orthovoltage energies are used, the dose correction (f factor) applied to compensate for the higher absorbed dose in bones from kilovolt range photons is not routinely recommended, particularly as these energies should be restricted to treatment of superficial bones such as ribs, sternum, and clavicle.

For spinal bone metastases, it is suggested that the radiation dose should be prescribed to the depth of the mid-vertebral body. This requires a lateral spine X-ray or a CT or MRI image to determine the depth. If it is not possible to obtain exact measurements of cord depth, an average depth of 5 cm may be chosen. Prescribing to mid-vertebra should give a relatively homogeneous dose across the vertebral body. If the shoulders can be positioned sufficiently low, cervical spine metastases should be treated with lateral opposed fields to reduce exit-dose toxicity to the larynx and oesophagus.

If not already prescribed, consideration should be given to the use of bisphosphonates in conjunction with radiotherapy since eight separate phase II studies (comprising just over 250 patients) have demonstrated an increase in bone density with the use of this combination (37).

Radiotherapy Toxicity

Pain flare (a temporary worsening of pain in the irradiated site) immediately after palliative radiotherapy has been well described with rates after treatment ranging from 2 to 44%. This wide range is probably accounted for by a variety of data capture methods in the literature. A study of dexamethasone at a daily dose of 8 mg for 3 days starting on the day of radiotherapy reported pain flare in 22% of patients compared to 36% in the same centre's registry study. This apparent reduction in flare occurred at the expense of greater insomnia, and the maximum flare occurred on day 5 (i.e. after dexamethasone had finished). A randomised trial of differing durations of dexamethasone is proposed (12).

The major toxic effect of bone radiotherapy is on bone marrow. This cannot be avoided, since a dose of radiation as low as 2 Gy will arrest mitosis in erythropoietic cells. For bone marrow regeneration, the amount of marrow included in the treatment volume seems to be a more important factor than the radiation dose delivered. If large volumes are treated with a single dose (as in wide-field radiotherapy), rapid compensation is observed. Normalisation of the full blood count does not necessarily indicate recovery of the irradiated marrow, however, since the response may occur within un-irradiated marrow. After irradiation of smaller volumes the stimulus to the uninvolved marrow may be less significant and, paradoxically, compensation may be slower (38).

Longer-term recovery of marrow depends on the age of the patient and sequencing of therapies. Breast cancer patients heavily pretreated with chemotherapy are likely to have slower haemopoietic recovery after radiation; indeed, experience suggests that many of these patients will experience clinically relevant falls in haemoglobin after palliative radiotherapy treatment.

Normal bone formation is a relatively radioresistant process and bone healing continues after radiation doses in the therapeutic range. Healing and re-ossification are seen in 65–85% of lytic lesions after radiotherapy in an unfractured bone (39). The process of reossification is relatively slow, however, and the radiological evidence of the process may not be present until at least 6 months (Fig. 1).

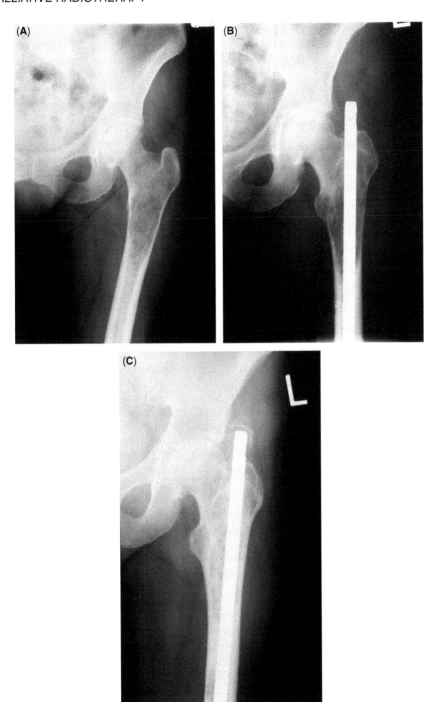

FIGURE 1 X-rays taken prior to (panel B) and 1 year after (right panel C) adjuvant radiotherapy following surgical fixation of a pathological fracture, showing new bone formation within the radiation field.

After higher doses of radiotherapy there are discrepancies in the literature. Radiation doses above 30 Gy may prevent long bone healing, yet doses above 40 Gy have been reported to assist the healing of vertebral fractures. These results are not necessarily inconsistent: long bones repair by a process of endochondral bone formation mediated by a relatively radiosensitive chondrogenic phase, whereas vertebrae depend on direct osteogenesis for intramembranous bone formation, a process which is more radioresistant.

Adjuvant Radiotherapy Following Surgical Fixation

Patients whose metastases involve the cortex of long bones preserve mobility for longer and with improved pain control if orthopaedic intervention is offered before pathological fracture occurs. The theory that radiotherapy interferes with osteogenesis (see the previous section) has been invoked to argue that adjuvant radiation should not be given after surgical fixation. It is clear, however, that failure to follow this practice leads to high rates of failure of the surgical fixation, regardless of theoretical considerations (40). Adjuvant radiation should therefore be considered standard and, since there is no evidence to suggest that it compromises post-surgical recovery, should be given as promptly as is practicable. There is anecdotal evidence that orthopaedic fixation may seed tumour along the length of the bone and therefore whenever practical the whole bone should be included in the post-operative radiation field (41,42).

Wide-Field Radiotherapy

In patients with multiple, widespread bone metastases, simultaneous irradiation of multiple areas of the skeleton is an attractive policy that reduces the overall number of treatments and offers prophylactic treatment for early lesions. As predicted by the gate theory of pain, restricting treatment to the most painful lesion in patients with multiple bony deposits often does not improve the patient's symptoms, as adequate local treatment simply "unmasks" pain from the other untreated lesions.

For these reasons the practice of wide-field radiotherapy (WFRT) has developed. The term WFRT is preferred to hemi-body irradiation, as it is often not the hemi-body that is covered by these treatment fields. Within the RTOG studies of this technique, in which the majority of patients were men with prostate cancer and the number of breast cancer patients was small, the approach was associated with appreciable haematological toxicity (12% of patients experienced grade 3–4), and even after premedication with steroids many patients experienced immediate and delayed emesis (43). Because of concerns over longer-term erythropoiesis in patients who may receive further multiple lines of chemotherapy, WFRT has become less popular in breast cancer than localised radiotherapy.

Radionuclide Therapy

An alternative to wide-field EBRT is the use of bone-seeking radiopharmaceuticals that concentrate in areas of increased bone turnover. These vectors are combined with beta-emitting radionuclides (e.g., [89]strontium and [153]samarium). Beta emitters produce ionising radiation of low energy that penetrates only a few millimetres of the surrounding tissue. The compounds accumulate in bone after intravenous injection and only the immediately adjacent tissue receives the dose. This offers the promise of whole skeleton treatment without visceral toxicity (although bone marrow toxicity with consequential thrombocytopenia and lymphopenia is common). Having established a clear treatment benefit in metastatic prostate cancer there is now an evidence base in breast cancer (44).

[186]Re-hydroxyethylidene diphosphonate (Re-186 HEDP) is a useful radiopharmaceutical with a shorter half-life than most other compounds (90 hours) and a

maximum beta emission of 1.07 MeV. It has 9% gamma emission of 137 KeV meaning that uptake can easily be visualised on a standard gamma camera. These characteristics allow for repeat treatments with less marrow toxicity and apparently faster onset of action than longer-acting agents such as [89]strontium (45). Rates of pain relief are similar and in some cases greater than those achieved with EBRT (44). As with EBRT data there is the promise of synergy in combination with bisphosphonates in early phase II work (46).

Another novel and promising development is the incorporation of [153]samarium-EDTMP into the cement used during vertebroplasty for patients with painful bone metastases. In a phase I trial at New York Methodist Hospital 26 patients have safely undergone the procedure, which has achieved technically satisfactory palliation with highly local radiation delivery (47).

RADIOTHERAPY IN THE TREATMENT OF LOCAL RECURRENCE AND FUNGATION
Local Recurrence in Breast/Chest Wall

Treatment of local recurrence or cutaneous metastasis to breast or chest wall presents particular problems in those cases where the area has previously been irradiated in the adjuvant setting (Fig. 2). Due to a legitimate concern about exceeding normal tissue tolerances and consequent ulceration or necrosis of underlying soft tissue, radiotherapy is often avoided and endocrine or chemotherapy treatment is preferred. If these options have been exhausted, radiotherapy may offer useful palliation of unpleasant fungation or malodorous recurrence and may "dry" the affected tissues, reducing the need for dressings and analgesia. Patients referred for re-irradiation within 12 months of the initial radiation course are unlikely to respond, with local failure being a marker of relative radioresistance of the tumour (48).

In order to reduce toxicity to underlying connective tissues from re-treatments, the beam may be delivered using electrons rather than photons. The physical properties of electrons are such that the energy required for cell kill is transferred over short distances so that deeper connective tissue and lung receive a much lower radiation dose. The technique is occasionally limited by the requirement to treat a relatively flat

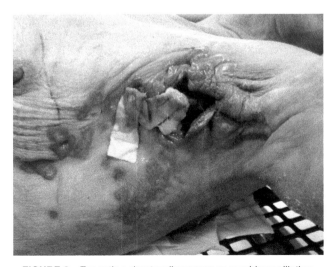

FIGURE 2   Fungating chest wall recurrence requiring palliation.

surface; where disease extends around the curvature of the chest wall, multiple fields (with problems of overlap) may be necessary to achieve coverage.

Photon fields may be delivered either directly or as a reprise of the previous tangential fields. In choosing a dose/fractionation schedule, there needs to be consideration of the likelihood of late effects of overdose becoming clinically significant within the patient's expected lifetime. The prescriber should also be aware that some radiobiological recovery of normal tissues takes place over years. Much of the data on re-irradiation in this setting lacks detailed toxicity data. A study of re-irradiation of 39 patients from Pittsburgh to a cumulative radiotherapy dose in the region of 100 Gy reported a "good to excellent" cosmetic result in 75% and an intact breast at death or censoring in 76.9% (49). A multi-institutional review of eight major US centres reported only a single case of grade 4 dermatitis and three instances of grade 3 toxicities in 81 patients re-irradiated to a cumulative median dose of 106 Gy (48).

Breast or chest wall radiotherapy may also be considered with or without surgery to maintain local control with minimal toxicity in patients presenting with oligometastatic disease and radical treatment of the primary disease may not be appropriate in them (50).

Hyperthermia

In an attempt to overcome the problems of normal tissue tolerance, hyperthermia has been used as a method of increasing the therapeutic ratio. Hyperthermia enhances the cytotoxic effects of radiotherapy and if delivered synchronously can increase cell kill. Since heating of tumour cells to 41–45°C is itself cytotoxic to both tumour and normal tissues, tumours must be selectively heated if the therapeutic ratio is to be increased.

Heating is usually achieved by methods that rely on the thermal absorbance of the soft tissue (electromagnetic current or ultrasound), with a cooling water bolus at the surface. All methods risk hot spots within the treatment field, which may affect the patient's ability to cope with the treatment or cause burns at the edge of the treated area. Current technology limits the amount of heat that can be effectively delivered to tumours deeper than 3 cm and most of the research show benefit for smaller tumour deposits (51).

Initial studies were small and therefore an international effort to randomise patients to larger studies was initiated. Unfortunately this failed to recruit; so, a combined analysis of 307 breast patients from multiple centres was performed in 1996 (52). All patients had locally recurrent breast cancer and the majority (68%) had previously received radiotherapy. Only half of them had evidence of metastatic disease.

The studies delivered radiotherapy doses in the order of 28–32 Gy in 8 fractions, treating twice a week with or without heating to 43°C, and showed a convincing benefit for hyperthermia in achieving local control (Table 3). No survival benefit was shown for the approach, and curiously no benefit for hyperthermia was observed in previously un-irradiated patients (where a biological rationale for radiosensitisation by hyperthermia still exists despite the higher radiation doses used).

In the collaborative study, only 28% of patients had received prior systemic hormone therapy and 9.8% prior chemotherapy. Developments in these areas have largely superseded hyperthermia and radiation as a treatment in this situation although there is some limited experience of successfully combining modern chemotherapies (capecitabine, vinorelbine, and paclitaxel) with hyperthermia and radiotherapy (53). Because of the practical and radiobiological concerns, the technique is rarely used in the United Kingdom, despite advocacy in Europe (54).

TABLE 3 Hyperthermia Trial Data

	Radiotherapy only	Radiotherapy with hyperthermia	Odds ratio (95% confidence intervals)
Number of patients	135	171	
CR overall	55 (41%)	101 (59%)	2.3 (1.4–3.8)
CR in an area not irradiated previously[a]	27/45 (60%)	32/51 (63%)	1.24 (0.46–3.32)
CR in a previously irradiated area[b]	28/90 (31%)	68/120 (57%)	4.7 (2.4–9.5)
Toxicities:			
Blistering	2%	11%	
Ulceration	2%	7%	

[a]Receiving "radical" closes in region of 40 Gy.
[b]Receiving palliative doses in the region of 28–32 Gy.
Abbreviation: CR, complete response rate.

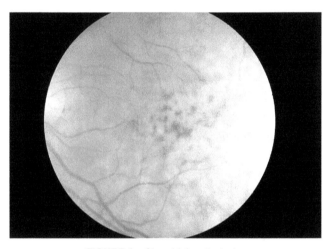

FIGURE 3 Choroidal metastasis.

RADIOTHERAPEUTIC MANAGEMENT OF CHOROIDAL METASTASES

Choroidal metastasis is a disabling complication of breast cancer (Fig. 3). In prospective studies asymptomatic disease has been documented in 5% of patients with metastatic breast cancer and symptomatic disease in 1–2% of patients. In 41% of these patients metastases were bilateral. Although the development of choroidal disease is associated with poor prognosis (median survival time 10 months) the complication of reduced visual acuity is devastating, and palliative treatment is warranted to prevent deterioration. Prior to the advent of highly active chemotherapies, radiotherapy was the treatment of first choice (55), with an 80% response rate and complete resolution in 25%. More recently, authors incorporating systemic therapies into their treatments (in 55% of cases) have reported complete regression in 57.8% of eyes treated (56). No chemotherapy study has reproduced the results of the early radiotherapy studies.

The authors know of no published randomised studies of radiation dose. The largest prospective series, the ARO-95-08 from Germany, recruited 56 patients (65 eyes), of whom 62% had breast cancer. Patients were treated with 40 Gy in 20 fractions. Visual acuity was stabilised (50%) or improved (36%) for the majority and no treated asymptomatic patients (n = 15) developed ocular symptoms during follow-up. 70% of patients in the study with unilateral disease were treated with a unilateral radiotherapy beam arrangement; that none of these patients developed contralateral disease suggests that a lower total dose may have been adequate for tumour control.

In delivering the treatment, CT-planned virtual simulation enables the application of a simple direct beam that targets the choroid and is angled posteriorly to avoid entering the lens of either eye. Where this is not available, a 4 cm × 4 cm field covering the bony orbit but sparing the lens anteriorly may simply be angled posteriorly by 5° to reliably spare the contralateral eye.

Radiotherapeutic Management of Cerebral Metastases

For patients with breast cancer, the development of cerebral metastases is associated with significant physical and psychological distresses. Quality of life may be severely affected by neurological symptoms and diminished independence, and the prognostic implications are bleak. Unfortunately, cerebral metastases are relatively common, and conventional treatments have limited efficacy.

According to population-based studies, brain metastases are diagnosed in approximately 5% of women with breast cancer. Postmortem examinations have suggested that the actual incidence may be as high as 20–30%, with many cases going unnoticed during the patient's lifetime. There is growing evidence that the incidence of cerebral metastasis is increasing, particularly in heavily treated patients who have lived with metastatic disease for a number of years. The incidence of cerebral metastases in women receiving combination chemotherapy for advanced disease has been estimated at between 25 and 48% (57,58), and the perception that patients with disease overexpressing HER2 are at increased risk of brain metastases is now supported by most of the published data. Two large studies with median follow-up periods of around 4 years have estimated the incidence of intracranial disease at between 1.3% and 2.1% in HER2-negative patients and 5.0–7.8% in patients with HER2-positive tumours (59,60). Patients with triple-negative tumours also had an elevated risk of developing brain metastases (59). Among patients with intracranial disease, there is some evidence that those with HER2-positive tumours have a better prognosis (61–63) but this is not a consistent finding.

These figures illustrate a number of issues. Firstly, the need for effective treatment is greater than ever. Secondly, cerebral metastases can develop and progress in the face of effective systemic treatment. Thirdly, management of disease in the brain has failed to keep pace with the remarkable improvements in systemic therapies that have taken place over the past 20 years. Another consequence of improved control of disease at other sites is that many patients with cerebral metastases survive long enough to experience the potentially devastating long-term effects of radiation on the normal brain. Care must therefore be taken to ensure that improvements in the efficacy of treatment do not occur at the expense of increased toxicity.

Whole-Brain Radiotherapy

For many years, the standard therapy for symptomatic brain metastases has been whole-brain radiotherapy (WBRT). Various factors underlie this approach: adenocarcinoma of the breast is generally radiosensitive; metastases are likely to be numerous and at multiple intracranial locations, even if not all can be detected by standard imaging; and most systemic treatments do not penetrate the blood–brain barrier effectively so are unlikely to be delivered to the target lesions at effective concentrations. Since the prognosis for this patient group is poor, attempts at radical dose treatments are rarely justified, so the dose of radiation applied is generally in the palliative range. In recent years, there has been a move towards intensifying local therapy in patients who are judged to have a better prognosis, while deferring whole-brain irradiation until absolutely necessary. The evidence underlying this approach will be discussed in more detail later in the chapter.

WBRT Technique

WBRT is delivered using parallel opposed, lateral fields encompassing the contents of the cranium but avoiding radiosensitive normal tissues, particularly the eyes. Megavoltage photon treatment using a linear accelerator has the advantage of reducing radiation dose to the scalp. Traditionally, patients have been immobilised using a personalised thermoplastic mask that is secured to the treatment couch and the treatment fields have been simulated fluoroscopically or by virtual simulation. Some patients find immobilisation claustrophobic, however; so in many centres the palliative nature of the treatment has been acknowledged and patients are treated without rigid immobilisation devices. Similarly, treatment fields may be planned on the treatment couch using anatomical landmarks—the accuracy of the set-up can then be checked at the first treatment session using electronic portal imaging (Fig. 4). Additional advantages of this more pragmatic approach are a reduction in the number of patient visits and the opportunity to minimise delays in starting treatment. Both factors may be helpful in alleviating patient anxiety at what is often an emotionally demanding time.

WBRT Radiation Dose

The delivered dose of radiotherapy varies widely between centres. In many countries, the standard dose for WBRT is 30 Gy in 10 daily fractions, but alternative regimens range from 12 Gy in 2 fractions to 45 Gy in 15 fractions. In many cases, the dose and duration of treatment will be determined by the patient's general condition and performance status. Outpatient treatment is entirely appropriate in most cases. In the United Kingdom, 20 Gy in 5 daily fractions is commonly delivered on the basis that a more prolonged course of treatment is not justified for patients whose life expectancy is a matter of weeks.

This array of treatment regimens reflects the paucity of evidence to support the use of any particular radiation schedule. Most studies have been retrospective and

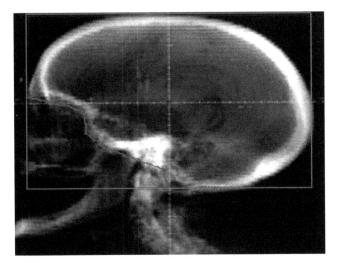

FIGURE 4   An electronic portal image showing lateral beam arrangement for the delivery of whole-brain radiotherapy for cerebral metastases. Field borders were determined using bony landmarks and verified by portal imaging at the time of the first treatment.

subject to the important confounding factor of patient selection. Generally, patients who are offered more aggressive regimens are those with better performance status, for whom prognosis is better regardless of treatment. Also, most of the published data are derived from heterogeneous groups of patients with various primary tumours, amongst which breast cancer patients are often in a minority. Very few randomised trials addressing radiation dose have been conducted. Hence, interpretation of the available data is problematic. However, the largest retrospective study published to date (1085 patients) showed no effect of radiation dose on survival (64).

Two retrospective studies have been published that focused specifically on breast cancer patients. The first involved 207 patients and found no difference in outcome among three regimens (20 Gy in 5 fractions, 30 Gy in 10 fractions, and 40 Gy in 20 fractions) (65). In a second study comprising 223 patients, however, radiation doses of 30 Gy or above were associated with a reduced risk of death (62).

Median survival rate from the time of diagnosis of brain metastases for patients receiving symptomatic treatment only has been reported as 4–6 weeks, whereas patients receiving WBRT have a life expectancy of 4–6 months. Rates of symptomatic response have been quoted as 60–85%, but clinical experience suggests that steroid treatment alone is often associated with a prompt improvement in neurological symptoms. In one study, 67% of patients were able to discontinue steroids shortly after completing radiotherapy, although 38% restarted this medication during the follow-up period (66). Perhaps more relevant was the observation that 30–40% of surviving patients showed an improved or a stable functional status (Karnofsky Performance Status) at 1 and 3-month follow-up. Radiological response rates are rarely reported, and the available data are often biased by preferential imaging of patients experiencing new or worsening neurological symptoms.

The majority of attempts to improve response rates and survival by increasing radiation dose have been unsuccessful. In those studies where a survival benefit was identified, this was attributable to beneficial effects of the higher dose on a small subgroup of patients displaying favourable prognostic features (67). The largest randomised controlled study of radiation dose was the RTOG 9104 study in which the control protocol was 30 Gy in 10 daily fractions and patients in the experimental arm received accelerated, hyperfractionated treatment to the whole brain of 32 Gy in 20 twice daily fractions and a boost of 22.4 Gy in 14 fractions to tumour sites. No difference in median or 1-year survival was demonstrated (68). Amongst the published data derived specifically from breast cancer patients, the only consistent predictors of improved survival are performance status and/or recursive partitioning analysis class (62,66,69,70) although the recent Dawood study did report a significant reduction in risk of death for patients receiving doses of 30 Gy or greater (62).

WBRT Toxicity

Acute toxicity associated with WBRT includes alopecia, which is inevitable but temporary; and fatigue and nausea, one or both of which occur in 8–12% of patients. The latter two may be ameliorated by corticosteroid and anti-emetic therapy. A rare but debilitating complication of WBRT in adults is "somnolence syndrome", a subacute consequence of cranial irradiation that occurs in up to 60% of children receiving such treatment for leukaemia. The clinical features are overwhelming fatigue and apathy, typically commencing 4–6 weeks after completion of radiotherapy. The syndrome is self-limiting and there is some evidence for a partial symptomatic response to steroids, but the development of this complication in a woman with a life expectancy of only a few months clearly represents a failure of palliative therapy. Unfortunately, there is very little data to inform any estimate of the risk of somnolence for an individual. In a small prospective study of patients receiving high-dose cranial radiotherapy for primary brain tumours, the incidence of somnolence symptoms was 84%

(71). In the setting of metastatic brain involvement, the dose of radiation delivered is generally lower, but the volume of brain irradiated is greater. Specific questioning for and reporting of symptoms of somnolence would be a useful component of any future study in this area. At present, it is perhaps wise to inform patients of the nature of this possible complication, since its occurrence is usually associated with marked anxiety about the possible implications of the symptoms.

Documentation of the late complications of WBRT has also been scanty, partly because of the poor prognosis of the patient group and partly because the symptoms of cerebral radiation toxicity overlap significantly with those of progressive intracranial disease. The most important manifestations of late radiation damage are white matter necrosis, which may occur as early as 6 months after treatment, and cerebral atrophy associated with vasculopathy, which becomes apparent after 1–10 years. Generalised clinical symptoms include lethargy, short-term memory loss, and impaired cognitive function. More specific symptoms may arise from areas that were subjected to a higher radiation dose, or to localised damage of vascular origin. Symptoms do not always correlate with the radiological features of white matter changes and cerebral atrophy. In one retrospective study of patients who had received WBRT, actuarial rates of cerebral atrophy and white matter abnormalities respectively were 50% and 25% after 1 year, and 84% and 85% after 2 years. Clinical symptoms of late radiation toxicity at these time points occurred in 32% and 49% of patients, rising to 83% at 5 years (72).

An important randomised trial comparing the neurocognitive effects of stereotactic radiosurgery (SRS) plus WBRT with SRS alone was published in 2009 (73). After 58 patients had been recruited, the study was halted by the data monitoring committee because a significant decline in learning and memory function was observed in the SRS plus WBRT patients at the 4-month time point. This effect was measured as "a significant deterioration (5-point drop compared with baseline) in Hopkins Verbal Learning Test-Revised (HVLT-R) total recall". While providing important evidence that WBRT has significant effects on cognition, the dependence on a single test at a single time point reduces the clinical significance of this result. Other reservations include the relatively small number of patients monitored, the early stopping up of the study, and the fact that freedom from CNS recurrence at 1 year was significantly higher in the SRS plus WBRT group (73% vs. 27%).

Another study that addressed specifically the effect of WBRT on neurocognitive function in patients with cerebral metastases demonstrated no significant change in Mini-Mental Status Examination (MMSE) scores compared with pre-treatment values. The capacity of this study to demonstrate an effect was limited by the short follow-up period (3 months). However, an important finding to emerge was that the average MMSE score of patients whose metastases were not controlled by treatment fell by a significant and clinically meaningful extent (74). Finding the correct balance between the efficacy and lack of toxicity remains the key challenge in the management of this patient group.

Useful information about neurotoxicity can be extrapolated from studies of prophylactic cranial irradiation (PCI) in 265 patients with small cell lung cancer. An RTOG trial compared WBRT doses of 25 Gy in 10 fractions with 36 Gy in 18 or 24 fractions and reported an increased risk of late neurotoxicity in the high-dose group (75). This trial was part of the large PCI Collaborative Group study (720 patients), which reported no difference in neurocognitive function between patients receiving 25 Gy and 36 Gy (76). In the collaborative study, patients were assessed by the EORTC QLQ-C30 questionnaire and the BN20 brain tumour module. The smaller RTOG study also included a battery of more sophisticated neurocognitive tests, the results of which accounted for the difference between the two arms of the study. While they do not demonstrate a clear effect of radiation dose on late neurotoxicity, these data illustrate that specific and time-consuming neurocognitive assessments are probably required to detect subtle but important changes in neurological status after cranial irradiation.

Intensifying Local Therapy

In spite of the generally disappointing overall results presented so far, it has long been apparent that a subgroup of patients with cerebral metastases has a substantially better outlook than the average, and that these patients might benefit from a more intensive therapy. Clinical experience and some of the published data indicate that patients with breast cancer are over-represented in this good prognosis group. The first data to support the potential value of a more aggressive approach arose from studies of neurosurgical intervention. A randomised trial comparing surgical excision plus WBRT against needle biopsy plus WBRT in the treatment of solitary brain metastases (various primary tumour types) reported overall survival and duration of functional independence to be significantly longer in the resected group (median survival 40 weeks vs. 15 weeks) (77). Considering breast cancer specifically, retrospective data suggest that surgical excision can be associated with median survival rates of around 16 months in this highly selected patient group (78).

WBRT and Surgery

In many centres, neurosurgical excision of cerebral metastases is followed routinely by adjuvant WBRT. This approach is supported by two retrospective analyses which showed, subject to the usual concerns about patient selection, that delivery of postoperative WBRT was associated with improved survival (79) and increased time to neurological relapse (80). A cautionary finding of the latter study was that 11% of irradiated patients surviving for more than one year developed severe radiation induced dementia.

While a cohort of neurosurgeons was acquiring expertise and enthusiasm for resecting cerebral metastases, technical developments in radiotherapy delivery were increasing the opportunities for non-surgical management of localised intracranial disease.

Stereotactic Radiotherapy

Stereotactic radiotherapy involves the precise delivery of radiation to a localised target volume by relating its anatomical location to a three-dimensional image data set using numerical coordinates. The aim of treatment is to achieve a relatively high radiation dose at the tumour target whilst delivering a minimal dose to the surrounding normal tissue. Patient immobilisation is critical and most techniques necessitate fitting a rigid stereotactic frame to the patient's head (Fig. 5). This frame is in place during the imaging and treatment phases and enables precise and reproducible localisation of the target relative to components of the frame, and hence to the radiotherapy delivery system.

For the treatment of brain metastases, the dose to the tumour deposit is usually delivered in a single fraction, a scenario that has led to the widespread use of the term "stereotactic radiosurgery" (SRS). It should be stressed that SRS is a non-invasive procedure that differs from stereotactic radiotherapy only in the magnitude of the dose delivered per treatment session. Two techniques are in general use: Linac-based stereotactic radiotherapy and Gamma Knife SRS. However, ongoing technical developments including real-time image guidance are enabling increasingly accurate planning and delivery of radiotherapy without the need for rigid frames, so the distinction between stereotactic and non-stereotactic treatments is beginning to blur.

Linac-based stereotactic radiotherapy exploits the capacity of a linear accelerator to move through a pre-defined arc around its isocentre whilst continuously delivering

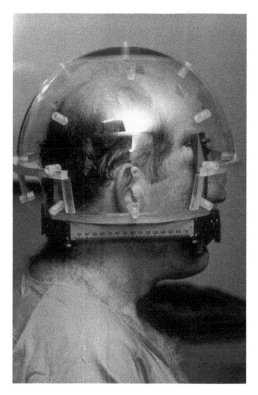

FIGURE 5   Stereotactic frame used in "Gamma Knife" treatment. *Source*: Courtesy of Dr. PN Plowman, London Radiosurgical Centre.

a collimated beam of x-rays (Fig. 6). "Gamma Knife" treatment utilises a stationary treatment device that houses around 200 small radioactive sources (Cobalt-60), the gamma radiation emissions from which are collimated into narrow beams that intersect at the site of the tumour (Fig. 7). Both methods are capable of accurately delivering therapeutic single doses of radiation to cerebral metastases. Differences between the two techniques affect the internal and external dose gradients achieved, and the number of lesions that can be treated in a single episode. Logistical considerations also mean that Linac-based treatments usually take place alongside conventional radiotherapy and may thus be subject to more stringent time restrictions than might apply in Gamma Knife treatment units. Perhaps because of this, the Gamma Knife facility has more often been used to treat multiple deposits in a single session, with some centres treating up to 10 metastatic lesions. This increases the number of patients eligible for treatment, and is often more convenient, but entails a lengthy period of immobilisation that requires sedation. At present, there is no evidence to suggest that either of these techniques is associated with a superior outcome, and it is extremely unlikely that a prospective, randomised study will ever be conducted.

Patient selection is clearly an important component of this treatment strategy. Patients with more deposits and a higher total volume of disease have a worse prognosis, even if treated with SRS (63,81), so the overall benefit of treating numerous lesions is questionable. Accuracy and homogeneity of the delivered dose fall as target volume increases; so many centres restrict treatment to tumour deposits that are no larger than 3 cm in diameter. Large or irregularly shaped lesions may be treated by using multiple isocentres. The radiation dose prescribed varies but is usually around

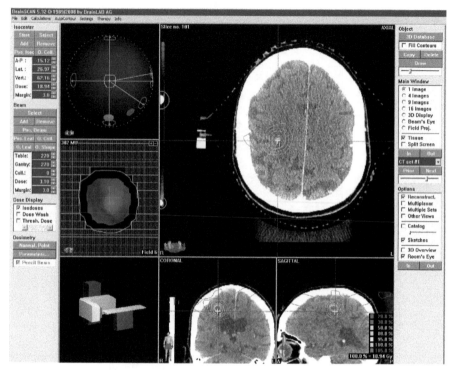

FIGURE 6 Radiation isodose contours generated during the planning of Linac-based stereotactic treatment for a solitary cerebral metastasis. *Source*: Courtesy of Dr. A. James and Ms. A. Williamson, Beatson West of Scotland Cancer Centre, Glasgow.

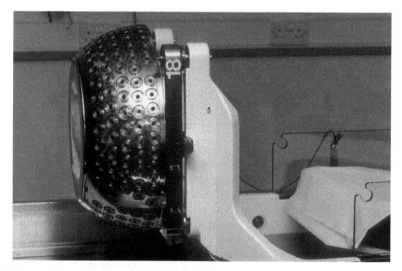

FIGURE 7 Multiple radioactive sources of the Gamma Knife machine and its treatment couch. *Source*: Courtesy of Dr. PN Plowman, London Radiosurgical Centre.

20 Gy, with more conservative doses used for larger lesions. The dose is usually prescribed to the 90% isodose, which corresponds to the tumour margin. Fractionated Linac-based stereotactic radiotherapy regimens delivering 24 Gy in 4 fractions have been employed in the treatment of larger metastases, and a recent non-randomised

study comparing single 20 Gy treatments with fractionated courses of 36 Gy in 6 fractions reported no difference in tumour control and reduced toxicity in the fractionated group, despite the fact that the tumours treated were larger or close to critical structures (82).

SRS Toxicity

The evidence to date suggests that the risk of late toxicity associated with the delivery of large radiation doses in single fractions is largely counterbalanced by the superior dose distribution achieved. Cerebral necrosis has been reported in between 3 and 17% of patients, of whom the majority experienced symptoms. In a large retrospective series of 350 breast cancer patients, symptomatic adverse events were recorded in 6% of cases (81). The risk of necrosis appears to rise with the volume irradiated: in one study the incidence at 5 years was 16% for tumours greater than 2 cm in diameter compared with 3.7% for smaller tumours (83). Haemorrhage is a rare complication, and long-term effects on cognition and memory have not been reported. Acute toxicity relates to the stereotactic frame, which can cause transient headaches and local irritation, and to radiation-induced oedema. The latter effect is minimised by the use of prophylactic high-dose steroids, but may cause nausea, vomiting, and drowsiness in a proportion of patients. Many oncologists report that a proportion of patients experience prolonged steroid dependency that can significantly reduce quality of life, but to date this has been poorly documented in the literature. The fact that SRS does not cause alopecia may be an important consideration.

SRS Efficacy

The stereotactic approach appears to yield impressive rates of control within the irradiated volume, with many studies quoting local control rates of over 90%. However, a randomised study comparing SRS plus WBRT with SRS alone (multiple primary tumour types) reported 12-month brain recurrence rates of 47% and 76% respectively (84). SRS enthusiasts consider the technique to be a valid alternative to neurosurgical excision: this view is supported by a retrospective study of 97 patients with solitary brain metastases treated either by surgery or SRS, which revealed no difference in survival, but significantly enhanced local control in the SRS group (85).

Combining and Scheduling Treatments

Patients treated with SRS remain vulnerable to relapse at other sites in the brain, so WBRT has been widely used as an adjunct to stereotactic treatment, or indeed as a first-line treatment option, with SRS reserved for recurrent disease. An important multicentre, randomised RTOG study interrogated whether upfront combination treatment improved outcomes, by allocating patients with one to three deposits (various primary malignancies) to receive WBRT alone or WBRT plus stereotactic boost(s). In this study, the addition of SRS was associated with a higher incidence of improved or stable performance status in all patients, and superior survival in patients who had good performance status at baseline (86). These data led to WBRT followed by SRS boost becoming standard therapy for suitable patients in many centres.

For many clinicians, however, concern about the longer-term neurocognitive effects of WBRT encouraged an alternative treatment philosophy according to which neurosurgical resection or SRS should be used as first-line treatment to achieve local tumour control while avoiding or delaying the use of WBRT. Whether the omission of WBRT impacted upon survival was initially assessed in a multi-institutional, retrospective study of 569 patients whose initial management was either SRS alone or WBRT and SRS (87). No difference in survival was detected, regardless of the performance status. A prospective study of patients with four or less metastases was conducted in which Linac-based SRS was given as first-line therapy and for treatable relapses: in this series only 29% of patients required salvage treatment with WBRT (88). More substantial evidence supporting this approach is provided by a large multicentre EORTC study in which 359 patients with one to three metastases managed initially by surgical resection or SRS were randomised to receive adjuvant WBRT (30 Gy in 10 fractions) or observation (89). Although WBRT reduced the incidence of intracranial relapse, there was no difference in overall survival (approximately 11 months in both arms) or in time to deterioration in performance status (approximately 10 months) and only 31% of patients in the observation arm went on to receive WBRT as salvage treatment.

In summary, SRS appears to be a useful addition to the treatment options for this patient group. Its suitability for an individual patient depends on the number and size of intracerebral deposits, the status of their extra-cranial disease, their performance status, and the local availability of Linac-based SRS or Gamma Knife facilities. Concerns over the financial implications of SRS treatment may be alleviated by the outcome of a cost utility analysis of surgery, WBRT and SRS, in which the combination of WBRT and SRS yielded the lowest cost per week of survival (90). Patients with a life expectancy of greater than 6 months may benefit from the first-line use of SRS to avoid the potential long-term complications of WBRT. Other roles are the palliation of patients whose intracranial disease has progressed after WBRT, or as part of a more aggressive approach in combination with WBRT.

New Treatment Strategies

The relative success of localised therapy for oligometastatic disease has encouraged efforts to intensify localised treatment. A number of small, non-randomised studies have reported prolonged local control when SRS has been delivered to the resection cavity(ies) after neurosurgical excision of cerebral metastases (91,92). Whether this combination provides any benefit over either individual modality remains to be seen, and definition of the post-operative volume at risk is unlikely to be straightforward in all cases.

Although SRS allows high-dose treatments to small-volume deposits while sparing the rest of the brain, many patients do not have access to this technology, and significant numbers are ineligible for SRS alone either because their deposits are too large or because they are at high risk of disease recurrence at other sites within the brain. Some of these patients might benefit from WBRT with intensification of treatment to gross sites of disease. Ongoing developments in intensity-modulated radiotherapy (IMRT) are enabling radiation oncologists to adopt a more flexible approach to the treatment of such patients, and examples of WBRT with simultaneous in-field boosts to one or more lesions are appearing in the literature. In one such study, 48 patients with one to three cerebral metastases were treated with WBRT (30 Gy in 10 fractions) and simultaneous boost(s) of 5 Gy–30 Gy (93). No dose-limiting toxicity was reported at 3 months after treatment, but longer term follow-up and a more detailed assessment of neurocognitive sequelae are needed to evaluate a more widespread application.

Many studies have illustrated that the most clinically relevant toxicity associated with WBRT is neurocognitive decline. An increasing body of research implicates specific areas of the brain in the pathogenesis of this devastating complication. Another potential role for IMRT in the treatment of multiple cerebral metastases is to deliver a therapeutic dose to the contents of the cranium while delivering a lower dose to these critical areas, which include the limbic system, hippocampus, and subventricular zones (reviewed in (94)). At the time of writing this approach is in its infancy, and the hypothesis itself remains largely unsubstantiated. However, the increasing sophistication of IMRT techniques is enabling researchers to contemplate and execute such novel strategies for the first time.

Drug and Radiation Combinations

The availability of a new generation of drug therapies with improved penetration of the central nervous system has increased the potential for drug/radiation combinations for patients with brain metastases. Agents under investigation include capecitabine (95), trastuzumab (96), and the oral EGFR/HER2 inhibitor lapatinib. At present the published data are insufficient to indicate how effective these radiation/drug combinations will be, or to evaluate whether neurotoxicity will be exacerbated. Poly(ADP-ribose) polymerase (PARP) inhibitors are another class of agents that are predicted to have tumour specific radiosensitising effects, have shown promising single agent activity against breast cancers with BRCA1 or BRCA2 mutations and are extremely well tolerated (97). Early-phase studies of PARP inhibitors in combination with WBRT in patients with multiple cerebral metastases are underway and the results are eagerly anticipated.

Radiotherapy for Cerebral Metastases: A Summary

In the treatment of cerebral metastases from breast cancer, WBRT increases survival but the extent and duration of palliation are limited, and toxicity may be significant. For patients with low-volume oligometastatic disease, stereotactic radiotherapy can be effective in palliating symptoms and achieving local control, and there is increasing evidence that WBRT can be safely deferred by the early use of this treatment modality. Novel radiation techniques and drug combinations must be considered as experimental at this stage, but they offer the prospect of improving outcomes for a broader spectrum of patients. Tools for measuring treatment-related neurotoxicity are improving and should be routinely employed in clinical studies of new treatment strategies.

REFERENCES

1. Leone BA, Romero A, Rabinovich MG, et al. Stage IV breast cancer: clinical course and survival of patients with osseous versus extraosseous metastases at initial diagnosis. The GOCS (Grupo Oncologico Cooperativo del Sur) experience. Am J Clin Oncol 1988; 11: 618–22.
2. Coleman RE. Metastatic bone disease: clinical features, pathophysiology and treatment strategies. Cancer Treat Rev 2001; 27: 165–76.
3. Theriault RL, Lipton A, Hortobagyi GN, et al. Pamidronate reduces skeletal morbidity in women with advanced breast cancer and lytic bone lesions: a randomized, placebo-controlled trial. Protocol 18 Aredia Breast Cancer Study Group. J Clin Oncol 1999; 17: 846–54.
4. Boyle WJ, Simonet WS, Lacey DL. Osteoclast differentiation and activation. Nature 2003; 423: 337–42.
5. Vassiliou V, Kalogeropoulou C, Petsas T, Leotsinidis M, Kardamakis D. Clinical and radiological evaluation of patients with lytic, mixed and sclerotic bone metastases from solid tumors: is there a correlation between clinical status of patients and type of bone metastases? Clin Exp Metastasis 2007; 24: 49–56.
6. Ben-Josef E, Shamsa F, Youssef E, Porter AT. External beam radiotherapy for painful osseous metastases: pooled data dose response analysis. Int J Radiat Oncol Biol Phys 1999; 45: 715–19.
7. Krempien R, Huber PE, Harms W, et al. Combination of early bisphosphonate administration and irradiation leads to improved remineralization and restabilization of osteolytic bone metastases in an animal tumor model. Cancer 2003; 98: 1318–24.
8. Hoskin PJ. Bisphosphonates and radiation therapy for palliation of metastatic bone disease. Cancer Treat Rev 2003; 29: 321–7.
9. Chow E, Wu JS, Hoskin P, et al. International consensus on palliative radiotherapy endpoints for future clinical trials in bone metastases. Radiother Oncol 2002; 64: 275–80.
10. Campos S, Presutti R, Zhang L, et al. Elderly patients with painful bone metastases should be offered palliative radiotherapy. Int J Radiat Oncol Biol Phys 2010; 76: 1500–6.

11. Kirou-Mauro A, Amanda H, Jennifer W, et al. Is response to radiotherapy in patients related to the severity of pretreatment pain? Int J Radiat Oncol Biol Phys 2008; 71: 1208–12.

12. Hird A, Zhang L, Holt T, et al. Dexamethasone for the prophylaxis of radiation-induced pain flare after palliative radiotherapy for symptomatic bone metastases: a phase II study. Clin Oncol (R Coll Radiol) 2009; 21: 329–35.

13. Steenland E, Leer JW, van Houwelingen H, et al. The effect of a single fraction compared to multiple fractions on painful bone metastases: a global analysis of the Dutch Bone Metastasis Study. Radiother Oncol 1999; 52: 101–9.

14. Wu JS, Wong R, Johnston M, Bezjak A, Whelan T. Meta-analysis of dose-fractionation radiotherapy trials for the palliation of painful bone metastases. Int J Radiat Oncol Biol Phys 2003; 55: 594–605.

15. Sze WM, Shelley MD, Held I, Wilt TJ, Mason MD. Palliation of metastatic bone pain: single fraction versus multifraction radiotherapy–a systematic review of randomised trials. Clin Oncol (R Coll Radiol) 2003; 15: 345–52.

16. van den Hout WB, van der Linden YM, Steenland E, et al. Single-versus multiple-fraction radiotherapy in patients with painful bone metastases: cost-utility analysis based on a randomized trial. J Natl Cancer Inst 2003; 95: 222–9.

17. Fairchild A, Elizabeth B, Sunita G, et al. International patterns of practice in palliative radiotherapy for painful bone metastases: evidence-based practice? Int J Radiat Oncol Biol Phys 2009; 75: 1501–10.

18. Hartsell WF, Konski AA, Lo SS, Hayman JA. Single fraction radiotherapy for bone metastases: clinically effective, time efficient, cost conscious and still underutilized in the United States? Clin Oncol (R Coll Radiol) 2009; 21: 652–4.

19. van der Linden YM, Lok JJ, Steenland E, et al. Single fraction radiotherapy is efficacious: a further analysis of the Dutch Bone Metastasis Study controlling for the influence of retreatment. Int J Radiat Oncol Biol Phys 2004; 59: 528–37.

20. Mithal NP, Needham PR, Hoskin PJ. Retreatment with radiotherapy for painful bone metastases. Int J Radiat Oncol Biol Phys 1994; 29: 1011–14.

21. Konski A, James J, Hartsell W, et al. Economic analysis of radiation therapy oncology group 97-14: multiple versus single fraction radiation treatment of patients with bone metastases. Am J Clin Oncol 2009; 32: 423–8.

22. Roos DE, Turner SL, O'Brien PC, et al. Randomized trial of 8 Gy in 1 versus 20 Gy in 5 fractions of radiotherapy for neuropathic pain due to bone metastases (Trans-Tasman Radiation Oncology Group, TROG 96.05). Radiother Oncol 2005; 75: 54–63.

23. NICE. Metastatic spinal cord compression: diagnosis and management of pateints at risk of or with metastatic spnal cord compression. UK: National Institute of Health and Clinical Excellence, National Collaborating Centre fro Cancer, 2008.

24. Prewett S, Venkitaraman R. Metastatic spinal cord compression: review of the evidence for a radiotherapy dose fractionation schedule. Clin Oncol (R Coll Radiol) 2010; 22: 222–30.

25. Rades D, Fehlauer F, Stalpers LJ, et al. A prospective evaluation of two radiotherapy schedules with 10 versus 20 fractions for the treatment of metastatic spinal cord compression: final results of a multicenter study. Cancer 2004; 101: 2687–92.

26. Rades D, Marisa L, Theo V, et al. Preliminary Results of Spinal Cord Compression Recurrence Evaluation (Score-1) Study comparing short-course versus long-course radiotherapy for local control of malignant epidural spinal cord compression. Int J Radiat Oncol Biol Phys 2009; 73: 228–34.

27. Rades D, Veninga T, Stalpers LJ, et al. Prognostic factors predicting functional outcomes, recurrence-free survival, and overall survival after radiotherapy for metastatic spinal cord compression in breast cancer patients. Int J Radiat Oncol Biol Phys 2006; 64: 182–8.

28. Rades D, Volker R, Theo V, et al. A score predicting posttreatment ambulatory status in patients irradiated for metastatic spinal cord compression. Int J Radiat Oncol Biol Phys 2008; 72: 905–8.

29. Patchell RA, Tibbs PA, Regine WF, et al. Direct decompressive surgical resection in the treatment of spinal cord compression caused by metastatic cancer: a randomised trial. Lancet 2005; 366: 643–8.

30. Rades D, Rudat V, Veninga T, et al. Prognostic factors for functional outcome and survival after reirradiation for in-field recurrences of metastatic spinal cord compression. Cancer 2008; 113: 1090–6.

31. Wong CS, Van Dyk J, Milosevic M, Laperriere NJ. Radiation myelopathy following single courses of radiotherapy and retreatment. Int J Radiat Oncol Biol Phys 1994; 30: 575–81.
32. Sahgal A, Christopher A, Dean C, et al. Stereotactic body radiotherapy is effective salvage therapy for patients with prior radiation of spinal metastases. Int J Radiat Oncol Biol Phys 2009; 74: 723–31.
33. Martin A, Gaya A. Stereotactic body radiotherapy: a review. Clin Oncol (R Coll Radiol) 2010; 22: 157–72.
34. Mancosu P, Piera N, Mario B, et al. Re-irradiation of metastatic spinal cord compression: a feasibility study by volumetric-modulated arc radiotherapy for in-field recurrence creating a dosimetric hole on the central canal. Radiother Oncol 2010; 94: 67–70.
35. Lo SS, Sahgal A, Hartsell WF, et al. The treatment of bone metastasis with highly conformal radiation therapy: a brave new world or a costly mistake? Clin Oncol (R Coll Radiol) 2009; 21: 662–4.
36. Williams MP, Cherryman GR, Husband JE. Magnetic resonance imaging in suspected metastatic spinal cord compression. Clin Radiol 1989; 40: 286–90.
37. Vassiliou V, Bruland O, Janjan N, et al. Combining systemic bisphosphonates with palliative external beam radiotherapy or bone-targeted radionuclide therapy: interactions and effectiveness. Clin Oncol (R Coll Radiol) 2009; 21: 665–7.
38. Sacks EL, Goris ML, Glatstein E, Gilbert E, Kaplan HS. Bone marrow regeneration following large field radiation: influence of volume, age, dose, and time. Cancer 1978 Sep; 42(3): 1057–65.
39. Garmatis CJ, Chu FC. The effectiveness of radiation therapy in the treatment of bone metastases from breast cancer. Radiology 1978; 126: 235–7.
40. Sim FH, Frassica FJ, Frassica DA. Metastatic bone disease: current concepts of clinicopathophysiology and modern surgical treatment. Ann Acad Med Singapore 1992; 21: 274–9.
41. Awan N, Azer A, Harrani K, Cogley D. Intramedullary spread of tumour cells during IM nailing: a histological diagnosis. Eur J Orthop Surg Traumatol 2002; 12: 53–5.
42. Esler C, Ashford R. Failure to irradiate the whole bone after surgery for skeletal metastasis may predispose to second metastasis formation. Clin Oncol (R Coll Radiol) 2010; 22: 618–19.
43. Salazar OM, Sandhu T, da Motta NW, et al. Fractionated half-body irradiation (HBI) for the rapid palliation of widespread, symptomatic, metastatic bone disease: a randomized Phase III trial of the International Atomic Energy Agency (IAEA). Int J Radiat Oncol Biol Phys 2001; 50: 765–75.
44. Liepe K, Runge R, Kotzerke J. Systemic radionuclide therapy in pain palliation. Am J Hosp Palliat Care 2005; 22: 457–64.
45. Sciuto R, Festa A, Pasqualoni R, et al. Metastatic bone pain palliation with 89-Sr and 186-Re-HEDP in breast cancer patients. Breast Cancer Res Treat 2001; 66: 101–9.
46. Liang JG, Jiang NY, Du JQ, et al. Clinical value of combined therapy with 188Re-HEDP and pamidronate in breast cancer with bone metastasis. Zhonghua Zhong Liu Za Zhi 2005; 27: 180–2.
47. Ashamalla H, Erico C, Mark M, et al. Phase I Trial of Vertebral Intracavitary Cement and Samarium (VICS): novel technique for treatment of painful vertebral metastasis. Int J Radiat Oncol Biol Phys 2009; 75: 836–42.
48. Wahl A, Rademaker A, Krystyna DK, et al. Multi-institutional review of repeat irradiation of chest wall and breast for recurrent breast cancer. Int J Radiat Oncol Biol Phys 2008; 70: 477–84.
49. Deutsch M. Repeat high-dose external beam irradiation for in-breast tumor recurrence after previous lumpectomy and whole breast irradiation. Int J Radiat Oncol Biol Phys 2002; 53: 687–91.
50. Bourgier C, Wassim K, Anne-Lise V, et al. Breast radiotherapy as part of loco-regional treatments in stage IV breast cancer patients with oligometastatic disease. Radiother Oncol 2010; 96: 199–203.
51. Li G, Mitsumori M, Ogura M, et al. Local hyperthermia combined with external irradiation for regional recurrent breast carcinoma. Int J Clin Oncol 2004; 9: 179–83.
52. Vernon CC, Hand JW, Field SB, et al. Radiotherapy with or without hyperthermia in the treatment of superficial localized breast cancer: results from five randomized controlled trials. International Collaborative Hyperthermia Group. Int J Radiat Oncol Biol Phys 1996; 35: 731–44.
53. Zagar TM, Higgins KA, Miles EF, et al. Durable palliation of breast cancer chest wall recurrence with radiation therapy, hyperthermia, and chemotherapy. Radiother Oncol 2010; 97: 535–40.

54. van der Zee J, van der Holt B, Rietveld PJ, et al. Reirradiation combined with hyperthermia in recurrent breast cancer results in a worthwhile local palliation. Br J Cancer 1999; 79: 483–90.
55. Thatcher N, Thomas PR. Choroidal metastases from breast carcinoma: a survey of 42 patients and the use of radiation therapy. Clin Radiol 1975; 26: 549–53.
56. Amer R, Pe'er J, Chowers I, Anteby I. Treatment options in the management of choroidal metastases. Ophthalmologica 2004; 218: 372–7.
57. Lai R, Dang CT, Malkin MG, Abrey LE. The risk of central nervous system metastases after trastuzumab therapy in patients with breast carcinoma. Cancer 2004; 101: 810–16.
58. Crivellari D, Pagani O, Veronesi A, et al. High incidence of central nervous system involvement in patients with metastatic or locally advanced breast cancer treated with epirubicin and docetaxel. Ann Oncol 2001; 12: 353–6.
59. Heitz F, Harter P, Lueck HJ, et al. Triple-negative and HER2-overexpressing breast cancers exhibit an elevated risk and an earlier occurrence of cerebral metastases. Eur J Cancer 2009; 45: 2792–8.
60. Musolino A, Ciccolallo L, Panebianco M, et al. Multifactorial central nervous system recurrence susceptibility in patients with HER2-positive breast cancer: epidemiological and clinical data from a population-based cancer registry study. Cancer 2011; 117(9): 1837–46.
61. Dawood S, Broglio K, Esteva FJ, et al. Defining prognosis for women with breast cancer and CNS metastases by HER2 status. Ann Oncol 2008; 19: 1242–8.
62. Dawood S, Broglio K, Buzdar AU, Hortobagyi GN, Giordano SH. Prognosis of women with metastatic breast cancer by HER2 status and trastuzumab treatment: an institutional-based review. J Clin Oncol 2010; 28: 92–8.
63. Matsunaga S, Shuto T, Kawahara N, et al. Gamma Knife surgery for metastatic brain tumors from primary breast cancer: treatment indication based on number of tumors and breast cancer phenotype. J Neurosurg 2010; 113(Suppl): 65–72.
64. Rades D, Bohlen G, Dunst J, et al. Comparison of short-course versus long-course whole-brain radiotherapy in the treatment of brain metastases. Strahlenther Onkol 2008; 184: 30–5.
65. Rades D, Lohynska R, Veninga T, Stalpers LJ, Schild SE. Evaluation of 2 whole-brain radiotherapy schedules and prognostic factors for brain metastases in breast cancer patients. Cancer 2007; 110: 2587–92.
66. Mahmoud-Ahmed AS, Suh JH, Lee SY, Crownover RL, Barnett GH. Results of whole brain radiotherapy in patients with brain metastases from breast cancer: a retrospective study. Int J Radiat Oncol Biol Phys 2002; 54: 810–17.
67. Priestman TJ, Dunn J, Brada M, Rampling R, Baker PG. Final results of the Royal College of Radiologists' trial comparing two different radiotherapy schedules in the treatment of cerebral metastases. Clin Oncol (R Coll Radiol) 1996; 8: 308–15.
68. Murray KJ, Scott C, Greenberg HM, et al. A randomized phase III study of accelerated hyper-fractionation versus standard in patients with unresected brain metastases: a report of the Radiation Therapy Oncology Group (RTOG) 9104. Int J Radiat Oncol Biol Phys 1997; 39: 571–4.
69. Lentzsch S, Reichardt P, Weber F, Budach V, Dorken B. Brain metastases in breast cancer: prognostic factors and management. Eur J Cancer 1999; 35: 580–5.
70. Rades D, Haatanen T, Schild SE, Dunst J. Dose escalation beyond 30 grays in 10 fractions for patients with multiple brain metastases. Cancer 2007; 110: 1345–50.
71. Faithfull S, Brada M. Somnolence syndrome in adults following cranial irradiation for primary brain tumours. Clin Oncol (R Coll Radiol) 1998; 10: 250–4.
72. Nieder C, Leicht A, Motaref B, et al. Late radiation toxicity after whole brain radiotherapy: the influence of antiepileptic drugs. Am J Clin Oncol 1999; 22: 573–9.
73. Chang EL, Wefel JS, Hess KR, et al. Neurocognition in patients with brain metastases treated with radiosurgery or radiosurgery plus whole-brain irradiation: a randomised controlled trial. Lancet Oncol 2009; 10: 1037–44.
74. Regine WF, Scott C, Murray K, Curran W. Neurocognitive outcome in brain metastases patients treated with accelerated-fractionation vs. accelerated-hyperfractionated radiotherapy: an analysis from Radiation Therapy Oncology Group Study 91-04. Int J Radiat Oncol Biol Phys 2001; 51: 711–17.
75. Wolfson AH, Bae K, Komaki R, et al. Primary analysis of a phase II randomized trial Radiation Therapy Oncology Group (RTOG) 0212: impact of different total doses and schedules of prophylactic cranial irradiation on chronic neurotoxicity and quality of life for patients with limited-disease small-cell lung cancer. Int J Radiat Oncol Biol Phys 2011; 81: 77–84.

76. Le Péchoux C, Laplanche A, Faivre-Finn C, et al. Clinical neurological outcome and quality of life among patients with limited small-cell cancer treated with two different doses of
prophylactic cranial irradiation in the intergroup phase III trial (PCI99-01, EORTC 22003-
08004, RTOG 0212 and IFCT 99-01). Ann Oncol 2011; 22: 1154–63.
77. Patchell RA, Tibbs PA, Walsh JW, et al. A randomized trial of surgery in the treatment of
single metastases to the brain. N Engl J Med 1990; 322: 494–500.
78. Pieper DR, Hess KR, Sawaya RE. Role of surgery in the treatment of brain metastases in
patients with breast cancer. Ann Surg Oncol 1997; 4: 481–90.
79. Wronski M, Arbit E, McCormick B. Surgical treatment of 70 patients with brain metastases
from breast carcinoma. Cancer 1997; 80: 1746–54.
80. DeAngelis LM, Mandell LR, Thaler HT, et al. The role of postoperative radiotherapy after
resection of single brain metastases. Neurosurgery 1989; 24: 798–805.
81. Kondziolka D, Kano H, Harrison GL, et al. Stereotactic radiosurgery as primary and salvage treatment for brain metastases from breast cancer. J Neurosurg 2010; 114: 792–800.
82. Kim YJ, Cho KH, Kim JY, et al. Single-dose versus fractionated stereotactic radiotherapy
for brain metastases. Int J Radiat Oncol Biol Phys 2010. [Epub ahead of print].
83. Varlotto JM, Flickinger JC, Niranjan A, et al. Analysis of tumor control and toxicity in
patients who have survived at least one year after radiosurgery for brain metastases. Int J
Radiat Oncol Biol Phys 2003; 57: 452–64.
84. Aoyama H, Shirato H, Tago M, et al. Stereotactic radiosurgery plus whole-brain radiation
therapy vs stereotactic radiosurgery alone for treatment of brain metastases: a randomized
controlled trial. JAMA 2006; 295: 2483–91.
85. O'Neill BP, Iturria NJ, Link MJ, et al. A comparison of surgical resection and stereotactic
radiosurgery in the treatment of solitary brain metastases. Int J Radiat Oncol Biol Phys
2003; 55: 1169–76.
86. Andrews DW, Scott CB, Sperduto PW, et al. Whole brain radiation therapy with or without stereotactic radiosurgery boost for patients with one to three brain metastases: phase
III results of the RTOG 9508 randomised trial. Lancet 2004; 363: 1665–72.
87. Sneed PK, Suh JH, Goetsch SJ, et al. A multi-institutional review of radiosurgery alone vs.
radiosurgery with whole brain radiotherapy as the initial management of brain metastases. Int J Radiat Oncol Biol Phys 2002; 53: 519–26.
88. Chitapanarux I, Goss B, Vongtama R, et al. Prospective study of stereotactic radiosurgery
without whole brain radiotherapy in patients with four or less brain metastases: incidence
of intracranial progression and salvage radiotherapy. J Neurooncol 2003; 61: 143–9.
89. Kocher M, Soffietti R, Abacioglu U, et al. Adjuvant whole-brain radiotherapy versus
observation after radiosurgery or surgical resection of one to three cerebral metastases:
results of the EORTC 22952-26001 study. J Clin Oncol 2010; 29: 134–41.
90. Mehta M, Noyes W, Craig B, et al. A cost-effectiveness and cost-utility analysis of radiosurgery vs. resection for single-brain metastases. Int J Radiat Oncol Biol Phys 1997; 39: 445–54.
91. Kelly PJ, Lin YB, Yu AY, et al. Stereotactic irradiation of the postoperative resection cavity
for brain metastasis: a frameless linear accelerator-based case series and review of the technique. Int J Radiat Oncol Biol Phys 2010. [Epub ahead of print].
92. Jensen CA, Chan MD, McCoy TP, et al. Cavity-directed radiosurgery as adjuvant therapy
after resection of a brain metastasis. J Neurosurg 2011; 114(6): 1585–91.
93. Rodrigues G, Yartsev S, Yaremko B, et al. Phase I trial of simultaneous in-field boost with
helical tomotherapy for patients with one to three brain metastases. Int J Radiat Oncol Biol
Phys 2011; 80(4): 1128–33.
94. Marsh JC, Gielda BT, Herskovic AM, Abrams RA. Cognitive sparing during the administration of whole brain radiotherapy and prophylactic cranial irradiation: current concepts
and approaches. J Oncol 2010; 2010: 198208.
95. Chargari C, Kirova YM, Dieras V, et al. Concurrent capecitabine and whole-brain radiotherapy for treatment of brain metastases in breast cancer patients. J Neurooncol 2009; 93: 379–84.
96. Chargari C, Idrissi HR, Pierga JY, et al. Preliminary results of whole brain radiotherapy
with concurrent trastuzumab for treatment of brain metastases in breast cancer patients.
Int J Radiat Oncol Biol Phys 2010. [Epub ahead of print].
97. Chalmers AJ, Lakshman M, Chan N, Bristow RG. Poly(ADP-ribose) polymerase inhibition
as a model for synthetic lethality in developing radiation oncology targets. Semin Radiat
Oncol 2010; 20: 274–81.

13 Management of neurological complications in metastatic breast cancer

Syed M. R. Kabir and Adrian T. H. Casey

INTRODUCTION

Breast cancer is now the most common cancer in the United Kingdom. In 2007, almost 45,700 women were diagnosed with breast cancer. The overall prognosis from breast cancer has improved significantly with a 5-year survival rate of 80% (1). Metastasis to the central nervous system (CNS) occurs in 14–20% of patients with breast cancer (2). In autopsy study this ranges from 18% to 30% (3). Current evidence suggests that the overall incidence of CNS metastasis is on the rise. This has been attributed to the selective destruction of non-brain metastasis by new chemotherapeutic agents. Many of these agents do not effectively cross the blood–brain barrier resulting in the subsequent development of brain metastasis (4). In this chapter; we have divided the management of CNS metastases according to their anatomical location. We discuss the neurological management, the latest advances in surgical techniques and other modalities of treatment including stereotactic radiosurgery and Cyberknife.

BRAIN METASTASIS

Lung and breast cancers are the most common tumours to present with brain metastasis (5,6) (Fig. 1). The median latency between the development of brain metastasis and the initial diagnosis of breast cancer is around 2–3 years (5,7). Brain metastasis is usually a late feature of the disease and develops after metastases have appeared systemically in the lungs, liver, and/or bone (8). Several factors have been identified that increase the risk of brain metastasis. These include young age (9,10), higher incidence in oestrogen receptor (ER) negative breast cancer, and human epidermal growth factor receptor-2 (HER-2) positive breast cancer (11). Brain metastases are thought to be haematogenous in origin (7). Around 14% of patients have a solitary intracerebral metastasis (10). Mean survival rate following the diagnosis of brain metastasis varies from 2 to 16 months, depending on CNS involvement, histopathological subtype, extent of extracranial disease, and treatment modality (7). The mean 1-year survival rate is around 20% (12).

Symptoms

Symptoms and signs associated with brain metastases result from the location of the tumour or the raised intracranial pressure resulting from the space occupying lesion, surrounding oedema, or obstruction to the cerebrospinal fluid (CSF) flow. Headache is the most frequent presenting symptom (40–50%). However, only 15–20% of these patients have papilloedema. Focal neurological deficits are present in 40% and seizures occur in 15–20% of the patients. Nausea and vomiting may develop with a further increase in the intracranial pressure and altered mental status or impaired cognitive function is often present (13). When patients with known metastatic breast cancer develop neurological symptoms, urgent diagnostic imaging studies are mandatory. The gold standard diagnostic study is a gadolinium-enhanced magnetic resonance imaging (MRI) scan of the brain which has been shown to be more sensitive than contrast-enhanced CT (14). MRI can detect lesions that are missed by CT, especially when lesions are situated in the posterior fossa

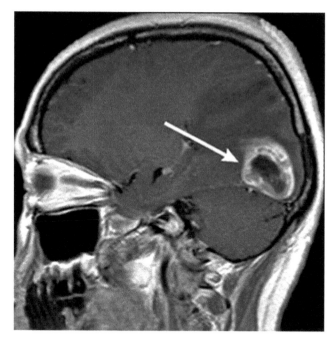

FIGURE 1   Metastasis of breast cancer to the occipital lobe.

and in the brain stem. It is also more sensitive in detecting multiple lesions (15), thereby influencing management.

Therapy
The therapy of brain metastasis is a subject of much debate. The prognosis is often dependent on disease activity at extra-cranial sites of disease. However, in breast cancer systemic therapy is superior to most solid tumours and consequently half of the patients with brain metastases will die due to neurological problems (16).

In order to preserve quality of life, treatment is important to control symptoms and reduce the risks or delay CNS relapse.

The mainstay of treatment includes corticosteroids, surgery, whole-brain radiotherapy (WBRT), and stereotactic radiosurgery.

Corticosteroids
Corticosteroids are given to reduce peri-tumoural oedema and to provide symptomatic relief. There is no class I evidence for the dosage in metastatic brain tumours, but in most studies dexamethasone 4 mg every 6 hours is used (17). During therapy it can be tapered to the patient needs.

Whole-Brain Radiotherapy
Whole-brain radiotherapy (WBRT) is the palliative treatment of choice for patients with multiple lesions or for patients with disease inaccessible to neurosurgical or radiosurgical approaches. WBRT alone improves survival and quality of life compared with corticosteroids alone and is still the mainstay of the treatment for a majority of patients. In a retrospective analysis of patients with brain metastases from breast cancer, the median survival following the start of radiotherapy is reported to be 4–5 months (18). Nausea, vomiting, headache, alopecia, fever, and transient

worsening of neurological symptoms can occur in the initial phase of therapy. WBRT is usually combined with corticosteroid therapy. The best clinical results are witnessed in patients less than 65 years, with good performance and in patients with the CNS as the only site of metastatic disease (19).

Surgery

Surgery is an important treatment modality in metastatic breast cancer for selected patients. Several studies have shown that surgery reduces symptoms quickly and increases the overall quality of life (20–22). In a recent Cochrane review (23), the authors concluded that there is currently no evidence that surgery extends survival. However, there is a clear benefit for the duration of functionally independent survival. This benefit is likely due to a direct lowering of the raised intracranial pressure following surgery and by reducing the need for long-term steroids. Studies have also shown that multiple metastases (up to three) can be removed surgically with risks similar to that of a single lesion, whilst simultaneously providing equivalent benefits (7,12). Surgery is currently followed by adjuvant radiotherapy. This combined approach has been shown to prolong median survival to 12 months, depending upon other factors (7,12). Surgery may also be helpful in selected patients with recurrent brain metastasis (7,12).

Surgery for superficial lesions is technically straightforward. The tumour is approached by a standard craniotomy. Surgery is often assisted by an image-guided system to reduce the craniotomy extent and to maximise safe removal of tumour (Fig. 2) (24).

Other developments like functional MRI and awake craniotomy will improve the safety of operating in eloquent areas (e.g. speech area or motor strip). In general the patients will require a stay of 4–5 days in hospital. Potential complications of surgery include post-operative haematoma formation, brain oedema, infection, and epilepsy. The rate of major complications is 12%, with neurological deficit occurring in 6% of patients (25). The mortality rate associated with such procedures is 2–3% (26).

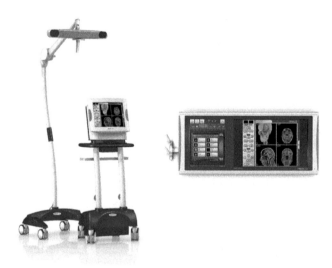

FIGURE 2 Use of neuronavigation such as the one above has made it easier to localise brain metastasis and made surgery safer.

Radiosurgery

Recently an increasing number of patients with single metastatic brain lesions were treated with stereotactic radiosurgery (SRS). Multiple lesions can also be treated but the risks of radionecrosis causing cerebral swelling and irritability increase. SRS is administered either by a linear accelerator or by multiple cobalt sources (Gamma Knife). Gamma Knife (Fig. 3) has the advantage of a sharply confined therapy field with a rapid dose fall-off, thereby minimising the risk to the surrounding brain tissue. In contrast to primary malignant brain tumours, brain metastases are well demarcated, minimally invasive lesions which make them ideal candidates for SRS.

This therapy is restricted to lesions smaller than 3–3.5 cm; with larger lesions there is an unfavourably high level of toxicity. Early complications due to oedema occur in 7–10% of patients within 2 weeks of treatment. Patients may report symptoms such as headache, nausea, vomiting, focal neurological deficits, and seizures. Normally they are well treated with corticosteroids. The major long-term complication is radionecrosis (5–11%), rarely requiring a further operation (13). The advantage of radiosurgery is that it is a non-invasive 1-day treatment and lacks many of the major complications of neurosurgery. In the authors opinion, neurological improvement with conventional surgery is perhaps more reliable and consistent.

With radiosurgery in highly selected patients with one to three lesions a very high level of 1-year local control can be achieved (80–90%), with a median survival comparable to surgical resection and WBRT (27–29). WBRT in combination with radiosurgery improves the CNS relapse rate, but has no effect in the median survival (30). SRS alone is now promoted with a careful follow-up and if necessary, a salvage therapy with WBRT or further stereotactic radiosurgery (31). Improved local control following SRS for brain metastases was associated with Karnofsky Performance Status ≥90, a radiation dose >15 Gy, and a planning target volume <13 cc (32).

The role of stereotactic radiosurgery in patients with more than three metastatic brain lesions has not been clearly defined. A recent study suggests radiosurgery in this category of patients is valuable, but randomised trials are necessary to confirm this (33). Other new forms of radiosurgery include the Cyberknife (Fig. 4) which unlike the Gamma Knife can be used for the spine as well. Cyberknife has been shown to provide promising results in certain types of brain metastasis (34).

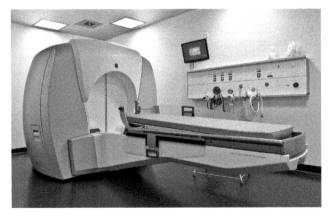

FIGURE 3 Stereotactic radiosurgery is delivered using the gamma knife machine. *Source*: Photo courtesy of Electa.

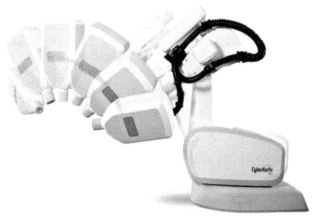

FIGURE 4 Focused radiotherapy using the Cyberknife machine. *Source*: Photo courtesy of Accuray Inc.

Chemotherapy

Due to the blood–brain barrier, chemotherapy is not generally a good treatment option for cancers that metastasise to the brain. However, in patients with human epidermal growth factor receptor-2 (HER2) overexpressing breast cancer with brain metastasis, treatment with trastuzumab has been shown to improve the outcome. This has been achieved through control and durable prolongation of systemic extracranial disease (35).

In breast cancer patients with brain metastasis, those with controlled extracranial tumour, age less than 65 years, and a favourable general performance (Karnofsky Performance Status ≥70) fare better compared to older patients with a Karnofsky score of <70. Patients who have solitary metastasis and a longer disease-free interval also tend to fare well (19,36).

LEPTOMENINGEAL METASTASIS

Leptomeningeal metastasis or meningeal carcinomatosis is an increasingly common manifestation of metastatic disease, probably due to the prolonged survival associated with improved systemic therapy. Breast cancer is the solid tumour associated most commonly with leptomeningeal metastasis (11). Leptomeningeal metastasis is more commonly seen in the lobular type of breast cancer compared to other histological types (5,37,38). In a series of 420 patients with breast cancer and CNS metastasis, Altundag et al. noted that 7% of patients presented with only leptomeningeal metastasis (11). Leptomeningeal metastases tend to arise in the pia and the arachnoid, or in the subarachnoid space (6). Leptomeningeal spread occurs through multiple routes including haematogenous, direct extension, transport through the venous plexus, and extension along nerves or perineural lymphatics (37). After reaching the leptomeninges, the tumour cells are thought to spread via the CSF (7).

Symptoms are related to the site and extent of tumour infiltration, to CSF flow disturbance with associated hydrocephalus, and to local inflammatory responses. The patient may suffer from raised intracranial pressure with associated headache and vomiting. Other symptoms include focal neurological deficits and seizures. The diagnosis is made by gadolinium-enhanced MRI and occasionally (multiple) lumbar punctures are required in the case of diagnostic uncertainty. The prognosis of meningeal carcinomatosis in general is very poor, with a median survival in untreated patients of 4–6 weeks and in treated patients of 4 months. In metastatic breast cancer the survival is slightly better due to improved chemosensitivity of the tumour, with reported median survival numbers between 5–7 months (39,40).

Radiotherapy

Radiotherapy of the whole brain and spinal cord is not possible due to bone marrow toxicity. Intrathecal chemotherapy is a possibility combined with local radiotherapy to space-occupying or symptomatic lesions. Systemic chemotherapy is sometimes also considered. Intrathecal chemotherapy can be administered by repetitive lumbar puncture or through an intraventricular route via a catheter with a subcutaneous reservoir (Ommaya catheter). An Ommaya is preferred because of the superior delivery of the drugs through the subarachnoid space and the achievement of adequate ventricular therapeutic drug concentrations. Early complications are common (10–20%) and include aseptic chemical meningitis, bacterial infections of the Ommaya, intracranial haemorrhage, and focal encephalopathy by leakage of CSF along the Ommaya reservoir. Late neurotoxicity includes necrotising leukoencephalopathy with a clinical picture of progressive ataxia and dementia and occurs in about half of the long surviving patients (41).

INTRAMEDULLARY METASTASIS
Overview

Intramedullary spinal cord metastasis is very rare indeed, with a reported incidence of 0.1–6% in metastatic disease with breast cancer, the second most common cause. The overall median survival is 3 months; however, in breast cancer it may be up to 13 months (42). The clinical presentation depends on the level of the tumour and consists of back pain with a partial or complete spinal cord lesion with motor, sensory, and autonomic deficits. The most common site is the cervical spinal cord. Clinically, there are no features which distinguish an intramedullary metastasis from an extradural lesion compressing the cord. The diagnosis is made by MRI with an isointense lesion on T1-weighted images and a nodular contrast enhancement on T1 and a pencil-shape hyperintensity on T2-weighted images. Therapy usually consists of steroids and radiotherapy (43). In selected cases, with patients of good performance status, stable systemic disease, and no evidence of leptomeningeal metastases surgery is an option. As the lesions tend to be well circumscribed, a gross total resection can be performed (44) with an improvement of the neurological deficit. The surgeon uses microsurgical techniques including an ultrasonic aspirator (CUSA EXcel™: Cavitron ultrasonic surgical aspirator, Integra radionics, inc.). Spinal cord monitoring using somatosensory and motor-evoked potentials (SSEPs and MEPs) is desirable. Stereotactic spine radiosurgery has recently been used for intradural and intramedullary metastasis with success (45). Promising results have also been reported with CyberKnife®, Accuray Inc (46).

EPIDURAL METASTASIS
Epidemiology and Clinical Presentation

In metastatic breast cancer, spinal epidural metastasis is a common problem and is considered critically important due to the devastating effect on the quality of life with ensuing spinal cord compression. The highly vascular posterior portion of the vertebral body is the place where vertebral metastases usually develop.

Epidural metastases occur most commonly in the thoracic (50–60%) and lumbar spine (30–35%) and less frequently in the cervical spine (10–15%), correlating with the volume of bone marrow in each region (47). Spinal cord compression may evolve due to direct extension of the tumour into the anterior epidural space. Less often, due to mechanical compromise, a vertebral collapse may occur, precipitating a spinal cord compression. About two-thirds of patients with breast cancer develop bone metastasis involving the vertebral column and in about 2-5% the clinical diagnosis of spinal epidural metastasis is made. Multiple lesions can be found in 20% of the patients with epidural metastasis (48). Symptoms result from spinal cord compression and instability of the spinal column.

For a majority of patients, back pain is the initial symptom. This is a red flag in a patient with breast cancer, particularly if the pain is in the thoracic spine. Radicular symptoms may develop after a few months. Myelopathic signs due to spinal cord compression may develop slowly, but can also present progressively over a few days. Sensory disturbances, weakness of arms or legs, spasticity, and autonomic dysfunction are all part of the myelopathy, depending on the spinal level of the tumour (49). Rapid recognition and treatment is the key to optimising outcome. The preferred diagnostic method is MRI of the whole spine. Conventional x-rays can be useful in evaluating the stability of the spine, but are not advocated as a screening method because a plain spinal radiogram will not demonstrate pathology until a 50% of the bone is destroyed (50). CT is useful in outlining the bony anatomy and is helpful prior to surgery.

Treatment

There are three goals of treatment in this palliative neurosurgical setting: to restore or preserve neurological function, to treat pain, and to restore or preserve spinal stability (51). The timing of therapy is of paramount importance. Several prognostic scoring systems are available in patients with spinal metastases (52). However, the pre-treatment ambulatory status is the strongest predictive factor of outcome. Most of the patients who are able to walk before therapy remain ambulatory. They have a shorter hospital stay, fewer complications, and a better functional outcome. Only 30% of non-ambulatory patients regain the ability to walk. The median survival with spinal epidural metastasis in breast cancer is approximately 6–9 months after the diagnosis of epidural disease. The survival of bed-ridden patients is approximately 6 weeks with complications of metastatic disease and the non-ambulatory state (53,54).

Dexamethasone is important in the early stage and is appropriate when there is symptomatic spinal cord compression. Normally an initial bolus of 10 mg is followed by a dosage of 4 mg four times a day during the first week which is then tapered of in 1 or 2 weeks (55).

Radiotherapy is traditionally the therapy of choice with a radiation area of one level above and below the affected vertebra. Ninety per cent of treated ambulatory patients remain ambulant with a local relapse rate of 10% after a median of 3–6 months (41). Radiotherapy on the other hand will not restore or preserve spinal stability.

There has been a long standing discussion whether surgery in metastatic epidural disease is of benefit. A great advantage of surgery is direct spinal decompression, with arguably a better neurological outcome. Early studies comparing the efficacy of radiotherapy and surgery (laminectomy) found no difference in neurological outcome and survival (56). However, metastatic epidural disease typically arises from the vertebral body, precipitating anterior compression, which *may not be helped* by a laminectomy. In patients with instability secondary to vertebral body destruction, laminectomy (removal of the last portion of healthy bone) will further compromise the spinal stability (57). This historical surgical error has now been recognised in most centres. Therefore, if a laminectomy is performed stabilisation is mandatory.

Surgery of metastatic epidural tumours has advanced significantly over the last 10 years due to the widespread availability of spinal stabilisation techniques. With anterior and posterolateral approaches, the goal is to remove the tumour, decompress the spinal cord, and stabilise the spinal column with instrumentation (58). The mortality rates in this kind of surgery are very low, with an acceptable morbidity rate of 10–20%, most of which result from wound complications (59). A recent randomised study by Patchell et al. comparing direct decompressive surgical resection with radiotherapy versus radiotherapy alone demonstrated an improved neurological outcome in the surgical cohort with less narcotic and steroid use (60).

Adjuvant radiotherapy should be given after surgery to prevent local relapse. We recommend delaying this for 3 weeks to facilitate safe wound healing. Radiotherapy before the operation is not advised because of the higher frequency of postoperative complications (61). There are many studies demonstrating a higher frequency of wound complications (2–3 folds) if radiotherapy precedes spinal surgery.

Surgery involves decompression. This may be anterior and involve a corpectomy (removal of vertebral body/tumour). For the cervical spine this is straightforward surgery (47). The spine is commonly reconstructed using a hollow titanium or carbon fibre cage (Figs. 5, 6). The cage is secured by an anterior locking plate. In the thoracic spine a thoracotomy is required to expose the spine. Reconstruction is afforded by a similar but larger titanium cage. In the lumbar spine a retroperitoneal approach is typically used and reconstructed with a cage supported by an anterior lateral plate or screw rod system. Expandable cages afford very good support and a tight fit.

Posterior decompression involves laminectomy (removal of lamina). This is a straightforward surgery but it will destabilise the spine. Fixation is therefore required. In the neck this is achieved by lateral mass screws connected to a titanium rod. In the thoracic and lumbar spine a similar result is achieved by pedicle screws (Fig. 7). Typically, screws are inserted two levels above and below the area of disease. This is based on detailed biomechanical testing.

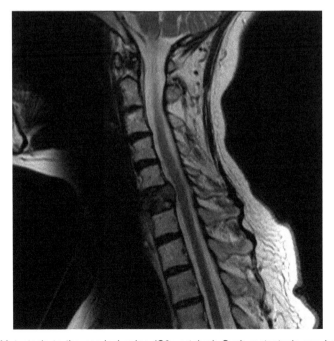

FIGURE 5   Metastasis to the cervical spine (C6 vertebra). Such metastasis can be treated with cervical corpectomy and reconstruction.

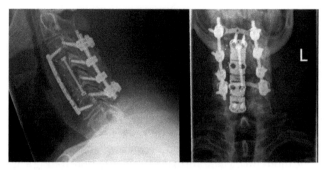

FIGURE 6   AP and lateral x-ray showing reconstruction following anterior cervical corpectomy. The reconstruction has been done using a carbon fibre cage to replace the removed vertebral body. Posterior reinforcement has been done using lateral mass screws.

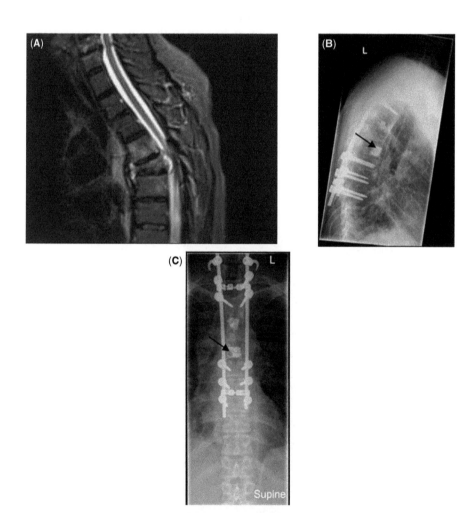

FIGURE 7   **A**: MRI scan showing metastatic involvement of the thoracic spine with wedge collapse of one of the vertebra causing kyphosis. Lateral (**B**) and AP(**C**) x-ray showing reconstruction and correction of the deformity via a posterior approach using pedicle screws. Cement has been injected into the adjacent involved vertebral body (arrow).

Spinal fixation facilitates reliable stability and aggressive tumour removal. However, it is relatively unusual for the surgeon to achieve a complete tumour removal. Surgery is palliative and reduces the risks of paralysis. Spinal fixation has a beneficial effect on reducing pain (reduced narcotics) and usually will significantly improve the quality of life.

New treatment modalities for spinal involvement include percutaneous vertebroplasty or kyphoplasty. These techniques involve injection of biological cement (methyl methacrylate) into the vertebral body, usually via the pedicle. It is a difficult technique and requires good radiological imaging either bi-planar fluoroscopy or CT fluoroscopy. Early results are promising in tumours. It helps pain mainly but the exothermic effect of the methyl methacrylate cement may kill some tumour. It has mainly been used for osteoporotic fractures. It is contraindicated if the posterior vertebral body wall is compromised by fracture or direct tumour infiltration. Risks include extravasation of the cement into the canal causing cord compression or through basivertebral venous system into the pulmonary tree causing pulmonary embolism. Vertebroplasty involves simple injection into the vertebral body. Kyphoplasty involves inflation of a balloon first which may restore sagittal balance and arguably decrease the risk of cement embolus.

Radiosurgical techniques have also been developed for the spine. Computer algorithms modified from intracranial computer guidance systems allow accurate delivery of high-dose radiotherapy to the mobile spine. Small percutaneous bony screws are required as fiducial markers for the radiotherapy planning, which co-registers and fuses CT scans with "real time" fluoroscopic images. Long-term results are not yet available. This technique shows promise in all osseous spine tumours. A recent study on the use of Cyberknife radiosurgery in metastatic spine tumour has reported promising results (62).

SUMMARY

Patients with metastatic breast cancer have a limited life expectancy and therapy is palliative. Systemic therapy in metastatic breast cancer is more effective compared with other solid tumours. With prolonged survival encountered with improved therapy, more neurological sequelae will be witnessed by physicians. Immediate and aggressive therapy in selected patients can improve outcome and preserve quality of life.

New developments in spinal fixation allow for safer and more reliable outcomes. Advances in stereotactic radiosurgery and Cyberknife are also promising. Recent developments with chemotherapeutic agents like trastuzumab will hopefully further improve the outcome in these patients.

REFERENCES

1. Cancer Research UK. Cancer Stats 2010.
2. Flowers A, Levin VA. Management of brain metastases from breast carcinoma. Oncology (Williston Park) 1993; 7: 21–6; discussion 31–24.
3. Tsukada Y, Fouad A, Pickren JW, Lane WW. Central nervous system metastasis from breast carcinoma. Autopsy study. Cancer 1983; 52: 2349–54.
4. Crivellari D, Pagani O, Veronesi A, et al. High incidence of central nervous system involvement in patients with metastatic or locally advanced breast cancer treated with epirubicin and docetaxel. Ann Oncol 2001; 12: 353–6.
5. Chang EL, Lo S. Diagnosis and management of central nervous system metastases from breast cancer. Oncologist 2003; 8: 398–410.
6. Lassman AB, DeAngelis LM. Brain metastases. Neurol Clin 2003; 21: 1–23, vii.
7. Weil RJ, Palmieri DC, Bronder JL, Stark AM, Steeg PS. Breast cancer metastasis to the central nervous system. Am J Pathol 2005; 167: 913–20.

8. Issa CM, Semrau R, Kath R, Hoffken K. Isolated brain metastases as the sole manifestation of a late relapse in breast cancer. J Cancer Res Clin Oncol 2002; 128: 61–3.
9. Lin NU, Bellon JR, Winer EP. CNS metastases in breast cancer. J Clin Oncol 2004; 22: 3608–17.
10. Evans AJ, James JJ, Cornford EJ, et al. Brain metastases from breast cancer: identification of a high-risk group. Clin Oncol (R Coll Radiol) 2004; 16: 345–9.
11. Altundag K, Bondy ML, Mirza NQ, et al. Clinicopathologic characteristics and prognostic factors in 420 metastatic breast cancer patients with central nervous system metastasis. Cancer 2007; 110: 2640–7.
12. Shaffrey ME, Mut M, Asher AL, et al. Brain metastases. Curr Probl Surg 2004; 41: 665–741.
13. Soffietti R, Ruda R, Mutani R. Management of brain metastases. J Neurol 2002; 249: 1357–69.
14. Schellinger PD, Meinck HM, Thron A. Diagnostic accuracy of MRI compared to CCT in patients with brain metastases. J Neurooncol 1999; 44: 275–81.
15. Akeson P, Larsson EM, Kristoffersen DT, Jonsson E, Holtas S. Brain metastases–comparison of gadodiamide injection-enhanced MR imaging at standard and high dose, contrast-enhanced CT and non-contrast-enhanced MR imaging. Acta Radiol 1995; 36: 300–6.
16. Bendell JC, Domchek SM, Burstein HJ, et al. Central nervous system metastases in women who receive trastuzumab-based therapy for metastatic breast carcinoma. Cancer 2003; 97: 2972–7.
17. Sarin R, Murthy V. Medical decompressive therapy for primary and metastatic intracranial tumours. Lancet Neurol 2003; 2: 357–65.
18. Mahmoud-Ahmed AS, Suh JH, Lee SY, Crownover RL, Barnett GH. Results of whole brain radiotherapy in patients with brain metastases from breast cancer: a retrospective study. Int J Radiat Oncol Biol Phys 2002; 54: 810–17.
19. Gaspar L, Scott C, Rotman M, et al. Recursive partitioning analysis (RPA) of prognostic factors in three Radiation Therapy Oncology Group (RTOG) brain metastases trials. Int J Radiat Oncol Biol Phys 1997; 37: 745–51.
20. Vecht CJ, Haaxma-Reiche H, Noordijk EM, et al. Treatment of single brain metastasis: radiotherapy alone or combined with neurosurgery? Ann Neurol 1993; 33: 583–90.
21. Patchell RA, Tibbs PA, Walsh JW, et al. A randomized trial of surgery in the treatment of single metastases to the brain. N Engl J Med 1990; 322: 494–500.
22. Mintz AH, Kestle J, Rathbone MP, et al. A randomized trial to assess the efficacy of surgery in addition to radiotherapy in patients with a single cerebral metastasis. Cancer 1996; 78: 1470–6.
23. Hart M, Grant R, Walker M, Dickinson H. Surgical resection and whole brain radiation therapy versus whole brain radiation therapy alone for single brain metastases. Cochrane Database Syst Rev 2005; (1): CD003292.
24. Tan TC, Mc LBP. Image-guided craniotomy for cerebral metastases: techniques and outcomes. Neurosurgery 2003; 53: 82–9; discussion 89–90.
25. Sawaya R, Hammoud M, Schoppa D, et al. Neurosurgical outcomes in a modern series of 400 craniotomies for treatment of parenchymal tumors. Neurosurgery 1998; 42: 1044–55; discussion 1055–1046.
26. Barker FG 2nd. Craniotomy for the resection of metastatic brain tumors in the U.S., 1988–2000: decreasing mortality and the effect of provider caseload. Cancer 2004; 100: 999–1007.
27. Lutterbach J, Cyron D, Henne K, Ostertag CB. Radiosurgery followed by planned observation in patients with one to three brain metastases. Neurosurgery 2003; 52: 1066–73; discussion 1073-1064.
28. Hasegawa T, Kondziolka D, Flickinger JC, Germanwala A, Lunsford LD. Brain metastases treated with radiosurgery alone: an alternative to whole brain radiotherapy? Neurosurgery 2003; 52: 1318–26; discussion 1326.
29. Vesagas TS, Aguilar JA, Mercado ER, Mariano MM. Gamma knife radiosurgery and brain metastases: local control, survival, and quality of life. J Neurosurg 2002; 97(5 Suppl): 507–10.
30. Sneed PK, Suh JH, Goetsch SJ, et al. A multi-institutional review of radiosurgery alone vs. radiosurgery with whole brain radiotherapy as the initial management of brain metastases. Int J Radiat Oncol Biol Phys 2002; 53: 519–26.

31. van den Bent MJ. Management of metastatic (parenchymal, leptomeningeal, and epidural) lesions. Curr Opin Oncol 2004; 16: 309–13.
32. Molenaar R, Wiggenraad R, Verbeek-de Kanter A, Walchenbach R, Vecht C. Relationship between volume, dose and local control in stereotactic radiosurgery of brain metastasis. Br J Neurosurg 2009; 23: 170–8.
33. Nam TK, Lee JI, Jung YJ, et al. Gamma knife surgery for brain metastases in patients harboring four or more lesions: survival and prognostic factors. J Neurosurg 2005; 102(Suppl): 147–50.
34. Hara W, Tran P, Li G, et al. Cyberknife for brain metastases of malignant melanoma and renal cell carcinoma. Neurosurgery 2009; 64(2 Suppl): A26–32.
35. Park YH, Park MJ, Ji SH, et al. Trastuzumab treatment improves brain metastasis outcomes through control and durable prolongation of systemic extracranial disease in HER2-overexpressing breast cancer patients. Br J Cancer 2009; 100: 894–900.
36. Lagerwaard FJ, Levendag PC, Nowak PJ, et al. Identification of prognostic factors in patients with brain metastases: a review of 1292 patients. Int J Radiat Oncol Biol Phys 1999; 43: 795–803.
37. Kesari S, Batchelor TT. Leptomeningeal metastases. Neurol Clin 2003; 21: 25–66.
38. Nussbaum ES, Djalilian HR, Cho KH, Hall WA. Brain metastases. Histology, multiplicity, surgery, and survival. Cancer 1996; 78: 1781–8.
39. Chamberlain MC, Kormanik PR. Carcinomatous meningitis secondary to breast cancer: predictors of response to combined modality therapy. J Neurooncol 1997; 35: 55–64.
40. DeAngelis LM. Current diagnosis and treatment of leptomeningeal metastasis. J Neurooncol 1998; 38: 245–52.
41. Boogerd W. Central nervous system metastasis in breast cancer. Radiother Oncol 1996; 40: 5–22.
42. Schiff D, O'Neill BP. Intramedullary spinal cord metastases: clinical features and treatment outcome. Neurology 1996; 47: 906–12.
43. Villegas AE, Guthrie TH. Intramedullary spinal cord metastasis in breast cancer: clinical features, diagnosis, and therapeutic consideration. Breast J 2004; 10: 532–5.
44. Kalayci M, Cagavi F, Gul S, Yenidunya S, Acikgoz B. Intramedullary spinal cord metastases: diagnosis and treatment - an illustrated review. Acta Neurochir (Wien) 2004; 146: 1347–54; discussion 1354.
45. Shin DA, Huh R, Chung SS, Rock J, Ryu S. Stereotactic spine radiosurgery for intradural and intramedullary metastasis. Neurosurg Focus 2009; 27: E10.
46. Gagnon GJ, Nasr NM, Liao JJ, et al. Treatment of spinal tumors using cyberknife fractionated stereotactic radiosurgery: pain and quality-of-life assessment after treatment in 200 patients. Neurosurgery 2009; 64: 297–306; discussion 306-297.
47. Heidecke V, Rainov NG, Burkert W. Results and outcome of neurosurgical treatment for extradural metastases in the cervical spine. Acta Neurochir (Wien) 2003; 145: 873–80; discussion 880-871.
48. Boogerd W, van der Sande JJ, Kroger R. Early diagnosis and treatment of spinal epidural metastasis in breast cancer: a prospective study. J Neurol Neurosurg Psychiatry 1992; 55: 1188–93.
49. Aebi M. Spinal metastasis in the elderly. Eur Spine J 2003; 12(Suppl 2): S202–13.
50. Perrin RG, Laxton AW. Metastatic spine disease: epidemiology, pathophysiology, and evaluation of patients. Neurosurg Clin N Am 2004; 15: 365–73.
51. Wu AS, Fourney DR. Evolution of treatment for metastatic spine disease. Neurosurg Clin N Am 2004; 15: 401–11.
52. Leithner A, Radl R, Gruber G, et al. Predictive value of seven preoperative prognostic scoring systems for spinal metastases. Eur Spine J 2008; 17: 1488–95.
53. Zaidat OO, Ruff RL. Treatment of spinal epidural metastasis improves patient survival and functional state. Neurology 2002; 58: 1360–6.
54. Helweg-Larsen S, Sorensen PS, Kreiner S. Prognostic factors in metastatic spinal cord compression: a prospective study using multivariate analysis of variables influencing survival and gait function in 153 patients. Int J Radiat Oncol Biol Phys 2000; 46: 1163–9.
55. Klimo P Jr, Kestle JR, Schmidt MH. Clinical trials and evidence-based medicine for metastatic spine disease. Neurosurg Clin N Am 2004; 15: 549–64.

56. Young RF, Post EM, King GA. Treatment of spinal epidural metastases. Randomized prospective comparison of laminectomy and radiotherapy. J Neurosurg 1980; 53: 741–8.
57. Findlay GF. The role of vertebral body collapse in the management of malignant spinal cord compression. J Neurol Neurosurg Psychiatry 1987; 50: 151–4.
58. Sundaresan N, Rothman A, Manhart K, Kelliher K. Surgery for solitary metastases of the spine: rationale and results of treatment. Spine 2002; 27: 1802–6.
59. Pascal-Moussellard H, Broc G, Pointillart V, et al. Complications of vertebral metastasis surgery. Eur Spine J 1998; 7: 438–44.
60. Patchell RA, Tibbs PA, Regine WF, et al. Direct decompressive surgical resection in the treatment of spinal cord compression caused by metastatic cancer: a randomised trial. Lancet 2005; 366: 643–8.
61. Ghogawala Z, Mansfield FL, Borges LF. Spinal radiation before surgical decompression adversely affects outcomes of surgery for symptomatic metastatic spinal cord compression. Spine 2001; 26: 818–24.
62. Tsai JT, Lin JW, Chiu WT, Chu WC. Assessment of image-guided CyberKnife radiosurgery for metastatic spine tumors. J Neurooncol 2009; 94: 119–27.

14   Thoracic complications

George Ladas

INTRODUCTION

One of the body compartments most commonly affected by metastatic breast cancer is the thorax. The thoracic surgeon has an important role as a member of the extended multidisciplinary breast cancer team and can help with diagnosis and staging, provide surgical palliation, but also occasionally perform potentially curative resection for localised metastatic disease. It is fair to say that with the significant progress in the systemic treatments of patients with advanced breast cancer in recent years, with resulting prolongation of their survival, the successful surgical palliation achieved by modern thoracic surgery has really transformed their quality of life.

The thoracic surgeon has a role in the management of the following:

- Surgical palliation of pleural effusions
- Surgical palliation of pericardial effusions
- Endoscopic palliation of airway obstruction including stents
- Pulmonary metastasectomy
- Metastatic involvement of the chest wall and sternum

SURGICAL PALLIATION OF PLEURAL EFFUSIONS

Pleural effusions are common during the course of malignant disease, with 16% of patients dying of malignancy found at autopsy to have a pleural effusion. Carcinomas of the lung and breast combined, account for 60% of all malignant pleural effusions. These effusions can cause significant morbidity, including dyspnoea in 96%, chest pain in 57%, and persistent cough in 44% of the patients (1). At the same time, the overall prognosis of patients with malignant pleural effusions is poor, with reported 1- and 6-month mortality rate of 54% and 85% respectively (2,3), so that quality of life is of paramount importance. Patients with malignant pleural effusions due to metastatic breast cancer had a longer life expectancy as a group, with a median survival of 7.1 months in our experience, even before the introduction of the newest systemic treatment modalities. Due to the effectiveness of modern systemic treatments for breast cancer, we would normally wait to see whether an effusion responds to such treatment initially before deciding to proceed to surgical palliation. Since dyspnoea in patients with advanced malignancy is often multifactorial, an initial needle aspiration will confirm diagnosis in 65% of the patients, but will also help define to what extent the pleural effusion itself is responsible for the symptoms. In frail patients with a very short life expectancy of 1–2 months, repeated processes of needle aspiration can be helpful in controlling the symptoms. In most of the patients with recurrent symptomatic malignant effusions, lasting palliation can be achieved by one of a spectrum of techniques used to achieve *chemical pleurodesis*, that is, fusion of the visceral and parietal pleura with the use of a "sclerosing agent". The basic prerequisite for a successful chemical pleurodesis by any technique is that the lungs can re-expand following drainage of the pleural effusion, so that the visceral and parietal pleura can remain apposed while adhesions are formed. However, the presence of a malignant restricting cortex on the visceral pleura prevents re-expansion of the lungs and apposition to the parietal pleura. The presence of such a *trapped lung* (Fig. 1A,B) means that any attempt at chemical pleurodesis is destined to fail. The treatment options in these circumstances are very

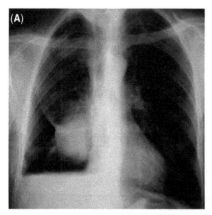 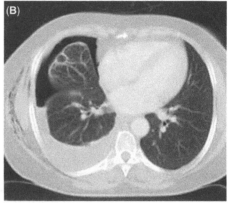

FIGURE 1   (A) Chest radiograph of a patient with a malignant right pleural effusion following insertion of chest drain. The presence of the trapped lung is obvious. (B) Computed tomography (CT) scan
appearances of the same patient. A right hydro-pneumothorax is present. Note the thickened, restricting visceral cortex overlying the right middle and lower lobes, preventing re-expansion of the lung; an
indication for immediate referral for insertion of a pleuro-peritoneal shunt. The drain should not be put
on suction, to avoid barotrauma.

few and most of them unattractive. Repeated aspirations require frequent hospitalisa-
tions and are painful, both detrimental to quality of life of the patients. Furthermore,
they carry the risk of the devastating complication of infection of the fluid and empy-
ema formation. This is the major concern which also limits the popularity of permanent
chest drain devices like PleurX® (Denver Biomedical Inc. Golden, Colorado). Thoracotomy and decortication of the lung, combined with chemical pleurodesis or pleurectomy on the other hand, involves a major surgery with very significant morbidity and
mortality, unacceptable for a palliative procedure (4). In contrast, pleuro-peritoneal
shunts provide an elegant, effective, and lasting solution to this difficult problem and
can be used with minimal morbidity and mortality in properly selected patients.

Sclerosing Agents
Sclerosing agents all act by triggering an intense inflammatory reaction of the pleura
by chemical irritation, the produced fibrin acting as the "glue". A wide variety of
substances have been used in the past for this purpose, for example adriamycin, bleo-
mycin, intrapleural tetracycline, or quinacrine. Currently, the most widely used agent
is talc. This consists of a powder containing 20% medical grade, asbestos-free iodised
talcum, mixed with starch. In frail patients, unfit for general anaesthesia, it is used as
sterile slurry via a tube thoracostomy. For the fitter patients, video-assisted thoracoscopy is used under general anaesthesia and an insufflation technique, which has been
shown to be effective in up to 93% of the patients (5).

Pleuro-peritoneal Shunts
Weese and Schouten in 1982 (6) first reported the use of a modified peritoneo-atrial
Holter valve (7) as a pleuro-peritoneal shunt. Since then, successful use of a purpose
built device has been reported for the treatment of benign (8) but also and mainly
malignant pleural effusions. The pleuro-peritoneal shunt (Denver Biomedical Inc.,
Denver, CO, U.S.A.; Fig. 2A) is made of inert silicone rubber. It is composed of a central pump body, which contains two unidirectional valves. The pressure gradient
required for the valves to open is 1 cm of water, and consequently a spontaneous flow

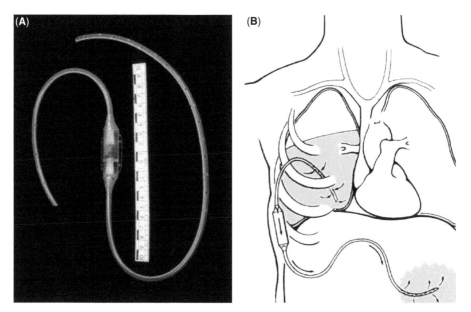

FIGURE 2 (A) The pleuro-peritoneal shunt. Note the central compressible pump chamber with the two unidirectional valves, and the thoracic and peritoneal limbs of the shunt. (B) A schematic diagram of the function of pleuro-peritoneal shunt.

occurs from the pleural to the peritoneal cavity at expiration or during cough. The presence of a pleural effusion increases the pressure gradient, which further enhances the flow. The stroke volume of the pump itself is about 1 mL, and so periodic compression ensures a minimum throughput but also clears the valve leaflets from deposited fibrin. The proximal catheter of the shunt is introduced into the pleural cavity and the distal one into the peritoneal cavity (Fig. 2B).

During the initial post-operative period, the nursing staff operate the pump every 3–4 hours for 2–3 minutes at a rate of around 30 strokes per minute. With the help of appropriate audio-visual training material the patients are able to assume responsibility for the shunt within 3–4 days postoperatively (Fig. 3).

We recently performed a retrospective review of 280 consecutive patients [109 male, median age 60 years (range 26–89)] undergoing 312 surgical procedures for palliation of malignant pleural effusions (MPE) over a 72-month period at the Royal Brompton Hospital. The commonest malignancies were breast (29%), mesothelioma (25%), lung (12%), ovary (9%) and adenocarcinoma of unknown primary (5%). Procedures performed were VATS talc pleurodesis 198, insertion of pleuro-peritoneal shunt 39, pleurodesis via an intercostal drain 37, pleural biopsy alone 28, and long-term drainage 9. The overall hospital mortality rate was 4.3% and complication rate 17%. Follow-up was 100% for a median of 1288 days (range 173–2329). Median post-operative survival was 210 days. Patients with breast cancer and mesothelioma had a significantly better median survival (258 and 297 days respectively) than those with ovarian cancer, adenocarcinoma of unknown primary, and lung cancer [133, 123, and 142 days respectively ($p = 0.02$)] (unpublished personal data).

Our series of patients, of the largest reported to date (9–11) show very low mortality and low treatment-related morbidity, combined with effective palliation in the vast majority of patients. Avoiding the need for repeated hospital admissions for thoracocentesis, not only dramatically improves the quality of life of these patients, but also reduces the overall cost of their care.

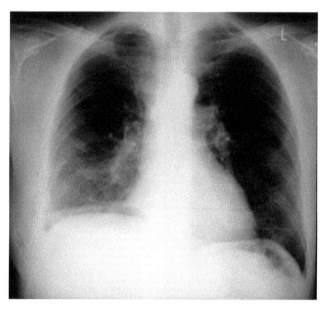

FIGURE 3   An early post-operative chest radiograph of a patient following the insertion of a shunt on the right. The proximal limb is clearly visible within the right hemithorax, with the pump body lying in the soft tissues overlying the costal margin. The limited pneumo-peritoneum resulting from air entering the peritoneal cavity intraoperatively, resolves within a few days.

PALLIATION OF PERICARDIAL EFFUSIONS

Pericardial effusions may develop in patients who develop metastatic implants on the serosa leading to exudation of fluid into the pericardial space. When the resorptive capacity of the pericardial serosa is exceeded, or when there is compromise of the venous or lymphatic drainage of the pericardium due to malignant infiltration, a significant effusion develops that may result in cardiac tamponade. Since the normal pericardium allows some distentibility, the rate of fluid accumulation can be as important as the total amount of fluid in defining the point at which cardiac function is compromised. Mild cardiac compression can be compensated and result only in an elevation of the central venous pressure with normal systemic blood pressure. Severe compression though results in serious compromise of diastolic filling, which cannot be compensated and leads to tamponade and cardiogenic shock.

Diagnosis

Even large pericardial effusions can be largely asymptomatic if compensated. A high level of suspicion is important. Diminished QRS voltages on the ECG or an enlarged cardiac silhouette and elevated central venous pressures in association with clear lung fields should point to the diagnosis. The classic triad of Beck (distended neck veins, muffled heart sounds, and hypotension) is characteristic and can be associated with pulsus paradoxus. Cardiac echocardiography is widely available, simple, non invasive, and highly accurate in diagnosing the problem.

Management

A pericardiocentesis is helpful in proving the malignant nature of the effusion as opposed to a reactive collection secondary to chemotherapy, radiotherapy, or other systemic reasons. In compromised patients with large effusions or tamponade it is appropriate to defuse the situation by introducing a catheter into the pericardial

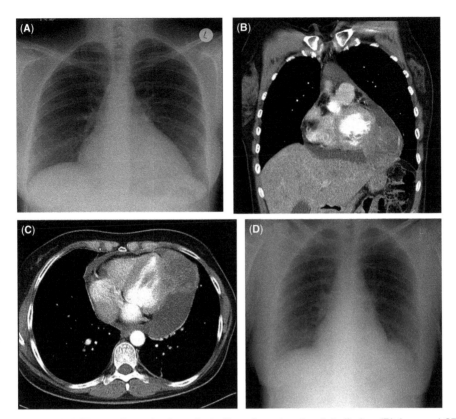

FIGURE 4 (A) Chest radiograph of a patient with malignant pericardial effusion. (B) A coronal CT scan image showing the effusion as well as large epicardial metastasis at the apex. (C) A cross-sectional CT scan image. (D) Chest radiograph of the same patient, immediately following sub-xiphoid pericardiectomy. Note the dramatic reduction of the cardiothoracic index, the transient pneumo-pericardium and the silhouette of the epicardial metastasis adjacent to the left heart border.

cavity under echocardiography guidance. This allows improvement in the clinical condition and ensures that a definitive procedure can be performed in safer circumstances.

An open pericardiotomy (pericardial window) can be performed in a variety of ways.

Video-assisted thoracoscopy or a *left anterolateral thoracotomy* can be used to create an opening towards either pleural cavity. Most of these patients though also have or will at some point in time develop concomitant malignant pleural effusions and will require a pleurodesis. Consequently, draining the pericardial effusion towards a pleural cavity is undesirable. Furthermore, these techniques result in respiratory compromise due to post-operative chest pain from the incisions and chest drains.

A sub-xiphoid pericardiotomy is the preferred technique in our practice. This involves a limited midline incision extending inferiorly for 5 cm from the tip of the xiphoid process. The linea alba is incised and the peritoneal sac is mobilised and displaced inferiorly, exposing the underside of the diaphragm. The peritoneal cavity is not entered. Next, a generous disc of the diaphragm with the attached overlying peri-cardium is resected and sent for histology. Fluid specimens are sent for cytology and microbiology. The effusion is therefore drained and a wide communication is created between the pericardial cavity and the compliant and resorptive pre-peritoneal space.

The wound is closed by simple re-approximation of the linea alba, without the need for any drains. This procedure provides lasting palliation, is tolerated extremely well by the patients, results in minimal post-operative pain, and leaves all options open regarding the management of any future pleural effusions (Fig. 4A–D).

ENDOSCOPIC PALLIATION OF AIRWAY OBSTRUCTION
Upper airway obstruction due to metastatic breast cancer is a relatively uncommon, but potentially serious problem. In an emergency, stridor and severe dyspnoea may be life threatening and demand immediate management.

Malignant disease may cause airway obstruction by (i) external compression due to mediastinal extension, usually due to nodal metastases (extraluminal component) or (ii) by direct growth of tumour in the lumen of the airway with resulting occlusion (intraluminal component), or (iii) a combination of both. Disobliteration of the airway lumen can be achieved by one of several methods, usually undertaken through the rigid bronchoscope under general anaesthesia. The Nd-YAG laser is widely used (12–18) and in the case of tumours in the distal bronchi can also be undertaken through the flexible bronchoscope under local anaesthesia. Cryo-ablation has also been used (19,20), but requires repeated treatment. In our (21–23) as well as others' (24) experience, diathermy resection through the rigid bronchoscope has proved to be a cheap, effective, and safe method of disobliteration, and can be easily combined with stenting when an extraluminal component of airway obstruction co-exists. Disobliteration can be valuable as a temporising measure to allow time for systemic treatment to act (25) (Fig. 5).

In a majority of patients the extraluminal component prevails or the intraluminal occlusion recurs rapidly following disobliteration. Radiotherapy is valuable, and external irradiation is the treatment of choice. If this is contraindicated, endobronchial irradiation via remote after-loading techniques is now available. It has the advantages of not exposing staff and other patients to irradiation, and of achieving high radiation doses locally during short out-patient sessions (26–28). When dealing with critical stenosis one has to secure the airway before irradiation, to allow for the tissue oedema which ensues.

Endobronchial stents and *T-tubes* are useful in several situations in which airway obstruction is due to malignant disease.

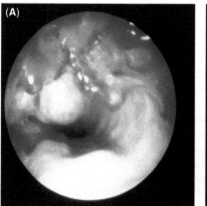
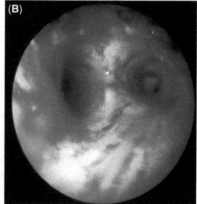

FIGURE 5   (A) Endoscopic appearances of airway obstruction due to intraluminal tumour growth. (B) The same patient following disobliteration using the diathermy resectoscope. The main carina and origin of the left and right main bronchus are visible and fully patent.

In intraluminal obstruction:

• When obstruction recurs during, or shortly after disobliteration

In extraluminal compression:

• When severe, extrinsic compression warrants immediate securing of the airway before further treatment.
• If after-loading therapy is not available and external radiotherapy is not possible, or the obstruction recurs following after-loading treatment.

An accurate evaluation of the extent of airway obstruction and the interplay of the various components is only possible with bronchoscopy, and the need for stenting may only become apparent after other steps have been taken (Fig. 6A–D).

TYPES OF STENTS
Silicone Stents
The silicone T-tube stent was described by Montgomery (29) to provide support for the upper trachea and the larynx. It consists of a length of silicone rubber with a side arm coming off at a right angle near the upper end, designed to emerge through a

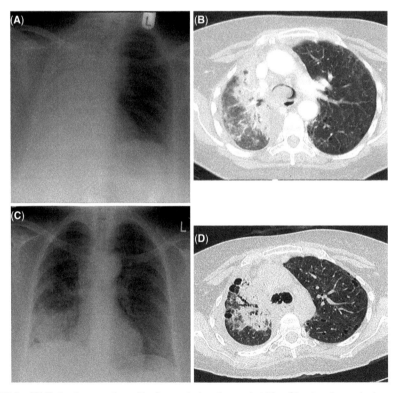

FIGURE 6   (A) Patient presenting with airway obstruction and stridor. Chest radiograph shows white-out due to atelectasis of the right lung. Note the mediastinal shift and tracheal deviation to the right. (B) A cross-sectional CT scan image. Note the tumour completely filling the right main bronchus and fungating into the lower trachea, obstructing the origin of the left main bronchus as well. (C) Chest radiograph immediately after rigid bronchoscopy, diathermy resection and insertion of self-expanding metal stent in the right main bronchus. (D) A post-operative cross-sectional CT scan image. Note metal strands at the proximal end of the stent.

tracheostomy incision, allowing easy access for bronchial suction. Normally, the external limb is spigotted when not being used for suction so that the patient can speak, cough, and humidify inspired gases normally. This type is still in regular use but there are now modifications in the form of T-Y stents (Fig. 7A). T-tubes require regular attention, and in common with all silicone tubes they tend to fur as sputum dries and forms concretions. If malignant disease regresses with subsequent treatment, these tubes can be removed.

Silicone endobronchial *stents* can be inserted through the bronchoscope without undertaking tracheostomy (22,30,31). They can be straight or bifurcated, and depending on the anatomy, a collar can be sutured to one or both ends prior to insertion, to prevent stent displacement (Fig. 7B). Such stents have advantages and disadvantages over other silicone stents and T-tubes. They are cheap, readily available, can be removed easily if no longer needed, or replaced with stents of different length and calibre as needed. They are impervious to the in-growth of granulation tissue or tumour. They have a relatively small internal diameter for the external size due to the thick wall, and tend to occlude slowly.

Wire Stents
Bucher in 1951 (32) was the first to report about the use of a stainless steel wire mesh in the treatment of tracheal and bronchial strictures. Since then, several patterns of expandable metal stents have been used in the airway (23,33,34). Self-expanding stents are widely used and several designs are available. They usually come stretched and constrained on a delivery catheter within a double sheath, the outer one released once in place (Fig. 7C). A combination of endoscopic and radiographic control is necessary to precisely position this type of stent. All patterns of wire stents must be regarded as permanent implants.

An inherent problem with all present patterns of wire stent is the presence of interstices, which allow tumour or granulation tissue in growth and recurrent airway

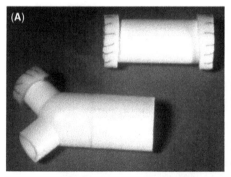
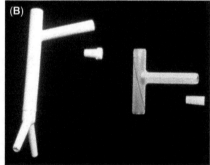
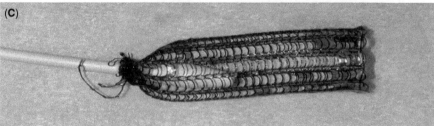

FIGURE 7 (**A**) Silicone straight and Y-type stents. (**B**) Silicone Montgomery T and T-Y tubes. (**C**) Self-expanding metal stent, partially deployed on the carrier catheter.

obstruction. They are therefore best suited for dealing with extraluminal compression where the airway wall is intact. To overcome this problem, new, covered wire stents, are now commercially available.

MANAGEMENT OF PULMONARY METASTASES

The first incidental resection of an isolated lung metastasis was performed by Weinlechner in 1882, in the course of intraoperative assessment for a chest wall sarcoma (35). In the following 50 years, surgery was offered only to a small number of patients who presented with a single-lung deposit or long disease-free interval (DFI) (36,37), mainly due to the view that pulmonary metastatic disease invariably represented a manifestation of generalised systemic spread. There was subsequent gradual recognition of the curative potential of the technique, largely due to the favourable results of work with metastatic sarcomas (38,39). In the last two decades, pulmonary metastasectomy has been systematically offered in properly selected patients with multiple or bilateral metastases from a variety of primaries, in major oncological centres in Europe and North America. More recently, the use of a special 1318 nm wavelength laser has been shown to greatly facilitate resection of multiple or large pulmonary metastases. We have recently reported our favourable initial experience with 44 laser metastasectomy procedures (40,41).

The advances in systemic treatment which can be potentially effective in micrometastases but not to eradicate bulky, clinically detectable deposits have further expanded the role of adjuvant or salvage surgery to excise residual tumour after induction chemotherapy or to confirm complete pathologic remission.

Basic Mechanisms

The basic mechanisms controlling the process of metastatic spread remain largely unknown. Recent research on angiogenesis and growth factors has provided new insight into some aspects of tumour progression but a full biologic explanation of the selectivity and specificity of distant metastases is still lacking.

Studies in large autopsy series have demonstrated that in 29% of patients who died of malignancies, lung was the second commonest metastatic site (42). Furthermore, in another series, lungs were the only site of detectable cancer in 20% of the autopsied patients (43).

Patient Selection

The clinical incidence of isolated lung metastases varies widely with the primary tumour site. In sarcomas and germ cell tumours many patients presenting with lung metastases will be candidates for metastasectomy. On the contrary, most patients with metastatic epithelial cancers have involvement of multiple organs and only a small fraction (1–2%) will be suitable for lung metastasectomy (44,45). This is usually the case for breast cancer patients, in whom an operation is considered normally only when there is a solitary lung lesion present.

In principle, following are the main prerequisites for any patient to be considered for pulmonary metastasectomy:

- Primary tumour is under control.
- Lung is the only site of metastasis (liver *and* lungs acceptable in colonic Ca).
- No better treatment method is available.
- Complete resection of all deposits is feasible.
- Patient is fit for the planned procedure.

In any patient with a history of previous malignancy and a new, solitary lung mass, a main consideration is whether this represents a new primary lung cancer.

This turns out to be the case in 63% of patients with previous breast cancer, compared with 58% when the previous malignancy was colonic Ca, 94% in head and neck tumours, and only 8% of patients with previous sarcoma (46). CT and positron emission tomography scan are invaluable when assessing the extent of disease.

In patients with breast cancer it is very important to type the metastatic tumour as the receptor profile often differs from that of the primary with significant treatment implications. Furthermore, since a lobectomy is the accepted minimum resection for primary lung cancer, distinguishing a new lung primary adenocarcinoma from a solitary breast metastasis is crucial in planning the appropriate resection. Up until recently, the only way was to perform a CT guided needle biopsy preoperatively, which was not popular due to concerns about inoculation. Up to 80% of primary lung adenocarcinomas stain positive for thyroid transcription factor-1 (TTF-1). We have recently reported successful use of intraoperative immunohistochemistry for TTF-1 on frozen section specimens at the Royal Brompton Hospital for making this distinction and help intraoperative decision making (47).

In a modern specialised thoracic surgical centre pulmonary metastasectomy is a very safe procedure. Multi-institutional data from the International Registry of Lung Metastases (IRLM) on 5206 patients, report complete resection in 88% of patients, and an overall 30-day mortality of 0.8% (48). In this author's personal series of more than 450 procedures over the last 12 years, the 30-day and in-hospital mortality was 0.2% ((49) and unpublished personal data).

In the experience of the IRLM the actuarial survival rate after complete metastasectomy was 36% at 5 years and 26% at 10 years, whilst the corresponding results following incomplete resection were 13% at 5 years and 7% at 10 years (45).

A number of independent prognostic indicators which apply universally in metastasectomy patients were identified from the International Registry of Lung Metastases data analysis (48) and are as listed below:

- Completeness of resection
- DFI more than 36 months
- Single deposit
- Tumour type

Long-term survival is possible even in patients with more than one deposit as long as complete resection is achieved, with no clear cut cut-off in the number of lesions. In contrast, the identification of multiple, miliary-type microdeposits on a CT scan or intraoperatively is a contraindication to metastasectomy.

In patients with metastatic breast cancer, pulmonary involvement often results from extension via the internal mammary or mediastinal lymph nodes rather than the limited haematogenous spread. Resection of isolated lung metastases represents less than 1% of all mammary carcinomas (50). There were 411 patients with metastatic breast cancer in the IRLM cohort, and the overall survival rates were 37% at 5 years and 21% at 10 years (median 37 months) (48).

METASTATIC INVOLVEMENT OF THE CHEST WALL AND STERNUM

When, rarely, in the context of pulmonary metastasectomy a direct extension of the tumour to the chest wall is encountered, then a complete en bloc resection is warranted and is still associated with good long-term survival (51).

Chest wall resection for breast cancer today is most often performed for recurrent local disease after failure of other forms of therapy (52,53).

Systemic recurrence is common, and chest wall resection is mainly directed towards relieving pain, removing fungating unsightly tumour, eliminating odour, and generally improving quality of life. Due to the scale of surgery involved, careful patient selection in terms of life expectancy is very important. Surgery should be part of a multimodality treatment approach, with pre- and post-operative chemotherapy and/or hormonal treatment playing a crucial role. Chest wall lesions often are the result of spread from involved internal mammary nodes, but we have seen the occasional patient with isolated, intramanubrial bone metastasis and no nodal disease. When previously irradiated lesions recur, the surgeon is presented with significant technical challenges.

The surgical principles include complete en bloc resection of all involved or previously irradiated and damaged skin, muscle, and part of chest wall including multiple ribs and sternum, as well as lung, pericardium, or diaphragm as required with wide clear margins (Fig. 8). The chest wall defect is then reconstructed with a prosthesis to avoid paradox and ensure protection of noble intrathoracic organs.

In our practice a composite polypropylene mesh and methyl-methacrylate resin (bone cement) prosthesis is the preferred option. Once the mesh is cut in shape, the two-part resin is mixed and applied in a paste form. This sets with an exothermic reaction to form a thin, yet robust, plate which is then secured at the edges of the chest wall defect (Fig. 9). In most cases, a soft tissue reconstruction to provide cover follows, usually in the form of myo-cutaneous pediclled rotation flaps of various origin, with rectus abdominis, latissimus dorsi, and pectoralis major muscles being popular donor choices. Occasionally, omentum in association with free skin grafts can also be used to cover large central sternal defects.

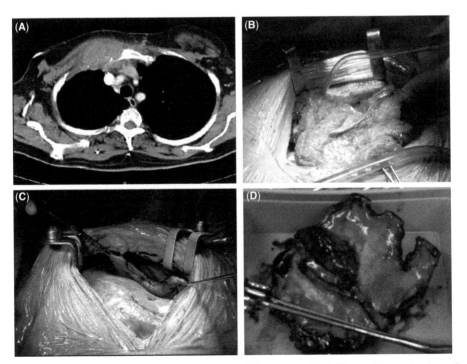

FIGURE 8 (A) Breast cancer metastatic to chest wall. A cross-sectional CT scan image showing soft tissue mass at the right anterior chest wall involving the sternum, ribs, overlying muscle, and lung. (B) Intraoperative photograph. Note en-bloc resection of skin eclipse, muscle, sternum and ribs and (C) wedge of underlying involved lung using staplers on this occasion. Note the size of residual chest wall defect. (D) The resected specimen (deep aspect) showing sternum, parts of 3 ribs bilaterally and attached wedge of the lung.

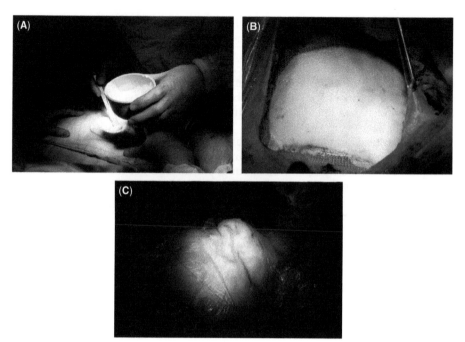

FIGURE 9 (**A**) Same patient as Fig 8. Preparation of the chest wall prosthesis. Application of the methyl-methacrylate resin (bone cement) to the polypropylene mesh. (**B**) When this sets hard, it is secured at the margins of the chest wall defect. (**C**) Appearances immediately after the end of the procedure. On this occasion primary soft tissue closure was possible.

Specialist input from a plastic surgeon is invaluable in providing a high quality service.

Breast tumours metastatic to the manubrium and the sternoclavicular area present formidable technical challenges for the thoracic surgeon due to their proximity to the noble structures of the thoracic inlet and superior mediastinum. We have recently reported excellent results on 18 women who underwent resection of such tumours between 1998 and 2007 (54), using complex surgical techniques developed for the management of Pancoast tumours of the lung (55,56). Twelve of these patients had total sternal resection, five patients had subtotal sternal resection, and one patient had resection of tumour and ribs. Seventeen patients required the insertion of a composite Marlex® methyl-methacrylate chest wall prosthesis, followed by soft tissue reconstruction with a pectoralis major or latissimus dorsi flap, in the majority of cases. In-hospital and 30-day mortality was 0%. One- and two-year overall survival was 87% and 80% respectively. The median recurrence-free survival was 18 months (95% CI 4–31 months). There was local and distant recurrence in one patient (5%), local recurrence in two patients (11%), and distant recurrence in eight patients (44%). Importantly, 15 out of 18 patients (77%) remained free from local recurrence at 5 years.

The proven safety of these complex procedures in our experience, in combination with the significant advances in systemic treatment and improved survival for patients with advanced breast cancer, makes them a very attractive option for the management of these very difficult problems in properly selected patients. The most gratifying aspect of these resections is the improved quality of life that they afford, with very efficient relief of pain and tenderness, and vastly improved cosmesis, and they are now routinely performed in our practice.

REFERENCES

1. Moragon EM, Aparicio J, Sanchis J, et al. Malignant pleural effusion:prognostic factors for survival and response to chemical pleurodesis in a series of 120 cases Respiration 1998; 65: 108–13.
2. Sahn AS. Malignancy metastatic to the pleura. Clin Chest Med 1998; 19: 351–61.
3. Wong PS, Goldstraw P. Pleuroperitoneal shunts: review. Br J Hosp Med 1993; 50: 16–21.
4. Martini N, Bains MS, Beattie EJ Jr. Indications for pleurectomy in malignant effusion. Cancer 1975; 35: 734–8.
5. Fentiman IS, Millis R, Sexton S, et al. Pleural effusion in breast cancer: a review of 105 cases. Cancer 1981; 47: 2087–92.
6. Weese JL, Schouten JT. Pleural peritoneal shunts for the treatment of malignant pleural effusions. Surg Gynaecol Obstet 1982; 154: 391–2.
7. Pollock AV. The treatment of resistant malignant ascites by insertion of a peritoneo-atrial Holter valve. Br J Surg 1975; 62: 104–7.
8. Milsom JW, Kron IL, Rheuban KS, Rodgers BM. Chylothorax: an assessment of current surgical management. J Thorac Cardiovasc Surg 1985; 89: 221–7.
9. Tsang V, Fernando HC, Goldstraw P. Pleuroperitoneal shunt for recurrent malignant pleural effusions. Thorax 1990; 45: 369–72.
10. Genc O, Petrou P, Ladas G, Goldstraw P. The long term morbidity of pleuroperitoneal shunts in the management of recurrent malignant effusions. Eur J Cardiothorac Surg 2000; 18: 143–6.
11. Little AG, Kadowki MH, Ferguson MK, Staszek VM, Skinner DB. Pleuroperitoneal shunting. Alternative therapy for pleural effusions. Ann Surg 1988; 208: 443–50.
12. Hetzel MR, Smith SGT. Endoscopic palliation of tracheobronchial malignancies. Thorax 1991; 46: 325–33.
13. Ross DJ, Mohsenifar Z, Koerner SK. Survival characteristics after neodymium: YAG laser photoresection in advanced stage lung cancer. Chest 1990; 98: 581–5.
14. Cavaliere S, Foccoli P, Farina PL. Nd: YAG laser bronchoscopy. A five-year experience with 1,396 applications in 1,000 patients. Chest 1988; 94: 15–21.
15. George PMJ, Garrett CPO, Hetzel MR. Role of neodymium YAG laser in the management of tracheal tumours. Thorax 1987; 42: 440–4.
16. Cortese DA. Endobronchial management of lung cancer. Chest 1986; 89: 234S–6S.
17. Dumon JF, Shapshay S, Bourcereau J, et al. Principles for safety in application of neodymium-YAG laser in bronchology. Chest 1984; 86: 163–8.
18. Vincent RG. Laser therapy for advanced carcinoma of the trachea and bronchus [editorial]. Chest 1983; 84: 509–10.
19. Vergnon JM, Boucheron S, Bonamour D, Emonot A. Cryotherapy or Nd-YAG laser in the treatment of tracheobronchial tumours? Chest 1987; 91: 473.
20. Walsh DA, Maiwand MO, Nath AR, et al. Bronchoscopic cryotherapy for advanced bronchial carcinoma. Thorax 1990; 45: 509–13.
21. Ledingham SJ, Goldstraw P. Diathermy resection and radioactive gold grains for palliation of obstruction due to recurrence of bronchial carcinoma after external irradiation. Thorax 1989; 44: 48–51.
22. Petrou M, Kaplan D, Goldstraw P. Bronchoscopic diathermy resection and stent insertion: a cost-effective treatment for tracheobronchial obstruction. Thorax 1993; 48: 1156–9.
23. Goldstraw P, Ladas G. Bronchial stenting. In: Sigwart U, ed. Endoluminal Stenting. London: W.B Saunders Co Ltd, 1996: 576–83.
24. Hooper RG, Jackson FN. Endobronchial electrocautery. Chest 1985; 87: 712–14.
25. Shankar S, George PJ, Hetzel MR, Goldstraw P. Elective resection of tumours of the trachea and main carina after endoscopic laser therapy. Thorax 1990; 45: 493–5.
26. Nori D, Hilaris BS, Martini N. Intraluminal irradiation in bronchogenic carcinoma. Surg Clin North Am 1987; 67: 1093–102.
27. Allen MD, Baldwin JC, Fish VJ, et al. Combined laser therapy and endobronchial radiotherapy for unresectable lung carcinoma with bronchial obstruction. Am J Surg 1985; 150: 71–7.
28. Burt PA, O'Driscoll BR, Notley HM, Barber PV, Stout R. Intraluminal irradiation for the palliation of lung cancer with the high dose rate micro-Selectron. Thorax 1990; 45: 765–8.
29. Montgomery WW. Reconstruction of the cervical trachea. Ann Otol 1964; 73: 5–9.

30. Tsang V, Goldstraw P. Endobronchial stenting for anastomotic stenosis after sleeve resection. Ann Thorac Surg 1989; 48: 568–71.
31. Cooper JD, Pearson FG, Patterson GA, et al. Use of silicone stents in the management of airway problems. Ann Thorac Surg 1989; 47: 371–8.
32. Bucher M, Burnett WE, Rosemond GP. Experimental reconstruction of tracheal and bronchial defects with stainless steel wire mesh. J Thorac Surg 1951; 21: 572.
33. Wallace MJ, Charnsangavej C, Ogawa K, et al. Tracheobronchial tree: expandable metallic stents used in experimental and clinical applications. Radiology 1986; 158: 309–12.
34. Irving JD, Goldstraw P. Tracheobronchial stents. Semin Int Radiol 1991; 8: 295–304.
35. Weinlechner JW. Tumoren an der Brustwand und deren Behandlung (resection der Rippen) Erroffnung der Brusthole und partielle Entfernung der Lunge. Wien Med Wschr 1882; 32: 590.
36. Barney JD, Churchill EJ. Adenocarcinoma of the kidney with metastasis to the lung. J Urol 1939; 42: 269.
37. Alexander J, Haight C. Pulmonary resection for solitary metastatic sarcomas and carcinomas. Surg Gynaecol Obstet 1947; 85: 129.
38. Martini N, McCormack PM, Bains MS. Indications for surgery for intrathoracic metastases in testicular teratoma. Semin Oncol 1979; 6: 99.
39. Vogt-Moykopf I, Krysa S, Bulzebruck H, et al. Surgery for pulmonary metastases: The Heidelberg experience. Chest Surg Clin North Am 1994; 4: 85.
40. Rolle A, Pereszlenyi A, Koch R, Richard M, Baier B. Is surgery for multiple lung metastases reasonable? A total of 328 consecutive patients with multiple-laser metastasectomies with a new 1318-nm Nd: YAG laser. J Thorac Cardiovasc Surg 2006; 131: 1236–42.
41. Okiror L, Qureshi S, Ladas G. Pulmonary metastasectomy using the 1318nm laser. Initial experience with 44 consecutive procedures. Annual Conference of the Society of Cardiothoracic Surgeons of Great Britain and Ireland. London, 2011.
42. Wills RA. Pathology of Tumors, 4th edn. London: Butterworth, 1967
43. Weiss L, Gilbert HA. In: Weiss L, Gilbert HA, eds. Pulmonary Metastasis. Boston: GK Hall, 1978: 142.
44. Mayo CW, Schlicke CP. Carcinomas of the colon and rectum. Dis Colon Rectum 1978; 22: 717.
45. McCormack PM, Attiyeh FF. Resected pulmonary metastases from colorectal cancer. Dis Colon Rectum 1979; 22: 583.
46. Cahan WG, Shah JP, Castro EB. Benign solitary lung lesions in patients with cancer. Ann Surg 1978; 187: 241.
47. Butcher DN, Goldstraw P, Ladas G, et al. Thyroid transcription factor 1 immunohistochemistry as an intraoperative diagnostic tool at frozen section for distinction between primary and secondary lung tumours. Arch Pathol Lab Med 2007; 131: 582–7.
48. Pastorino U, Buyse M, Friedal G, et al.; for The International Registry of Lung Metastases. Long term results of lung metastasectomy: Prognostic analysis based on 5206 cases. J Thorac Cardiovasc Surg 1997; 113: 37.
49. Negri F, Musolino A, Cunningham D, et al. Retrospective study of resection of pulmonary metastases in patients with advanced colorectal cancer: the development of a preoperative chemotherapy strategy. Clin Colorectal Cancer 2004; 4: 101–6.
50. Morrow CE, Vassilopoulos PP, Grage TB. Surgical resection for metastatic neoplasms of the lung :Experience at the University of Minnesota Hospitals. Cancer 1980; 45: 2981.
51. Pastorino U, Grunenwald D. Pulmonary Metastases. In: Pearson FG, Cooper JD, Deslauriers J, Ginsberg RJ, Hiebert CA, Patterson GA, Urschel HC, eds. In Thoracic Surgery. Philadelphia: Churchill Livingstone, 2002: 962–73.
52. Ryan MB, Mc Murtrey MJ, Roth JA. Current management of chest wall tumors. Surg Clin North Am 1989; 69: 1061.
53. Seyfer AE, Graeber GM, Wind GG. Resection and debridement of the chest wall. In: Seyfer AE, ed. Atlas of Chest Wall Reconstruction. Rockville, MD: Aspen Publishers, 1986.
54. Noble J, Sirohi B, Ashley S, Ladas G, Smith I. Sternal/para-sternal resection for parasternal local recurrence in breast cancer. Breast 2010; 19: 350–4.
55. Dartevelle P, Chapelier A, Macchiarini P, et al. Anterior transcervical-thoracic approach for radical resection of tumours invading the thoracic inlet. J Thorac Cardiovasc Surg 1993; 105: 1025.
56. Grunenwald D, Spaggiari L. Transmanubrial osteomuscular sparing approach for apical chest tumors. Ann Thorac Surg 1997; 63: 563–6.

15

Orthopaedic complications

Kuldeep K. Stöhr and Stuart C. Evans

Bone is the most common site of metastasis for breast cancer; 60–80% of patients will have bony lesions. One study found that approximately one-third of patients with metastatic breast cancer developed structurally significant bone destruction (1) and that only half of these patients were referred to an orthopaedic surgeon. Possible reasons for failure to refer include patient frailty, poor life expectancy, and the effectiveness of medical management (2); however, lack of awareness of the potential benefits of orthopaedic surgery may also play a part.

The basic aims of orthopaedic surgery are to relieve pain and restore function. Circumstances in which surgical intervention should be considered include the following:

- Pain due to bony metastases
- Fracture
- Risk of impending fracture
- Spinal metastases causing spinal instability
- Spinal metastases causing nerve root compression

In recent years improvements in medical management have reduced the need for orthopaedic surgery. Perhaps the most notable advance has been the widespread use of bisphosphonates which have significantly reduced the complications of bony metastases (3).

Bisphosphonates not only reduce the effect of metastases but also their occurrence, in addition they can offset some of the generalised bone loss that frequently accompanies cancer treatment. Unfortunately, prolonged use of bisphosphonates appears to be associated with subtrochanteric femoral fractures although the incidence is low, the aetiology unclear but may be the result of altered bone remodelling, a consequence of suppression of osteoclasts. Other risks include renal toxicity (necessitating the monitoring of renal function) and osteonecrosis of the jaw, a rare but well-documented complication.

Bisphosphonates not only bind to the bone matrix and slow down the rate of resorption by osteoclasts, they also enter the osteoclast and ultimately cause apoptosis reducing osteolysis and so the effect of metastases (4).

Monoclonal antibodies that bind specifically to the RANK ligand of the osteoclast offer further hope for medical management.

PRESENTATION

In a study of 498 patients with breast cancer 65% of those known to have metastases had a major bone-related complication (5). Patients with bony metastases can present with pain (although not invariably so), fracture, hypercalcaemia, and neurological symptoms secondary to nerve root compression (6,7). Almost all patients who suffer a pathological fracture have had pain that deteriorated over the weeks that preceded the fracture, therefore pain should be investigated expediently (8). Pelvic and femoral metastases frequently cause pain on weight-bearing that is usually relieved by rest. Night pain is characteristic although not always present.

INVESTIGATIONS (9)
Plain x-ray

Plain x-rays play a vital role in diagnosis, surgical planning, and monitoring response to treatment. Breast cancer metastases tend to be mixed or lytic in character although predominantly sclerotic lesions are not unknown (Fig. 1); the variation reflects the balance between osteoclastic and osteoblastic activity. The radiolucency of lytic lesions usually renders them more readily identifiable than the whiter sclerotic appearance of blastic lesions (Fig. 2).

Fractures are identified by areas of cortical discontinuity and are more apparent in the presence of deformity, displacement, and bone loss. Metastases, particularly mixed lesions, preceding a fracture can easily be missed. Plain x-rays tend to underestimate the degree of bone destruction. A 30–50% loss of bone mineral density (more for primarily trabecular bone lesions) has to occur before radiolucency can be seen. Thus, while having a high specificity, plain x-rays lack the sensitivity of other imaging modalities. Even amongst experienced orthopaedic surgeons there is

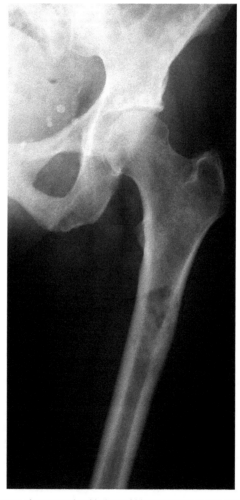

FIGURE 1   This x-ray image shows a mixed lytic and blastic lesion in the left femur below the lesser trochanter. Breast metastases are commonly of this type.

a significant inter-observer variation in the assessment of the size of lytic lesions on plain films (8). Despite these flaws x-rays remain a vital tool being inexpensive and easily accessible.

Biplanar x-rays (anteroposterior and lateral views) should be the first investigation. Any lesions identified in the long bone lesions on radionuclide scanning should be x-rayed. The whole length of the long bone must be imaged to exclude the possibility of other metastases. Similarly for vertebral metastases the whole spine should be visualised. The location and extent of a lesion will determine the relative indication for surgery and its nature. The appearance of sclerosis and new bone formation can signify response to treatment.

Nuclear Medicine Scanning

Radionuclide scanning utilises the property of technetium-99m to bind to various diphosphonates; these diphosphonates are taken up by osteoblasts and so scintigraphy can reflect metabolic bone activity. Nuclear medicine scanning is more sensitive than plain x-rays and the whole skeleton can be included in one study. It has been estimated that radionuclide scanning can detect skeletal metastases approximately 3 months earlier than plain x-rays. In addition, whilst plain x-rays can detect only lesions that are approximately 1 cm or larger in diameter, radionuclide scanning can identify those that are as small as 2 mm. With a specificity of 78–100% radionuclide

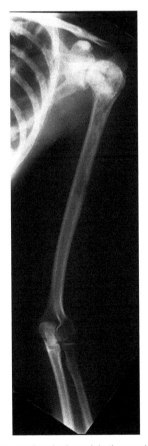

FIGURE 2 This x-ray image shows a sclerotic deposit in the proximal humerus. There is a lytic lesion in the midshaft.

imaging is more prone to false positives than plain x-rays, a misdiagnosis can be caused by trauma, inflammation, and arthritis. False negatives can occur with metabolically inactive metastases typically avascular lytic lesions with a slow bone turnover. Whole-body images are relatively inexpensive and form part of the work-up and surveillance of symptomatic breast cancer patients. Suspicious areas must be investigated with plain x-ray.

Computed Tomography Scanning
Computed tomography (CT) scanning is useful in quantifying and delineating a lesion that has already been revealed by other modalities. The bony window setting is highly sensitive for skeletal changes, particularly cortical destruction. Metastases can be detected in the early bone marrow deposition stage that precedes bone destruction. CT has particular value in the imaging of spinal metastases where the surrounding soft tissue can impair the definition of plain x-rays. Unfortunately, the advantage of high sensitivity is offset by the relatively small size of the imaging field (limited by cost and radiation dose).

Magnetic Resonance Scanning
Magnetic resonance (MR) is the gold standard for assessing bony metastases with accompanying soft tissue involvement, most notably in spinal cord and nerve root compression. Like CT, MR can detect metastases at the bone marrow deposition stage, but it is inferior to CT (and often plain x-rays) in quantifying cortical loss.

AXIAL METASTASES
In descending order of frequency the most common sites for skeletal breast cancer metastases are as follows (6):

- Vertebrae (primarily thoracolumbar)
- Pelvis
- Ribs
- Femur (mostly proximal)
- Humerus (mostly proximal)
- Other bony sites (e.g., scapula, tibia, skull)

Although the axial skeleton is involved predominantly, lesions in the appendicular skeleton are more likely to require operative fixation. This partly reflects the scope of surgical treatment and partly the relative success of local radiation for the axial skeleton. There are, however, circumstances in axial disease where orthopaedic intervention can be beneficial.

Spinal Metastases
It has been estimated that between 30 and 70% of patients with breast cancer have spinal metastases at the time of death (10). This predilection for the spine is believed to be due to the breast's venous drainage. Cancer cells may seed via lymphatics and the azygos vein into the paravertebral venous plexus of Batson where they deposit most frequently into the anterior and middle columns of the thoracolumbar spine (Fig. 3) (11).

Although spinal metastases can remain asymptomatic, approximately 95% are painful, a few will also cause deformity, and some will impair neurological function. The osteoclastic activity of breast metastases creates osteolysis which can lead to fracture, collapse, and kyphosis; the consequent pain can give rise to paraspinal muscle spasm and scoliosis. Nerve root and spinal cord compression can occur as a result of fracture fragments and soft tissue tumour. Pain can result from all these phenomena,

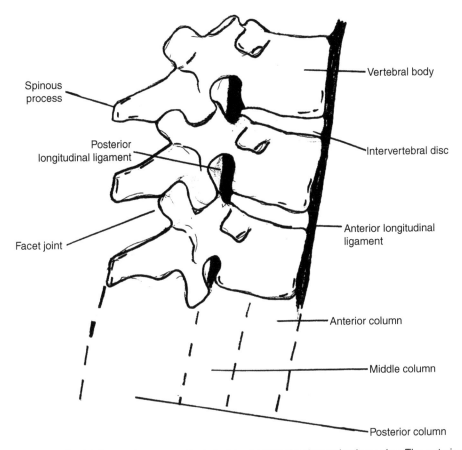

Spinous
process

Posterior
longitudinal ligament

Facet joint

Vertebral body

Intervertebral disc

Anterior longitudinal
ligament

Anterior column

Middle column

Posterior column

FIGURE 3   Denis' three columns are illustrated here using the thoracolumbar spine. The anterior column consists of the longitudinal ligament, the anterior part of the vertebral body, and the anterior portion of the annulus fibrosis. The middle column consists of the posterior longitudinal ligament, posterior part of the vertebral body, and posterior portion of the annulus fibrosis. The posterior column consists of the bony and ligamentous posterior elements; the latter are not shown in this diagram. *Source*: Ref. 11.

but in addition may be caused by mechanoreceptor stimulation in the periosteum, direct stimulation of nociceptors by the tumour, and the local release of chemical mediators such as substance P, bradykinin, and histamine (12).

In summary pain from spinal metastases can be as a result of the following:

1. enlarging tumour mass
2. bone defect leading to pathological fracture
3. bone defect leading to deformity—kyphosis, scoliosis, or a combination of both
4. nerve root compression—secondary to tumour mass, accompanying tissue reaction or fracture fragments
5. compression of spinal cord—secondary to tumour mass, accompanying tissue reaction or fracture fragments

Some spinal metastases remain asymptomatic, and only a few that cause symptoms require surgery. In 1986, Harrington (13) described a scheme for choosing between medical and surgical management (Table 1).

TABLE 1 Managing Spinal Metastases (13)

Class	Description	Management
I	No neurologic involvement	Chemotherapy and/or local radiation
II	Bone involvement but no collapse	Chemotherapy and/or local radiation
III	Neurologic impairment without body involvement	Local radiation and/or steroids
IV	Vertebral collapse or instability without significant neurological involvement	Surgical stabilisation via anterior approach
V	Vertebral collapse with major neurologic impairment	Surgical stabilisation and decompression via anterior approach

Although Harrington's scheme holds true, a more recent algorithm has been recommended that, for neurological impairment, takes into account the emerging preference for combining surgical spinal cord decompression with radiotherapy rather than radiotherapy alone (Fig. 4). This has been supported by a prospective, randomised, multicentre trial (14,15). Wherever possible surgery should precede radiation as the reverse order is accompanied by an almost three times greater incidence of wound healing problems (16).

The other group of patients considered for surgery are those with instability or impending instability, essentially those with defects in the anterior and middle vertebral columns as described by Denis (Fig. 3) (11). Spinal surgery can be a major undertaking with many attendant risks therefore it is important to have an understanding of indications, methods and outcomes.

The goals of spinal surgery include these:

- neural decompression
- spinal stability
- correction of spinal deformity

Frequently two or more of these aims have to be addressed in the same procedure. The general principles are to replace lost bone, to stabilise the spine in order to maintain height and alignment, and to decompress the spinal cord and nerve roots. Bone defects can be filled with bone cement (polymethacrylate) or a prosthesis (such as a metal cage); bone grafting is rarely indicated as the defects are generally too large and factors of both the disease and the treatment impair healing. Supplementary instrumentation is almost invariably required to prevent recurrent deformity and should extend to unaffected bone or disc above and below the lesion. The instrumentation (generally in the form of rods and pedicle screws) distracts or compresses the vertebral bodies and can promote fusion. The choice of device depends on the size of the lesions and the number of levels involved.

Surgical stabilisation generally necessitates an anterior or a combined anterior–posterior approach. The anterior approach to the cervical spine is through the soft tissues of the anterolateral aspect of the neck, to the thoracic spine is via the chest, and to the lumbar spine is through the abdomen. The posterior approach is through the midline followed by a laminectomy to access the foramen, spinal canal, and vertebral bodies. In the presence of bony metastases laminectomy can destabilise an already collapsing vertebral body, therefore, the outcome of surgical decompression is twice as good with an anterior approach as a posterior approach (17). Despite this increased risk, access to metastases affecting only the posterior half of the vertebral body may necessitate a posterior approach and patients with multilevel involvement

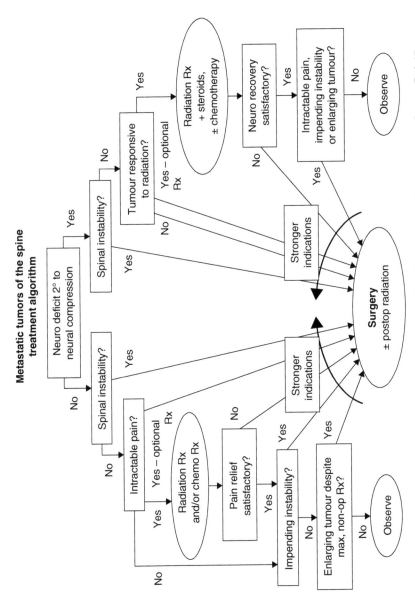

FIGURE 4 A spinal algorithm to direct appropriate patients towards surgical management. *Source:* Ref. 17.

requiring extensive internal fixation may require a combined anterior and posterior procedure.

Spinal surgery through an anterior approach is clearly a major undertaking and so spinal surgery has traditionally been reserved for those patients presenting with cord/nerve root compression or instability and who are also surgically fit and have a good prognosis—usually taken to mean a life expectancy greater than 6 months. However, this view is beginning to change with the advent of minimally invasive spinal surgery which is proliferating in three main areas:

- Biopsy
- Replacing bone loss: vertebroplasty and kyphoplasty
- Reconstruction and stabilisation, especially through endoscopic procedures

Tissue Diagnosis
With the advent of screening programmes and improved imaging techniques metastatic spinal disease is being detected earlier, bringing an increased need for minimally invasive and targeted bone sampling. Interventional radiology can be employed reducing the need for open or core biopsies and the associated risks of bleeding and nerve damage. CT or fluoroscopic guidance can access the posteriorly located lesions or those in the far lateral area of the vertebral body through the paravertebral approach, while lesions in the central or anterior parts of the vertebral body (where metastases typically emerge first) are more amenable to the transpedicular approach. The transpedicular approach in particular has brought about an earlier diagnosis, and open biopsies of deep vertebral lesions are almost obsolete.

Percutaneous Vertebroplasty (18)
Percutaneous vertebroplasty entails the injection of polymethyl methacrylate (PMMA) cement directly into a collapsed vertebral body. The technique has become established in the treatment of some osteoporotic vertebral fractures where it can result in relief of pain within 2 weeks and that can be sustained up to 1 year. PMMA confers an improvement of more than 195% in the compressive strength of an untreated isolated osteoporotic vertebral body. It is being increasingly used for metastatic lesions associated with vertebral collapse where it offers a rapid pain relief and return to function (19). The key appears to be the restoration of vertebral height.

The presence of cortical osteolysis and the associated increased risk of PMMA leakage reduce the effectiveness of vertebroplasty and kyphoplasty may be more appropriate for these patients. The technique entails inflation with saline of a balloon introduced at the tip of the needle into the vertebral body thereby restoring the height. The newly created void is then filled with PMMA cement. The balloon is removed once the cement hardens. Complications include cement leakage and infection although in a systematic review of 877 patients the risks of both appeared to be low (20). Results of published series are encouraging but there is still relatively little data, particularly for long-term follow-up.

Table 2 shows the current contraindications for vertebroplasty. As techniques improve and high-viscosity cements are developed, percutaneous vertebroplasty and kyphoplasty are likely to have a wider application.

Endoscopic Spinal Surgery
Video-assisted thoracoscopic surgery (VATS) is more commonly used by thoracic than orthopaedic surgeons but is finding application in the access of metastases in thoracic vertebrae.

VATS allows the surgeons to reach the vertebral bodies, discs, and pedicles and can be used to perform procedures such as decompression, tumour resection, and stabilisation with anterior plating and bone grafting. Exposure can be enhanced by the deflation of the relevant lung for the duration of the operation. In a few centres, laparoscopic techniques are also employed to access the lumbar vertebrae via the retroperitoneal approach. Reduced hospital stay and an earlier return to activity have been reported in comparison to open surgery and the techniques offer the hope of reduced chest complications and fewer traumas to the ribs and shoulder girdle. Endoscopic spinal surgery is however not widely available and entails specialist training that incurs a steep learning curve.

Hip and Pelvis Metastases (21)

Pelvic involvement in metastatic breast cancer is common and a frequent cause of immobility and loss of function. At present lesions in the femora and in the acetabuli are amenable to reconstruction while lesions in the pubic rami, sacrum, sacroiliac joint, superior ilium, and ischia are currently managed medically (Fig. 5). There have been some reported cases of solitary metastatic lesions being treated by excision; this is a difficult undertaking with a high morbidity and mortality. Preservation of the femoral artery, vein, and nerve; maintenance of the integrity of the bladder and

TABLE 2 Relative and Absolute Contraindications to Percutaneous Vertebroplasty and Kyphoplasty

Relative Contraindications	Absolute Contraindications
Epidural cortical osteolysis: danger of cement leak compromising the spinal cord	Coagulopathy
70% or greater loss of height: danger of fracture fragments displacing with cement injection	Osteomyelitis and discitis in the affected area
	Lack of surgical back-up in the event of complications

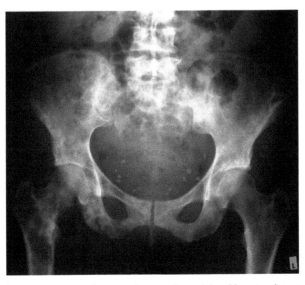

FIGURE 5 This is an anteroposterior x-ray image of a pelvis with extensive metastatic disease. Metastatic deposits are seen in the right pubic rami, right acetabulum, and in the right proximal femur.

TABLE 3 Managing Acetabular Metastases (21)

Class	Description	Reconstruction
I	Lateral cortices, superior and medial walls remain structurally intact	Conventional cemented total hip replacement
II	Deficient medial wall	Protrusio cup, cemented total hip replacement
III	Deficient lateral and superior acetabulum	Protrusio cup with fixation (e.g., screws or Steinmann pins) with cemented total hip replacement
IV	Solitary metastasis	Resection of lesion: super Girdlestone, saddle prosthesis, or custom-made prosthesis

rectum; and preservation of the sciatic nerve are the key to an acceptable outcome (22), but the risks of complications including infection, pain, thromboembolism, and poor post-operative mobility are high.

In this region the acetabulum is most commonly involved and surgical management is essentially total hip replacement accompanied by a resection of the tumour and its substitution with implants appropriate to deficiency. If complex acetabular reconstruction is required, the procedure can be a major undertaking. Careful selection of patients is needed taking into account their physiological and psychological ability to tolerate the operation, the rehabilitation, and the potential complications. Although no specific criteria exist, reasonable pre-operative function and more than 6 months' life expectancy are usually felt to be necessary.

The pattern and extent of acetabular bone loss influence the nature of reconstruction (Table 3); options include a conventional total hip replacement with a cemented cup, a protrusio cup with a cemented total hip replacement, a custom-made protrusio cup with pin and screw fixation into the pelvis. Uncemented prostheses are generally not appropriate due to impaired bone in-growth.

A protrusio cup is a specially reinforced acetabular component that extends into the pelvic cavity to rest on a disease-free bone; it is indicated in cases of extensive bone loss in the floor and walls of the acetabulum (Fig. 6). Tumour infiltration of the greater part of the acetabular walls is an indication for the use of devices to fix the cup to the pelvis; these include Steinmann pins, threaded rods, and screws. In addition, the acetabular components may need reinforcement with rings, bone graft, PMMA cement or silastic, and wire meshes.

An anatomical guideline to the choice of acetabular reconstruction in metastatic bone disease was formulated by Harrington based on plain x-rays. Although this is the most frequently used classification it must be remembered that it is a guide for *all* metastatic disease and not just breast cancer, this is particularly pertinent for Class IV lesions where excision of the hip joint (Girdlestone procedure) is one of the recommendations for solitary, symptomatic lesions, a situation that is rarely encountered in metastatic breast cancer.

Although total hip replacement is common, when undertaken for metastatic breast cancer the procedure can be technically demanding and should generally be performed only by a surgeon with a specialist interest in the field. Meticulous pre-operative planning and patient preparation is essential. Intraoperative bleeding is generally greater than in comparable procedures in the absence of tumour and the surgeon must be ready to act swiftly in the curettage of the deposit and the employment of PMMA cement, bone wax, absorbable sponge, and thrombin as necessary. The risk of major complications, including neurovascular injury, infection, thromboembolism, and death, has been shown to be as high as 30%. However, despite these

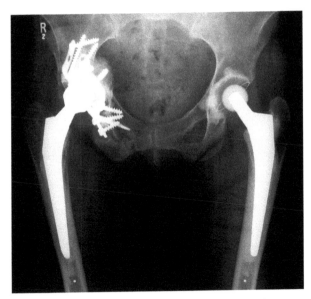

FIGURE 6 This x-ray image shows bilateral total hip replacements. There is a conventional cemented total hip replacement on the left. The right shows a total hip replacement which has been modified to accommodate acetabular bone loss. There is a protrusio cup which is held into the pelvis with screws, plates, and methyl methacrylate cement.

concerns, for the correct patient, total hip replacement can result in a marked reduction of pain and improvement in function.

Recently, cadaveric allografts have been employed to replace metastases in the pubic rami, ischia, or iliac crests that have been treated with en bloc bone excision. In a series of 24 patients (23), five cases with solitary metastatic lesions underwent resection of the deposit and replacement using un-irradiated cadaveric allograft that had been dipped in rifampicin. The complication rate is exceptionally high (approximately 83%) and the procedure has generally been limited to the treatment of young patients with primary bone tumours.

APPENDICULAR SKELETON
Long Bone Metastases

Although axial metastases predominate, surgical fixation is undertaken more frequently for deposits in the appendicular skeleton. Appendicular metastases may present with pain or fracture. Fractures often occur with minimal or no trauma and as a consequence the accompanying soft tissue injury, including bruising or swelling, can be minimal.

The occurrence of any fracture is associated with a poor prognosis. Observational data (24) demonstrated a median life expectancy of 12 months after fracture; approximately half that of patients with bony metastases who do not sustain a fracture. Long bone fracture causes pain and loss of function. An upper limb fracture imposes a significant loss of independence; for patients with co-existent pathology the loss of an upper limb with which they would otherwise use a stick or crutch can prove crucial. Thus a fracture is an extremely serious event and the aim across all specialties should be to address it's risk and prevention. From the surgeon's point of view an intact bone, however weak, is easier to stabilise than a broken one; from a

TABLE 4   Mirels' Scoring System for Appendicular Metastases (26)

	Points		
	3	2	1
Location	Peri-trochanteric	Lower extremity	Upper extremity
Lesion type	Lytic	Mixed: lytic and blastic	Blastic
Amount of cortical loss	>2/3	1/3–2/3	≤1/3
Pain	Functional	Functional, moderate	Moderate

patient's point of view a broken bone can mean a longer hospital stay (25), a more painful and protracted post-operative period, and a reduced life-expectancy.

Most patients will report pain in the weeks preceding fracture and x-rays may demonstrate localised bone loss (as previously noted, a 30–50% loss in bone mineral density has to occur before a metastatic lesion is visible on plain films). Numerous attempts have been made to describe the radiological changes that signify significant weakening of bone. We know that osteolytic lesions are more likely to result in fracture than sclerotic lesions. When the loss involves cortical bone a surprisingly small area (0.5 cm diameter) can cause significant weakening and may be the origin of a fracture when that bone is subjected to forces a little greater than those encountered in normal activity.

Fidler believed that a metastasis causing 50% reduction in the thickness of cortical bone on plain x-rays signifies an impending fracture; therefore, an osteolytic lesion ≥2.5 cm is also considered significant (9). These observations have been supported by others but less bone loss can prove critical in areas where the forces are greater.

Mirels drew all these factors together to create a system that can help in deciding for or against prophylactic fixation, his scheme was based on his observations of 78 metastatic lesions undergoing radiation therapy (26) (Table 4). Using his system a score of 8 points or above is considered an indication for surgery.

Mirels' scheme though widely accepted, should be treated more as a guideline than an edict when applied to breast cancer. In breast disease most lesions are mixed (lytic and blastic) and as such tend to respond well to radiation therapy though a new bone can take 2–3 months to reconstitute. The ability of a particular patient to tolerate pain and restricted activity (e.g., partial weight-bearing) for an extended period needs to be considered. Despite the generally favourable response to radiotherapy if fracture is believed to be imminent fixation should precede expediently (27). The conclusions of the 1997 Working Party on Metastatic Bone Disease in Breast Cancer in the UK (28) are helpful in this respect; this multidisciplinary group, comprising of breast surgeons, orthopaedic surgeons, and oncologists, recommended prophylactic fixation *before* commencing radiotherapy for those lesions with a score 9 or above, provided the patient is able tolerate the surgery.

GENERAL SURGICAL CONSIDERATIONS
Physiological
Absolute contraindications to fixation include imminent death and severe comorbidities. Two-thirds of patients undergoing orthopaedic surgery for skeletal metastases have cardiovascular or respiratory compromise (29). Other contraindications are relative and should be considered on an individual basis, these include coagulopathy,

infection (particularly when present in the surgical field), thromboembolic disease, severe neurovascular impairment, and the inability to comprehend or cooperate with rehabilitation. Post-operative survival is difficult to predict; a retrospective study showed that functional ability, the number of bony metastases, the presence of visceral metastases, and the level of haemoglobin are the most useful prognostic indicators but these still only resulted in accuracy in 33% of cases (30).

Technical
Fractures due to metastases may fail to unite. There should be secure fixation above and below the lesion; it is important to obtain images of the whole length of the involved limb to ensure that all deposits will be spanned by the implant. The chosen device should be rigid and load-bearing. The bone-metalwork interface must be secure; this necessitates securing the implant to the bone either employing the inherent qualities of the implant (such as locking screws with an intramedullary nail) or with cement. The aim is to achieve a rapid mobilisation; in the lower limb this means the capacity to withstand full weight-bearing immediately after the operation. Intramedullary nails most readily achieve these objectives; open plating can create more problems with the management of the bone defect and necessitates a greater exposure and extensive soft tissue stripping all of which hamper rehabilitation and increase the risk of impaired wound healing. Improvements in nail design with more options in introduction and locking have rendered open plate and screw fixation almost obsolete in this field.

Femoral Metastases (31)
The femur is the long bone most frequently involved. The majority of metastases occur proximally and most will cause pain on weight. Avulsion of the lesser trochanter as seen on plain x-rays is a stark warning of impending fracture.

Lesions confined to the femoral head and neck are usually treated with a cemented total hip replacement, with close attention being paid to lesions in the pelvis that may dictate the choice of the acetabular component. Peri-trochanteric lesions and metastases in the femoral shaft are generally treated with intramedullary nails. Nailing has largely supplanted the older techniques of curettage (packing of the defect with methyl methacrylate cement or bone graft) and plate fixation. The surgical approach required by conventional plating imposes slow rehabilitation and is associated with a high risk of failure due to poor healing and the inability of the implant to sustain the high forces demanded for long periods. Procedures using intramedullary devices, such as standard intramedullary nails, retrograde nails, and cephalomedullary nails are less invasive and are familiar to most trauma surgeons.

Cephalomedullary nails enable the femoral head to be secured to the whole length of the shaft thus bridging the whole length of the bone (Fig. 7). Commonly used examples are the long Gamma and Recon nails and are increasingly used in the place of the spiral blade devices (32).

Intramedullary nails should cover the whole length of the femur and should be locked proximally and distally to prevent axial rotation and shortening both of which can become an increasing problem if the tumour enlarges and causes further loss of bone integrity. Intramedullary nails can be reamed or unreamed; reamed nails are usually of larger diameter and although hollow generally have a greater load bearing capacity than unreamed nails. Reaming enlarges the medullary cavity with successive drills of increasing diameter to accommodate the nail. The reaming process adds time to the operation and causes high transient intramedullary pressures that result in a small but significant incidence of thromboembolism and fat embolism. Contrary to popular belief, studies that compare reamed with unreamed femoral nails in

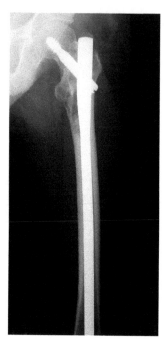

FIGURE 7   This x-ray image demonstrates a third-generation intramedullary femoral nail with a screw providing added neck fixation (the "Gamma" nail). The entry point is in the greater trochanter. In addition to the proximal screw in the femoral neck, there are distal locking screws (not seen in this view) which provide rotational stability. This nail occupies the whole length of the femur and thus allows for further bone weakening from a future tumour growth or subsequent fracture. Furthermore, as it acts as an internal splint, immediate weight-bearing is possible.

metastatic disease have not shown a significantly higher incidence of embolism in the reamed group (33). Due to their greater strength most surgeons choose a reamed nail unless it is important to keep the surgical time to a minimum.

It is known that reaming causes seeding of tumour cells throughout the medullary cavity (34,35) and theoretically may embolise tumour cells into systemic circulation. For this reason if there is any doubt about the diagnosis, a full tumour work-up including biopsy is indicated before nailing is performed. The radiotherapy that follows nail insertion must include the whole length of the bone.

Significant bone loss can be managed by filling the defect around the nail with PMMA cement. The cement, bone, and nail create a solid construct that should permit immediate weight-bearing (36). Smaller degrees of bone loss cause less structural impairment and can be treated with radiotherapy alone. Currently, bone grafting does not have a role.

In advanced disease an intramedullary nail may be insufficient to address widespread and severe bone loss, and excision of a segment of femur and implantation of a tumour prosthesis may be required. These are typically very large prostheses that necessitate an extensive tissue dissection, these so-called "mega prostheses" may need to be custom-made and are currently the realm of more specialised tumour and arthroplasty surgeons (Fig. 8). Due to the soft tissue disruption, function after the insertion of these prostheses is rarely as good as with an intramedullary nail. In exceptional circumstances amputation may be the only option; while this can reduce pain, rehabilitation is protracted.

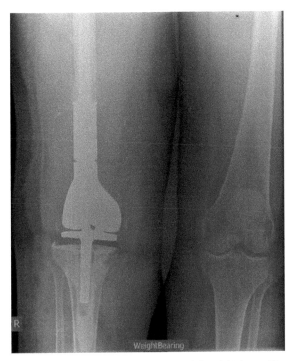

FIGURE 8 This x-ray image shows a mega-prosthesis of the right knee. The whole of the distal femur has been replaced with a metal prosthesis which is cemented into intact bone. With acknowledgements to Mike Hanlon, Consultant Orthopaedic Tumour Surgeon, Auckland City Hospital.

Humeral Fractures (37)

The humerus is the second most common site for breast metastases in the appendicular skeleton. Both diagnosis and management can be challenging and the clinician should be sure that they are treating a breast metastasis before embarking on surgery, and biopsy should be performed if doubt exists (38). Deposits greater than 2.5–3 cm in diameter with 50% destruction or more of the cortex and ongoing functional pain after radiotherapy should benefit from fixation.

The proximal third of the humerus is most frequently involved. Lesions in this area, if relatively small, are treated with curettage and packing with methyl methacrylate cement, larger metastases may require hemiarthroplasty. Surgery around the shoulder can be challenging due to the risk of neurovascular injury and difficulty in balancing soft tissues if extensive excision is required. Shoulder hemiarthroplasty, regardless of the indication, is dependent on sound reconstruction of the rotator cuff and prolonged rehabilitation. Even with several months of physiotherapy the functional results can be disappointing; as a result, shoulder replacement is rarely performed in these patients.

For diaphyseal lesions at or below the insertion of deltoid, the surgical options are of intramedullary nailing or plate fixation. Intramedullary devices include antegrade nails, retrograde nails, Enders nails, or Rush rods. Intramedullary nailing generally requires only limited surgical exposure, is relatively quick, and provides immediate stabilisation (Fig. 9). The choice of antegrade or retrograde insertion is determined by the location of the lesion and the preference of the surgeon, but both methods have drawbacks. Antegrade insertion can disrupt the rotator cuff, thus impairing shoulder function and retrograde insertion can increase the risk of supracondylar fractures.

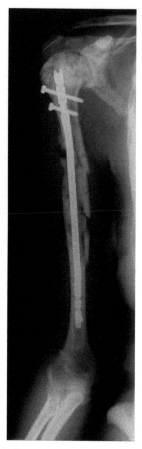

FIGURE 9   This x-ray image is of a humerus with extensive metastatic disease which has been treated with a reamed intramedullary humeral nail. This is an antegrade nail with the entry point in the proximal humerus. Proximal and distal locking screws have been used to provide rotational stability—the distal screws are seen "end-on" in this image. There is a fracture which has occurred intraoperatively at the mid-shaft, a risk when reaming bone is weakened by tumour deposit.

Occasionally, the site and size of a lesion may dictate the use of flexible intramedullary devices. In these situations, Enders nails or Rush rods may be inserted into the lesion and passed proximally and then pushed distally to span the lesion. For this more than one nail is required and cement augmentation may be necessary. Enders nails and Rush rods are more likely to be used for large, distal lesions. Their insertion can be challenging, the hold on the bone is less secure than with conventional nails, and there is a significant risk that the device will migrate post-operatively; as a result they are now rarely used.

The disadvantages of plate fixation of the humerus are similar to those of the femur. A large exposure is required, the soft tissue disruption can be extensive, and the risks of neurovascular injury are high. Healing and rehabilitation can be problematic and failure of the implant or the bone is more likely than with intramedullary devices. Despite these drawbacks lesions in the distal humerus (within 12 cm of the elbow joint) are usually treated with plates as the proximity of the elbow and the geometry of the intramedullary canal preclude adequate hold with a nail. A triceps splitting approach is required and PMMA cement augmentation is often required. More extensive bone destruction may demand a custom-made elbow prosthesis.

In circumstances where the amount of diaphyseal bone destruction precludes fixation but long-term survival of the patient is anticipated a salvage procedure using a modular segmental prosthesis may be used. Similarly, a custom-made shoulder or elbow prosthesis may be required for extensive proximal or distal lesions. Such situations are uncommon and when encountered require the expertise of a surgeon specialising in tumour surgery.

In general, rigid intramedullary fixation of diaphyseal lesions will result in good pain control and early restoration of function. The outcome of treatment of proximal and distal humeral lesions is less predictable.

CONCLUSION

The relief of pain and the restoration of function imparted by orthopaedic surgery, particularly through the stabilization of the long bones of the lower limbs, can be life-altering. Much benefit can also be gained by the surgical treatment of peri-articular metastases, particularly at the hip, elbow, and shoulder, and in cases of extensive bone loss.

It is recommended that a member of the orthopaedic or trauma service be designated to manage the relatively common appendicular metastases and that a specialist orthopaedic oncology team is identified to address the more demanding cases that can require "mega" or custom-made prosthesis (28). The 1997 Working Party (28) advised liaison between breast surgeons, oncologists, radiologists, and orthopaedic surgeons with combined clinics if justified by the workload.

The average life-expectancy of patients with breast cancer presenting with bone-only metastases has improved from 24 to 36 months; 20% of these patients will be alive at 5 years. As the medical management of metastatic breast cancer improves and screening programmes identify patients at an earlier stage of their disease, less invasive orthopaedic surgery will be needed and fewer patients will suffer the pain and disability of skeletal failure.

REFERENCES

1. O'Donaghue DS, Howell A, Walls J. Orthopaedic management of structurally significant bone destruction in breast cancer bone metastases. J Bone Joint Surg Br 1997; 79-B: 98–9.
2. Ali SM, Harvey HA, Lipton A. Medical management of bone metastases. Clin Ortho 2003; 415S: S132–7.
3. Pavlakis N, Schmidt R, Stockler M. Bisphosphonates for breast cancer. Cochrane Database Syst Rev 2005; (3): CD003474
4. Coleman R. The use of bisphosphonates in cancer treatment. Ann NY Acad Sci 2011; 1218: 3–14. doi:10.111/j.1749-6632.201005766
5. Coleman RE, Rubens RD. The clinical course of bone metastases from breast cancer. Br J Cancer 1987; 55: 61–6.
6. Hage W, Aboulafia A, Aboulafia D. Incidence, location, and diagnostic evaluation of metastatic bone disease. Orthop Clin North Am 2000; 31: 515–28.
7. Coleman RE. Metastatic bone disease: clinical features, pathophysiology and treatment strategies. Cancer Treat Rev 2001; 27: 165–76.
8. Rougraff BT, Frassica FJ. Presentation and staging of metastatic bone disease. Clin Orthop 2003; 415S: S129–31.
9. Fidler M. Prophylactic internal fixation of secondary neoplastic deposits in long bones. Br Med J. 1973; 1: 341–3.
10. Wetzel FT, Phillips FM. Management of metastatic disease of the spine. Orthop Clin North Am 2000; 31: 611–21.
11. Denis F. The three-column spine and its significance in the classification of acute thoracolumbar spinal injuries. Spine 1983; 8: 817–31.

12. Aaron AD. Treatment of metastatic adenocarcinoma of the pelvis and the extremeties. J Bone Joint Surg Am 1997; 79-A: 917–32.
13. Harrington KD. Metastatic disease of the spine. J Bone Joint Surg Am 1986; 68: 1110.
14. Patchell RA, Tibbs PA, Regine WF, et al. Direct decompressive surgical resection in the treatment of spinal cord compression caused by metastatic cancer: a randomised trial. Lancet 2005; 366: 643–8.
15. Simmons ED, Zheng Y. Vertebral tumours: surgical vs. nonsurgical treatment. Clin Orthop Relat Res 2006; 443: 233–47.
16. Biermann JS, Holt GE, Lewis VO, Schwartz HS, Yaszemski MJ. Metastatic bone disease: diagnosis, evaluation, and treatment. J Bone Joint Surg Am 2009; 91: 1518–30.
17. Walker M, Yaszemski MJ, Kim CW, et al. Metastatic disease of the spine: evaluation and treatment. Clin Orthop 2003; 415S: S165–75.
18. Binning MJ, Gottfried ON, Klimo P, Schmidt MH. Minimally invasive treatments for metastatic tumours of the spine. Neurosurg Clin N Am 2004; 15: 459–65.
19. Dalberyrak S, Onen MR, Yilmaz M, Naderi S. Clinical and radiographic results of balloon kyphoplasty for treatment of vertebral metastases and multiple myelomas. J Clin Neurosci 2010; 17: 219–24.
20. Mendel E, Bourekas E, Gerszten P, Golan D. Percutaneous techniques in the treatement of spine tumours: what are the diagnostic and therapeutic indications and outcomes? Spine 2009; 34(22 Suppl): S93–100.
21. Patterson FR, Peabody TD. Operative management of metastases to the pelvis and acetabulum. Orthop Clin North Am 2000; 31: 623–31.
22. Enneking W. Local resection of malignant lesions of the hip and pelvis. J Bone Joint Surg Am 1966; 48: 991–1007.
23. Delloye C, Banse X, Brichard B, Docquier P. Cornu :pelvic reconstruction with a structural pelvic allograft after resection of a malignant bone tumour. J Bone Joint Surg Am 2007; 89: 579–87.
24. O'Donaghue DS, Howell A, Bundred NJ, Walls J. Implications of fracture in breast cancer bone metastases. J Bone Joint Surg Br 1997; 79-B: 97–8.
25. Ward WG, Holsenbeck S, Dorey FJ, Spang J, Howe D. Metastatic disease of the femur: surgical treatment. Clin Orthop Relat Res 2003; 415(Suppl): S230–44.
26. Mirels H. Metastatic disease in long bones: A proposed scoring system for diagnosing impending pathologic fractures. Clin Orthop 1989; 249: 258.
27. Rougraff B. Indications for operative treatment. Orthop Clin North Am 2000; 31: 567–75.
28. Tillman RM. The role of the orthopaedic surgeon in metastatic disease of the appendicular skeleton. J Bone Joint Surg Br 1999; 81-B: 1–4.
29. Bibbo C, Patel D, Benevenia J. Perioperative considerations in patients with metastatic bone disease. Orthop Clin North Am 2000; 31: 577–93.
30. Nathan S, Healey J, Mellano D, et al. Survival in patients operated on for pathologic fracture: Implications for end-of-life orthopaedic care. J Clin Oncol 2005; 23: 6072–82.
31. Ward WG, Spang J, Howe D. Metastatic disease of the femur. Orthop Clin North Am 2000; 31: 633–45.
32. Gibbons CE, Pope SJ, Murphy JP, Hall AJ. Femoral metastatic fractures treated with intramedullary nailing. Int Orthop 2000; 24: 101–3.
33. Cole AS, Hill GA, Theologis TN, et al. Femoral nailing for metastatic disease of the femur: a comparison of reamed and unreamed femoral nailing. Injury 2000; 31: 25–31.
34. Awan N, Azer A, Harrani K, Cogley D. Intramedullary spread of tumour cells during IM nailing: a histological diagnosis. Eur J Orthop Surg Trauma 2002; 12: 53–5.
35. Roth SE, Rebello MM, Kreder H, Whyne CM. Pressurization of the metastatic femur during prophylactic intramedullary nail fixation. J Trauma 2004; 57: 333–9.
36. Bickels J, Dadia S, Lidar Z. Surgical management of metastatic bone disease. J Bone Joint Surg Am 2009; 91: 1503–16.
37. Bashore CJ, Temple HT. Management of metastatic lesions of the humerus. Orthop Clin North Am 2000; 31: 597–609.
38. Beauchamp CP. Errors and pitfalls in the diagnosis and treatment of metastatic bone disease. Orthop Clin North Am 2000; 31: 675–85.

16

Thermal ablation of hepatic metastases

Andy Adam

INTRODUCTION

Two-thirds of women with metastatic breast cancer eventually have disease involving the liver, which is the third most common site of metastases from carcinoma of the breast after the bone and lung. A few patients with metastatic breast cancer have isolated hepatic metastases (12–16%). A larger group of patients have stable bone metastases and hepatic metastases. There is a trend towards a more aggressive treatment for this patient group.

The best-established method of local treatment of hepatic metastases is surgical resection. The most extensive experience with this type of surgery is in patients with colorectal metastases. Approximately 25% of patients with liver metastases from colorectal cancer have no other site of metastasis and can be treated with regional therapies directed towards their liver tumours. Hepatic resection results in survival rates ranging from 55 to 80% at 1 year and 25–50% at 5 years (1). However, because of advanced disease, unfavourable location of the metastases, or poor physical condition, less than 20% of patients are eligible for hepatic resection (2–7). In general, only patients with fewer than four or five metastases, limited to one lobe and with no evidence of extrahepatic disease, are eligible for surgery. Without resection, patients with hepatic metastases from colorectal carcinoma have a medium survival of less than 1 year (8–10).

Hepatic resection is less well established in patients with carcinoma of the breast. Many surgeons have been reluctant to operate in such patients because of the high risk of undetected extrahepatic disease. However, some patients with apparently isolated hepatic metastases have been operated on with good results. Yoshimoto et al. conducted a study on 25 patients with breast cancer treated with hepatic resection (11). Fourteen had solitary lesions and 11 had multiple metastases. Eight patients had extrahepatic disease. All of the metastases were resected and all but one patient also received chemotherapy. After the hepatectomy, recurrent tumours were detected in 18 of the patients, being located in the liver in 12 (67%) of them. Overall, however, hepatectomy ensured that the liver was clinically recurrence-free for a median of 24 months (range 2–132 months). The 2- and 5-year cumulative survival rates after hepatectomy were 71% and 27%, respectively, and the median survival duration was 34.3 ± 3.2 months, much better than the period of 8.5 months for another series of patients treated with standard or non-surgical therapies at the author's institution. The number and the size of hepatic metastases, the interval between treatment of the primary lesion and hepatectomy, and the existence of extrahepatic metastases were not adverse prognostic factors. In another study, Pocard et al. examined 65 patients with breast cancer liver metastases (12). The selection criteria for surgery were normal performance status and liver function tests; radiological objective response to chemotherapy and/or hormone therapy; in cases of non-isolated hepatic metastases, patients were included if there had been complete response of the associated metastatic site (usually bone) and no brain metastases. The median follow-up was 41 months (6–100 months). The survival rate after surgery was 90% at 1 year, 71% at 3 and 46% at 4 years. Thirteen patients were alive at 4 years. The recurrence rate in the liver remnant at 36 months differed according to the lymph node status of the initial breast cancer: 40% for N0-N1 versus 81% for N1b-N2 (p = 0.01) and according to the type of liver resection: 45% for minor liver resection versus 73% for major (p = 0.02). These and other similar studies, although limited and highly selective, suggest that surgical treatment of hepatic metastases from breast cancer may be beneficial in certain subgroups of patients. Whether surgery prolongs survival in the setting of metastatic disease is not conclusively proven. There are no randomised trials showing that resection of any metastatic site prolongs survival compared with systemic treatment alone. Moreover, it is unlikely that such data will be forthcoming, as the number of eligible patients is small, and accrual of patients into surgery versus no surgery trials is extremely difficult.

At least three observational studies directly comparing outcomes of surgically treated patients with pulmonary or hepatic metastases with those receiving chemotherapy alone suggest a significant survival advantage for surgery (13–15).

Minimally invasive techniques for local ablation of hepatic metastases may provide reasonable alternatives for patients who are not candidates for surgery. Such techniques include cryotherapy and thermal ablation with microwaves or radiofrequency (RF). This chapter focuses mainly on radiofrequency ablation, the most widely used method of percutaneous local therapy.

RF ABLATION

RF radiation produces local heat in tissues. Needle-like electrodes are placed percutaneously directly into the tumour, with the guidance of ultrasound (US), computed tomography (CT), or magnetic resonance imaging (MRI). The third modality offers the possibility of monitoring with MR thermometry; however, this has not shown to be clinically useful. MRI guidance is cumbersome and expensive and is used rarely. US guidance is inexpensive and widely available. However, many interventional radiologists prefer CT guidance because of its greater accuracy.

The RF electrode typically is comprised of a metal shaft, which is insulated except for an exposed conductive tip that is in direct electrical contact with the targeted tissue volume. The RF generator supplies RF power to the tissue through the electrode. It is connected both to the shaft(s) of the RF electrode and to the reference electrode, usually a large conductive pad in contact with the patient's skin in an area of relatively good electrical thermal conductivity (such as the thigh). The RF generator produces RF voltage between the active electrode and the reference electrode, thereby establishing lines of electric field within the patient's body between the two electrodes. At the low RFs used for this procedure (less than 1 MHz), the electric field pattern is governed essentially by electrostatic equations. The electric field oscillates with the alternating RF current, which causes oscillatory movement of ions in the tissue in proportion to the field intensity. The mechanism of tissue heating for RF ablation is frictional, or resistive, energy loss caused by the motion of the ionic current (16,17). All RF generators are operated at 460 kHz at a power setting of 50–200 W.

There are several different types of RF generators and electrodes on the market, employing different methods of producing an area of coagulation sufficiently large to destroy the tumour being treated. Some electrodes are shaped like a straight needle, whereas others are shaped like an umbrella. The choice largely depends on operator preference.

Patient Selection and Procedural Technique

Initially, most investigators were limiting treatment with RF ablation to patients with four or fewer and 5 cm or smaller, primary or secondary malignant hepatic tumours, with no evidence of extrahepatic disease. However, more recently, patients with a small number of pulmonary metastases or with stable bone metastases are increasingly being offered treatment; as such metastases do not usually have a significant impact on survival. Ideal tumours are smaller than 3 cm in diameter, completely surrounded by hepatic parenchyma, 1 cm or more deep to the liver capsule, and 2 cm or more away from large hepatic or portal veins. Subcapsular liver tumours can be ablated, but their treatment is usually associated with greater procedural and post-procedural pain. Tumours adjacent to large blood vessels are more difficult to ablate completely because the blood flow in the vessels causes loss of heat, thus limiting the extent of the ablation (Fig. 1). Ablation of tumours adjacent to the large portal triads causes increased pain and poses the risk of damage to the associated bile duct. Contraindications to treatment include sepsis, severe debilitation, and uncorrectable coagulopathies.

Percutaneous RF ablation is often carried out with the use of conscious sedation alone although some investigators routinely employ general anaesthesia. The procedure can be performed on an outpatient basis, but most interventional radiologists prefer to keep the patients in hospital overnight, partly in order to treat any discomfort and partly because of the small risk of haemorrhage accompanying the procedure.

The goal of RF thermal ablation is to destroy the tumour as well as a 5–10 mm-circumferential cuff of adjacent normal hepatic parenchyma. Each ablation requires an exact placement of the electrode tip in the tumour. A single ablation treatment raises local tissue temperatures to 60–100°C and produces a spherical thermal injury approximately 3–5 cm in diameter (Fig. 2). If the procedure is performed

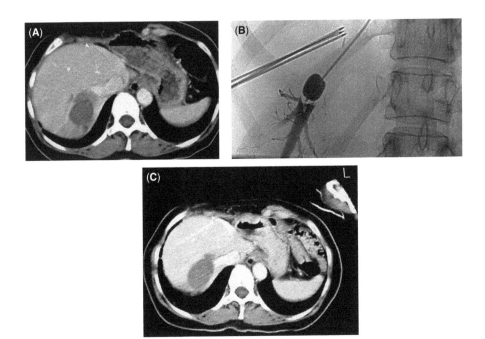

FIGURE 1 (**A**) Residual tumour adjacent to the right hepatic vein. The fast-flowing blood carried away some of the heat and thus prevented complete coagulation. (**B**) The procedure was repeated after occluding the vein with an occlusion balloon inserted via the right internal jugular vein. (**C**) Successful coagulation of the residual disease.

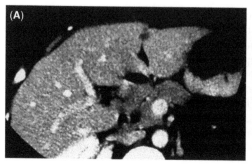
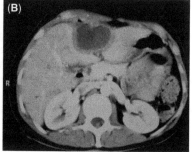

FIGURE 2 (A) CT shows a small metastasis from carcinoma of the breast, at the junction of the lateral segments and the quadrate lobe of the liver. (B) Large area of coagulation following treatment with radiofrequency. Coagulated areas are of lower attenuation than viable tumour or normal liver.

under US guidance, the size of each ablation is delineated sonographically by echogenic microbubbles that are produced during the ablation.

Tumours smaller than 3 cm in diameter can be treated with one or two ablations. Tumours greater than 3 cm require several overlapping ablations. Each ablation usually lasts 12–15 minutes and two or three ablations can be carried out during the same session.

Major complications are unusual. The main ones are intraperitoneal haemorrhage, liver abscess, and seeding along the tumour tract. There is often some pain after the procedure, but this usually settles within 24 hours. Approximately 10–20% of patients have a 1–3°C rise in temperature, as a response to tumour necrosis; this mild pyrexia usually begins the day after the procedure and can last up to a week. However, prolonged, marked pyrexia should always raise the suspicion of infection and merits further investigation.

Assessment of Treatment Effectiveness

CT and US cannot demonstrate the result of the procedure at the time of treatment. MR has the potential of measuring temperature and providing "online" monitoring, but this capability is limited by several other practical considerations, including the difficulty of using RF in an MR machine.

In practice, patients are followed up with contrast-enhanced CT or MR carried out the day after the procedure or later. Remaining viable tumours appear as an enhancing area, which can be targeted at a subsequent session of treatment.

Patient Outcomes

Most studies have focused on patients with colorectal metastases, although some have included a mixture of tumours, including metastases from carcinoma of the breast. The results of several clinical series, which have used different methods of RF ablation (18–23) appear promising, with a 52–67% complete ablation rate at 1 year and survival rates of 96%, 64%, and 40% at 1, 3, and 5 years respectively. Approximately 39% of lesions develop local recurrence following treatment (23). The frequency and time to local recurrence are related to the size of the lesion. In a recent series of 117 patients, survival was not found to be influenced by the number of metastases at the time of initial therapy (23). This is contrary to the results of some surgical series which reported (24–26) that tumour recurrence and/or survival following surgical treatment was negatively influence by the number of metastases removed. However, authors of larger and/or more recent reports (27–40) have failed to confirm this correlation and have suggested that—in the range of the analyses (generally one to eight metastases removed)—survival following surgical resection is not correlated with the number of metastases removed. These findings suggest that the decision to treat should be guided more by the likelihood of achieving tumour control than the number of lesions present.

RF ablation was used by Livraghi et al. to treat 24 patients with 64 hepatic metastases from carcinoma of the breast (37). The treatment was carried out with 17-gauge, internally cooled electrodes, with the patient under conscious sedation and analgesia or general anaesthesia. A single lesion was treated in 16 patients, and multiple lesions were treated in eight patients. Follow-up with serial CT ranged from 4 to 44 months (mean, 10 months; median, 19 months). Complete necrosis was achieved in 59 (92%) of 64 lesions. Among the 59 lesions, complete necrosis required a single-treatment session in 58 lesions (92%) and two-treatment sessions in one lesion (2%). In 14 (58%) of 24 patients, new metastases developed during follow-up. Ten (71%) of these 14 patients developed new liver metastases. Ten (63%) of 16 patients whose lesions were initially confined to the liver were free of disease at the time of publication of this study. One patient died of progressive brain metastases. No major complications occurred. The authors concluded that RF ablation appears to be a simple, safe, and effective treatment for focal liver metastases in selected patients with breast cancer.

Some surgeons have advocated delaying resection of liver metastases to allow additional metastases, which may be present but undetected, to be identified. This "test-of-time" approach can limit the number of resections performed on patients who ultimately will develop additional metastases. Livraghi et al. evaluated the potential role and possible advantages of performing RF ablation during the interval between diagnosis and hepatic resection as part of a "test-of-time management approach" (38). They treated 88 consecutive patients who were potential candidates for surgery and who had 134 colorectal carcinoma liver metastases. Complete necrosis was obtained in 53 of 88 patients (60%) and in 85 of 134 lesions (63%). During a follow-up of these 53 patients, 16 (30%) remained free of disease and 37 (70%) developed new metastases. New lesions were intrahepatic in 26 of 37 patients (70%), extrahepatic in 4 patients (11%), and both intrahepatic and extrahepatic in 7 patients (19%). Of the 26 patients whose new lesions were intrahepatic only, 15 (58%) were re-treated with RF and 7 were free of disease at the time of last follow-up (median follow-up, 28 months). Ten additional patients with only intrahepatic new lesions were deemed untreatable and one patient underwent resection. Overall, among the 53 patients in whom complete tumour necrosis was achieved after RF ablation therapy, 52 (98%) were spared from surgical resection: 23 (44%) because they have remained free of disease and 29 (56%) because they developed disease progression. Among all 88 patients, 21 (24%) underwent resection after RF ablation (8 were free of disease at the time of last follow-up), 23 (26%) remained free of disease after successful RF ablation, and 56 (64%) developed untreatable disease progression (44 after RF alone, 12 after RF and surgery). Lesions in 35 of 88 patients (40%) demonstrated local tumour recurrence on follow-up imaging studies. Twenty of these 35 patients (57%) underwent surgical resection, whereas the remaining 15 patients (43%) developed additional, untreatable metastases. Of the 15 patients, new lesions were intrahepatic in 9 (60%), extrahepatic in 1 (7%), and both intrahepatic and extrahepatic in 5 (33%). No patient who had been treated with RF ablation became unresectable due to the growth of metastases and there was no evidence of needle track seeding in any patient after RF ablation. Overall, among the 35 patients in whom complete tumour necrosis was not achieved after RF ablation therapy, 15 (43%) were spared from surgical resection. This important study suggests that current RF ablation techniques, when used as part of a test-of-time management approach, can decrease the number of resections performed. The approach used by these authors provides an interval for others who ultimately will develop new intrahepatic and/or extrahepatic metastases to do so. Surgery may be offered in combination with systemic therapy to those patients with breast cancer who have macroscopically resectable hepatic metastases. However, when compared with surgical resection, RF ablation is less invasive, less expensive, and has fewer contraindications. Moreover, since many patients will develop liver metastases after surgery, the test-of-time approach described above could be used in patients with breast cancer liver metastases. This approach will help avoid unnecessary surgery in patients who develop new metastases.

Meloni et al. (41) used RF ablation to treat 87 breast cancer liver metastases (mean diameter, 2.5 cm) in 52 female patients (median age, 55 years). Inclusion criteria were as follows: fewer than five tumours, maximum tumour diameter of 5 cm or smaller, and disease either confined to the liver or stable with medical therapy. Of the 50 patients 45 had (90%) previously had chemotherapy, hormonal therapy, or both, and had no response or an incomplete response to the treatment. Complete tumour necrosis was achieved in 97% of tumours. Median time to follow-up from the diagnosis of liver metastasis and from RF ablation was 37.2 and 19.1 months, respectively. Local tumour progression occurred in 25% of the patients. New intrahepatic metastases developed in 53% of them. From the time of first RF ablation, overall median survival time and 5-year survival rate were 29.9 months and 27%, respectively. From the time the first liver metastasis was diagnosed, overall median survival time was 42 months and the 5-year survival rate was 32%. Patients with tumours 2.5 cm in diameter or larger had a worse prognosis than those with tumours smaller than 2.5 cm in diameter. The above survival rates in selected patients with breast cancer liver metastases treated with RF ablation are comparable with those reported in the literature, which were achieved with surgery.

Other ablative therapies have been used to treat breast cancer liver metastases. To date, the largest study on the use of ablative therapies to treat breast cancer metastases was preformed by Mack et al. (42), who treated 578 liver metastases from breast cancer in 232 female patients with MR-guided laser thermotherapy. The exclusion criteria were the same as those adopted in this study. Mack et al. achieved 3- and 5-year survival rates of 66% and 38%, respectively, from the time of treatment, with 1.5% of patients experiencing clinically relevant complications. In the subset of patients eligible for surgery, Mack et al. reported a median survival time of 3.7 years from the diagnosis of the MR-guided laser thermotherapy–treated metastasis. MR-guided ablative therapy is more expensive than other techniques. RF ablation is generally performed with CT and/or US guidance, both of which are more readily accessible than open interventional MR imagers and do not require non-ferromagnetic ablation devices.

Microwave ablation has also been used to treat breast cancer liver metastases. Abe et al. (43) assessed the feasibility and efficacy of using MR-guided microwave thermocoagulation therapy in eight patients with liver metastasis from breast cancer, including patients with a maximum of five liver metastases smaller than 3 cm in diameter. Half of the patients had bone metastases, lung metastases, or both at enrollment. At the end of the study, after a mean observation period of 25.9 months, five (62%) of the eight patients were alive, and all of them had new metastases. No procedure-related deaths or major complications were encountered. While Abe et al. found that MR-guided microwave ablation appeared to be a safe and feasible method for use in these patients, more experience is needed.

CONCLUSIONS

When attempting to evaluate the benefits of percutaneous radiofrequency ablation for hepatic metastases, the following questions must be asked:

1. Is it safe?
2. Can it reliably ablate liver metastases?
3. Can it improve survival?

Interpreting the results of ablation is more difficult than assessing the outcome of hepatic resection. RF treatment can ablate metastases in 50–90% of cases and is much safer than hepatic resection. With respect to overall survival, there has been no randomised comparison to show that radiofrequency treatment alters long-term survival compared with chemotherapy alone. However, this may be related to the fact that most patients being referred for ablative treatment are considered unsuitable for hepatic resection and have more extensive disease that can be difficult to eradicate. The ideal patient for ablative therapy would be one who, several years after resection of the primary neoplasm for an early-stage well-differentiated cancer develops a small metastasis in the middle of a lobe of the liver. Such a patient is, however, also ideally suited to surgical treatment and for such a patient the long-term results of surgery are good. Interventional therapy tends to be used in patients who are otherwise considered to be beyond the scope of conventional surgical treatment. It is possible that ablative therapy would achieve similar results to surgery if only similar patients were referred for this method of treatment.

In view of the rarity of use of hepatic resection in patients with hepatic metastases from carcinoma of the breast, it is unlikely that a randomised comparison with radiofrequency ablation will ever be carried out. It seems appropriate to employ thermal ablation in patients with a small number of hepatic metastases. A study comparing chemotherapy alone with radiofrequency treatment plus chemotherapy in patients with more extensive disease would require careful planning; however, such a study would help to define the role of thermal ablation in this large group of patients.

REFERENCES

1. Nagorney DM, van Heerden JA, Ilstrup DM, Adson MA. Primary hepatic malignancy: surgical management and determinants of survival. Surgery 1989; 106: 740–9.
2. Adson MA, VanHeerden JA, Adson MH, Wayner JS, Ilstrup DM. Resection of hepatic metastases from colorectal cancer. Arch Surg 1984; 119: 647–51.
3. Foster JH. Survival after liver resection for secondary tumors. Am J Surg 1978; 135: 390–94.
4. Cobourn CS, Makowka L, Langer B, Taylor BR, Falk RE. Examination of patient selection and outcome for hepatic resection for metastatic disease. Surg Gynecol Obstet 1987; 165: 239–46.
5. Nordlinger B, Parc R, Delva E, et al. Hepatic resection for colorectal liver metastases. Ann Surg 1987; 205: 256–63.
6. Steele G, Bleday R, Mayer RJ, et al. A prospective evaluation of hepatic resection for colorectal carcinoma metastases to the liver: gastrointestinal tumour study group protocol 6584. J Clin Oncol 1991; 9: 1105–12.
7. Fong Y, Blumgart LH, Cohen AM. Surgical treatment of colorectal metastases to the liver. CA Cancer J Clin 1995; 45: 50–62.
8. Baden H, Andersen B. Survival of patients with untreated liver metastases from colorectal cancer. Scand J Gastroenterol 1975; 10: 221–3.
9. Wood CB, Gillis CR, Blumgart LH. A retrospective study of the natural history of patients with liver metastases from colorectal cancer. Clin Oncol 1976; 2: 285–8.
10. Bengtsson G, Carisson G, Hafstrom L, Jonsson PE. Natural history of patients with untreated liver metastases from colorectal cancer. Am J Surg 1981; 141: 586–9.

11. Yoshimoto M, Tada T, Saito M, et al. Surgical treatment of hepatic metastases from breast cancer. Breast Cancer Res Treat 2000; 59: 177–84.
12. Pocard M, Pouillart P, Asselain B, Falcou MC, Salmon RJ. Liver resections from breast cancer metastasis: results and prognosis factors after hepatic resection in 65 cases. Ann Chir 2001; 126: 413–20.
13. Staren ED, Salerno C, Rongione A, Witt TR, Faber LP. Pulmonary resection for metastatic breast cancer. Arch Surg 1992; 127: 1282–4.
14. Murabito M, Salat A, Mueller MR. Complete resection of isolated lung metastasis from breast carcinoma results in a strong increase in survival. Minerva Chir 2000; 55: 121–7.
15. Schneebaum S, Walker MJ, Young D, Farrar WB, Minton JP. The regional treatment of liver metastases from breast cancer. J Surg Oncol 1994; 55: 26–31.
16. Cosman ER, Naswhold BS, Ovelman-Levitt J. Theoretical aspects of radiofrequency lesions in the dorsal root entry zone. Neurosurgery 1984; 15: 945–50.
17. Organ LW. Eelctrophysiologic principles of radiofrequency lesion making. Appl Neuro-physiol 1976; 39: 69–76.
18. Solbiati L, Lerace T, Goldberg SN, et al. Percutaneous US-guided radiofrequency tissue ablation of liver metastases: treatment and follow-up in 16 patients. Radiology 1997; 202: 195–203.
19. Livraghi T, Goldberg SN, Monti F, et al. Saline-enhanced radiofrequency tissue ablation in the treatment of liver metastases. Radiology 1997; 202: 205–10.
20. Rossi S, Stasi MD, Buscarini E, et al. Percutaneous RF interstitial thermal ablation in the treatment of hepatic cancer. AJR Am J Roentgenol 1996; 167: 759–68.
21. Rossi S, Buscarini E, Garbangnati F, et al. Percutaneous treatment of small hepatic tumors by an expandable RF needle electrode. AJR Am J Roentgenol 1998; 170: 1015–22.
22. Solbiati L, Goldberg SN, Ierace T, et al. Hepatic metastases: percutaneous radiofrequency ablation with cooled-tip electrodes. Radiology 1997; 205: 367–73.
23. Solbiati L, Livraghi MD, Goldberg N, et al. Percutaneous radiofrequency ablation of hepatic metastases from colorectal cancer: long-term results in 117 patients. Radiology 2001; 221: 159–66.
24. Cady B, NMonson DO, Swinton NW. Survival of patients after colonic resection for carcinoma with simultaneous liver metastases. Surg Gynecol Obstet 1970; 131: 697–700.
25. Ekberg H, Tranberg KG, Andersson R, et al. Pattern of recurrence in liver resection for colorectal secondaries. World J Surg 1987; 11: 541–7.
26. Gayowski TJ, Iwatsuki S, Madariaga JR, et al. Experience in hepatic resection for metastatic colorectal cancer: analysis of clinical and pathologic risk factors. Surgery 1994; 116: 703–10.
27. Adson MA, van Heerden JA, Adson MH, Wayner JS, Ilstrup DM. Resection of hepatic metastases from colorectal cancer. Arch Surg 1984; 199: 647–51.
28. Butler J, Attiyek FF, Daly JM. Hepatic resection for metastases of the colon and rectum. Surg Gynecol Obstet 1986; 162: 109–13.
29. Fortner JG, Silva JS, Golbey RB, Cox EB, Maclean BJ. Multivariate analysis of a personal series of 247 consecutive patients with liver metastases from colorectal cancer. Ann Surg 1984; 199: 306–16.
30. Nordlinger B, Prc R, Delva E, et al. Hepatic resection for colorectal liver metastases. Ann Surg 1987; 205: 256–63.
31. Scheele J, Stangl R, Altendorf-Hofmann A, Gall FP. Indicators of prognosis after hepatic resection for colorectal secondaries. Surgery 1991; 110: 13–29.
32. Rosen CB, Nagorney DM, Taswell HF, et al. Perioperative blood transfusion and determinants of survival after liver resection for metastatic colorectal carcinoma. Ann Surg 1992; 216: 493–505.
33. Fon Y, Cohen AM, Fortner JG, et al. Liver resection for colorectal metastases. J Clin Oncol 1995; 15: 938–46.
34. Petrelli N, Gupta B, Piedmonte M, Herrera L. Morbidity and survival of liver resection for colorectal adenocarcinoma. Dis Col Rectum 1991; 34: 899–904.
35. Gillams AR, Lees WR. Five-year survival in 309 patients with colorectal liver metastases treated with radiofrequency ablation. Eur Radiol 2009; 19: 1206–13.
36. Sorensen SM, Mortensen FV, Nielsen DT. Radiofrequency ablation of colorectal liver metastases: long-term survival. Acta Radiol 2007; 48: 253–8.

37. Livraghi T, Goldberg N, Solbiati L, et al. Percutaneous radio-frequency ablation of liver metastases from breast cancer: initial experience in 24 patients. Radiology 2001; 220: 145–9.

38. Livraghi T, Solbiati L, Meloni F, et al. Percutaneous radiofrequency ablation of liver metastases in potential candidates for resection: the 'test-of-time' approach. Cancer 2003; 15: 3027–35.

39. Iwatsuki S, Esquivel C, Gordon RD, Starzl TE. Liver resection for metastatic colorectal cancer. Surgery 1986; 100: 804–10.

40. Hughes KS, Simon R, Songhorabodi S, et al. Resection of the liver for colorectal carcinoma metastases: a multi-institutional study of patterns of recurrence. Surgery 1986; 100: 278–84.

41. Meloni MF, Andreano A, Laeseke PF, et al. Breast cancer liver metastases: US-guided percutaneous radiofrequency ablation—intermediate and long-term survival rates. Radiology 2009; 253: 861–9.

42. Mack MG, Straub R, Eichler K, et al. Breast cancer metastases in liver: laser-induced interstitial thermotherapy—local tumor control rate and survival data. Radiology 2004; 233: 400–9.

43. Abe H, Kurumi Y, Naka S, et al. Open-configuration MR-guided microwave thermocoagulation therapy for metastatic liver tumors from breast cancer. Breast Cancer 2005; 12: 26–31.

17 Palliative care and metastatic breast cancer

Jayne Wood and Anna-Marie Stevens

"To cure sometimes
To relieve often
To comfort always".
(Anonymous, 15th Century A.D.)

INTRODUCTION

This chapter begins by discussing the role of palliative care, recent developments, and its application to treating patients with metastatic breast cancer. The chapter further discusses the management of common symptoms that such a patient might experience including pain, nausea and vomiting, constipation, and breathlessness. The chapter concludes with a discussion of management of the terminal phase and the future of palliative care in this setting.

THE ROLE OF PALLIATIVE CARE

The World Health Organisation (WHO) has defined palliative care as:

> ...an approach that improves the quality of life of patients and their families facing the problem associated with life-threatening illness, through the prevention and relief of suffering by means of early identification and impeccable assessment and treatment of pain and other problems, physical, psychosocial and spiritual (1)

Historically, the provision of palliative care has focused on improving the quality of life for patients in the terminal phase of their illness. However, recent developments in the field of palliative care supported by various national strategies have promoted the importance of ensuring that palliative care is available to patients at all stages of disease and not simply because active treatment is no longer available. The American Society for Clinical Oncology firmly endorses a holistic model of support for the patient during all phases of care (2). Figure 1 demonstrates a model of oncological care/palliative care as endorsed by the WHO (1). Table 1 (1) demonstrates the characteristics of palliative care as described by the WHO which can be as easily applied to those patients at the beginning of their treatment (which maybe with curative or palliative intent) as to those nearing the end of their treatment or indeed when further anti-cancer treatment is no longer available.

The provision of palliative care is grounded in a holistic approach in which physical symptoms are addressed as equally as those that are spiritual, psychological and social.

The World Health Organisation promotes this approach:

> ...management of pain and other symptoms and provision of psychological, social and spiritual support is paramount. The goal of palliative care is achievement of the best quality of life for patients and their families (1)

Indeed, the majority of palliative care is provided by the multidisciplinary team (MDT). To name but a few, the members of the Palliative Care MDT may include

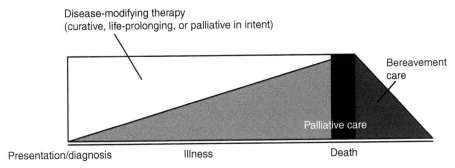

Disease-modifying therapy
(curative, life-prolonging, or palliative in intent)

Bereavement care

Palliative care

Presentation/diagnosis   Illness   Death

FIGURE 1   Model of palliative care (1). *Source*: From Ref. (1).

TABLE 1   Characteristics of Palliative Care

- Provides relief from pain and other distressing symptoms.
- Affirms life and regards dying as a normal process.
- Intends neither to hasten nor postpone death.
- Integrates the psychological and spiritual aspects of patient care.
- Offers a support system to help patients live as actively as possible until death.
- Offers a support system to help the family cope during the patient's illness and in their own bereavement.
- Uses a team approach to address the needs of patients and their families, including bereavement counselling, if indicated.
- Will enhance quality of life, and may also positively influence the course of illness.
- Is applicable early in the course of illness, in conjunction with other therapies that are intended to prolong life, such as chemotherapy or radiation therapy, and includes those investigations needed to better understand and manage distressing clinical complications.

Source: Adapted from Ref. (1).

physicians and nurses specialising in palliative medicine, occupational therapists, physiotherapists, speech and language therapists, dieticians, pharmacists, social workers, discharge coordinators and those that may attend to pastoral and spiritual needs such as a Chaplaincy team. Essential to the provision of optimal palliative care to the patient with a diagnosis of metastatic breast cancer is the close working of the palliative care MDT with the breast care unit. Frequently, the role of the palliative care team will be to support the breast care unit in addressing symptom issues and maximising the quality of life for the patient. In many circumstances, the unit will have the skills to perform a palliative care assessment and construct an effective management plan. When the circumstances are more complex, the specialist palliative care team may be involved. There is now an extensive network of palliative care providers within the primary and secondary care settings which can be accessed to facilitate ongoing symptom control. The palliative care team may be involved to ensure that continuity of care is seamless irrespective of the setting in which the patients find themselves to be.

As previously mentioned, various national strategies have promoted the importance of involving palliative care services as early as possible in the management of patients with a potentially life threatening illness. In the United Kingdom, alongside reducing the risk of cancer and waiting times, the NHS Cancer Plan (3) aimed to increase the provision of palliative care services to those with a diagnosis of cancer. The Department of Health National Cancer Survey, carried out between 1999 and 2000, had revealed a wide variation in the care given to patients with cancer. Reasons proposed for this inequality were cited to be secondary to poor communication and coordination, the unrecognised needs of professionals involved, and the fact that services are not universally available. The NHS Cancer Plan and their subsequent guidance on "Improving Supportive and Palliative Care for Adults with Cancer" (4) published by the National Institute for Clinical Excellence (NICE) in 2004 promoted palliative care as a way of improving upon this variation. Guidance on "Advanced Breast Cancer: Diagnosis and Treatment" published by NICE in 2009 (5) referred to existing guidance {"Improving Supportive and Palliative Care for Adults with Cancer" [NICE cancer service guidance 2004 (4)] and "Improving Outcomes in Breast Cancer: Manual Update" [NICE cancer service guidance 2002 (5)]} to recommend the following with regards to supportive care:

> Assessment and discussion of patients' needs for physical, psychological, social, spiritual and financial support should be undertaken at key points (such as diagnosis at commencement, during, and at the end of treatment: at relapse; and when death is approaching)
>
> Mechanisms should be developed to promote continuity of care, which might include the nomination of a person to take on the role of "key worker" for individual patients

Achievement of these recommendations may be facilitated by close liaison between the breast care unit and palliative care MDT.

MANAGEMENT OF PHYSICAL PROBLEMS

Cancer patients often experience a number of different physical problems. Portenoy et al. (6) reported that the median number of symptoms experienced by a mixed group of cancer patients was 11. There was no difference in the number of symptoms experienced by patients with different tumour types (breast, colon, ovary, and prostate), or different tumour stages (unknown, no disease, local disease, and metastatic disease). However, there was a difference in the number of symptoms experienced by patients with differing performance status, that is, the worse the performance status, the more symptoms experienced (and vice versa).

The aetiology of physical symptoms includes the following:

1. A direct effect of the underlying cancer
2. An indirect effect of the underlying cancer
3. An effect of the cancer treatment
4. An effect of a concomitant physical disease
5. An effect of concomitant psychological problems
6. A combination of the aforementioned factors

Assessment

The management of physical symptoms involves the following:
Assessment
Treatment of the underlying cause of the symptom
Treatment of the symptom and (if necessary)
Reassessment

As previously discussed, assessment is essential to determine the underlying aetiology of the symptom so that treatment may be targeted. Assessment is also essential to determine the response of the symptom to treatment. The assessment of response should take into account both the efficacy and tolerability of the treatment. If the treatment proves ineffective, the patient should be re-assessed and an alternative treatment is considered. In cases of continued poor efficacy and/or poor tolerability, alternative therapeutic options should be considered as might a second opinion.

The key to managing any symptom is in the clinical assessment. Lack of attention to general principles is the largest cause of misdiagnosis which may inhibit the correct treatment being selected. A comprehensive evaluation involves taking a careful history, performing a medical and psychological examination.

PAIN

Pain is not a simple sensation but a complex phenomenon having both a physical and an affective (emotional) component. To reflect this, the International Association for the Study of Pain (IASP) (7) published the following definition of pain:

> An unpleasant sensory and emotional experience associated with actual or potential tissue damage, or described in terms of such damage.

There are several ways to categorise pain, for example, acute or chronic, nociceptive (somatic or visceral) or neuropathic. It is increasingly recognised that acute and chronic pain may represent a continuum rather than distinct separate entities, combine different pain mechanisms, and vary in duration (8).

History taking should include the following (9):

- The site of the pain
- Quality of the pain
- Exacerbating and relieving factors
- The temporal pattern
- The exact onset
- Associated signs and symptoms
- Interference with activities of daily living
- Impact on the patients psychological state
- Response to previous analgesic therapies

Chronic pain is defined as pain that exists for more than 3 months lasting beyond the usual course of the acute disease or expected time of healing (7). It is often associated with major changes in personality, lifestyle, and functional ability (9). Chronic pain occurs as a result of both cancer and non-malignant chronic conditions such as neuropathic, musculoskeletal, and chronic postoperative pain syndromes. The prevalence of chronic pain is approximated at being between 30% and 50% among patients with cancer who are undergoing active treatment for a solid tumour and between 70% and 90% among those patients with advanced disease (10). Approximately two-thirds of patients with advanced cancer will also complain of anorexia, one-half will have a symptomatic dry mouth and constipation, and one-third will suffer nausea, vomiting, insomnia, dyspnoea, cough, or oedema (11).

A diagnosis of cancer does not necessarily mean that the malignant process is the cause of the pain. Pain may be secondary to the following (12):

- the cancer itself
- the treatment
- the result of debilitating disease such as a pressure ulcer
- a process unrelated to either the cancer or the treatment

The WHO Analgesic Ladder

The Analgesic Ladder (13) was designed as a framework for the management of chronic pain. There are several drugs available to manage chronic pain and the Analgesic Ladder allows the flexibility to choose from the range according to the patient's requirements and tolerance (14). The guidelines promote five main principles with regard to the use of analgesic agents:

1. "By mouth": drugs should be given orally (where possible)
2. "By the clock": drugs should be given regularly
3. "By the ladder": drugs should be given in a step-wise manner (Fig. 2)
4. "For the individual": opioid drugs should be individually titrated
5. "Attention to detail"

Step 1: Non-Opioid Drugs

Examples of non-opioid drugs include paracetamol, aspirin, and non-steroidal anti-inflammatory drugs (NSAIDs). They are effective for mild to moderate pain. These drugs are especially effective for musculoskeletal and visceral pain (12).

Step 2: Opioids for Mild to Moderate Pain

Examples of opioids for mild to moderate pain include codeine, dihydrocodeine, tramadol, and oxycodone (steps 2 and 3). These drugs are used when adequate pain management is not achieved with the use of non-opioids and are usually used in combination formulations. It is not recommended to administer another analgesic from the same group if the drug being used is not controlling the pain. Uncontrolled pain requires assessment and further titration of an opioid by movement up the Analgesic Ladder. The exception to this would be if the patient was experiencing intolerable side effects on the weaker opioid when an alternative drug may be beneficial.

In recent studies tramadol has been recognised as being efficacious in the management of chronic cancer pain of moderate severity (15). It is uncertain whether tramadol is more effective in neuropathic pain than other opioids for mild to moderate pain although one report (12,16) suggests a reduction in allodynia (pain from stimuli which is not normally painful). Circumstantial reports suggest tramadol lowers the seizure threshold and, therefore, care needs to be taken in those patients who have a history of epilepsy, as well as any other medications that may contribute to the lowering of the seizure threshold, for example tricyclic antidepressants and selective

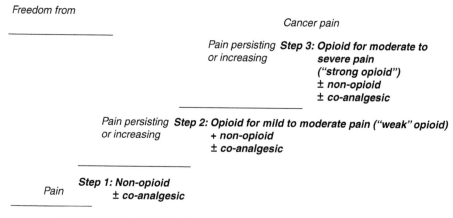

FIGURE 2   The WHO "Analgesic Ladder". *Source*: Adapted from Ref. 13.

serotonin reuptake inhibitors (12). A few patients with severe pain will achieve a satisfactory level of pain control with tramadol. It is available in immediate and modified release preparations.

Step 3: Opioids for Moderate to Severe Pain

Examples of opioids for moderate to severe pain include morphine, oxycodone, fentanyl, diamorphine, methadone, buprenorphine, hydromorphone, and alfentanil.

Non-Opioid Analgesics

Paracetamol and Paracetamol Combinations

The use of non-opioid analgesics such as paracetamol or paracetamol combined with a weak opioid such as codeine is recommended for managing pain following minor surgical procedures or when the pain following a major surgery begins to subside (McQuay et al.) (17). Paracetamol can also be given rectally if the oral route is contraindicated. An intravenous preparation of paracetamol is now available and can provide effective analgesia after surgical procedures (Romsing et al.) (18). It is more effective and of faster onset than the same dose given enterally. The use of the intravenous form should be limited to patients in whom the enteral route is considered not appropriate. Paracetamol taken in the correct dose of not more than 4 g per day is relatively free of side effects. When used in combination with codeine preparations, the most frequent side effect is constipation.

Non-Steroidal Anti-Inflammatory Drugs

NSAIDs have been shown to provide better pain relief than paracetamol combinations for acute pain (McQuay et al.) (17). These drugs can be used alone or in combination with both opioid and non-opioid analgesics. Two commonly used NSAIDs are diclofenac, which can be administered by the oral, parenteral, enteral, or rectal route, and ibuprofen, which is available only in an oral preparation. The presence of a coagulopathy, renal impairment and/or, gastrointestinal disturbance limits the use of NSAIDs. The newer COX 2-specific NSAIDs, which are associated with similar analgesia and anti-inflammatory effects (19) as the non-specific types mentioned earlier, have no effect on platelet function or the gastric mucosa (20). However, several of these drugs have recently been withdrawn from the market due to long-term cardiovascular side effects and it will take time for newer products with an improved safety profile to re-establish themselves in practice (8).

Opioid Analgesics

Opioids are the first-line treatment for pain that follows major surgery (21) and can also be prescribed for cancer and non-cancer related chronic pain. Opioid doses need to be titrated carefully to achieve pain relief to suit each individual patient while minimising any unwanted side effects (17).

Evidence for the concept of opioid rotation when patients have intolerable opioid-related side effects originate from cancer pain studies (22) but it may be a useful strategy to consider in the management of acute pain as well.

Opioids for Mild to Moderate Pain

Tramadol

Tramadol has been shown to be an effective analgesic for the management of mild to moderate pain postoperative pain (19,23). Although tramadol does have some side effects, which include nausea and dizziness, it is free of NSAID side effects and causes less constipation than codeine preparations and opioids (24). The combination of tramadol with paracetamol is more effective than either of the two components administered alone (25).

Codeine

Codeine is a naturally occurring derivative of an opium alkaloid, it is a "true" opiate (26) and is a relatively weak opioid used most commonly for mild to moderate pain. WHO analgesic guidelines recommend codeine as a step-2 drug on the analgesic ladder. Codeine is available in tablet, liquid, and parenteral preparations.

Opioids for Moderate to Severe Pain

Morphine

A large amount of information and research is available concerning morphine as an analgesic agent and therefore tends to be the drug of choice within this category (27,28). It is available in oral, rectal, parenteral, and intraspinal preparations. A recent study of 43 European Palliative Care Units showed that morphine was the most frequently used opioid for moderate to severe pain, with over 50% of patients taking oral or parenteral preparations (29). All strong opioids require careful titration from an expert practitioner. It is advisable to begin with a small dose, usually one that is equivalent to the previous medication, and titrate gradually in conjunction with careful assessment of its effectiveness (27). Titration begins with the immediate-release form which is available in tablet (sevredol) or elixir (oramorph) preparations, and once pain control is achieved the patient can be converted to a modified release preparation that acts over a 12-hour period (e.g., zomorph).

Breakthrough analgesia is administered using the immediate-release preparation at the equivalent 4-hourly dose. This dose can be given as required (hourly) and subsequent adjustments can be made to the modified form if the patient is requiring more than three breakthrough doses in a 24-hour period (27). Patients should be informed of potential side effects such as constipation, nausea, and increased sleepiness, in order to allay any fear. The patient should also be told that nausea and drowsiness are transitory and normally improve within 48 hours, but that constipation can be an ongoing problem. It is recommended that a laxative should be prescribed when commencing an opioid therapy. The most effective laxative for this group of patients is a combination of both a softening and a stimulating laxative (15).

Patients often have many concerns about commencing strong opioids. Frequent fears centre around addiction and believing that its use signifies the terminal phase of the illness (30). Time should be taken to reassure patients and their families and provide verbal and written information. Although morphine is still considered to be the opioid drug of choice for moderate to severe pain (27) alternative opioids are also available which vary in their action dependent upon patient and drug factors. This enables the patient to experience optimal analgesic effect and tolerability.

Oxycodone

Oxycodone is a useful opioid as an alternative to morphine (31). It has similar properties to morphine and can be administered orally, rectally, and parenterally. Oxycodone is available as an immediate or modified release preparation and titration should occur in the same way as morphine. Oxycodone has an analgesic potency of 1.5–2.0 times higher than morphine and although has similar side effects it has been found to cause less nausea (32) and significantly less itchiness (33).

"Targinact" is a combination of modified release oxycodone and naloxone. The naloxone component aims to counteract the negative effects that oxycodone (and other opioids) has on bowel function. It is suggested that approximately 97% of the naloxone is eliminated by first pass elimination in the healthy liver preventing it from significantly affecting any analgesic effect (34).

Fentanyl

Fentanyl is a strong opioid, available as a transdermal patch recommended in the management of stable pain. It is reported to have an improved side-effect profile in comparison to morphine (35) although some patients experience nausea and mild drowsiness (36) and occasionally a reaction to the adhesive in the patch (37). Use of the patch allows a reduction in tablet burden.

The patch should be changed every 72 hours with steady plasma levels achieved between 8–16 hours (38), although it may be necessary to change the patch more frequently. The patch should be applied to skin that is free from excess hair and any form of irritation and should not be applied to irradiated areas. The site of the patch should be rotated to avoid an adverse skin reaction. Occasionally, difficulties arise relating to the titration of the patch as each patch is equivalent to a range, rather than a specific dose, of morphine.

Although available in a parenteral preparation, administration via this route is limited due to the large volumes incurred. In such circumstances, alfentanil may be a useful alternative (39).

Hydromorphone

Hydromorphone is similar to morphine in its pharmacokinetic profile but is approximately 5.0–7.5 times more potent. It is available in an immediate- and sustained-release preparations and titration occurs in a similar manner (40). The side effects are similar to those of morphine (41).

Other alternative strong opioid agents include buprenorphine, alfentanil, methadone, and diamorphine. Newer routes of delivery have been developed to improve on the analgesic effect such as the transmucosal delivery of fentanyl which aims to hasten the speed of onset.

Table 2 illustrates an approximate guide to the recommended equivalent doses of the strong opioids. As the dose of morphine escalates the recommended equivalent doses will become progressively more erroneous.

Breakthrough Analgesia

Breakthrough pain refers to a transitory exacerbation of pain experienced by the patient who has relatively stable and adequately controlled background pain (42). There should not be a time limit on this type of prescription because it will need to be given when the patient demonstrates any signs of discomfort or pain (with the exception of renal failure where dosages need to be limited). If several rescue doses are required within a 24-hour period, the background analgesia should be increased (43). It is important to be aware that various classifications of breakthrough pain exist, which guide the prescriber as to the best agent to use. Increasing the background dose will not always be indicated. For example, a patient who only experiences breakthrough pain when lying on a radiotherapy table might experience intolerable side effects from the strong opioid if the regular dose was simply increased rather having available immediate acting analgesic to be given to cover that specific incident.

Ideal properties of an analgesic for the management of breakthrough pain is one with good efficacy, a rapid onset of action, a short duration of action, and one associated with minimal adverse effects.

Use of Opioids in Renal Impairment

Renal failure can cause significant and dangerous side effects due to the accumulation of the drug. Basic guidelines for pain management in renal failure include the following:

- Reduce analgesic dose and/or dose frequency (6-hourly instead of 4-hourly)
- Select a more appropriate drug (non-renally excreted) such as alfentanil

- Avoid modified release preparations
- Seek advice from a specialist pain/palliative care team and/or pharmacist (44)

Adjuvant Drugs (Co-Analgesics)

Adjuvant drugs are a miscellaneous group of drugs whose primary indication is for conditions other than pain which may, however, relieve pain in specific circumstances (12). Examples of this category of drugs include NSAIDs, steroids, antibiotics, antidepressants, anti-epileptics, N-methyl-d-aspartate receptor channel blockers, antispasmodics, and muscle relaxants (12).

TABLE 2 An Approximate Guide to Conversion Between Alternative Opioids

Drug	Dose	Route	Approximate equivalent oral morphine dose (mg)
Morphine sulphate IR (oramorph/sevredol)	10 mg	po	10
Morphine sulphate MR (zomorph)	10 mg	po	10
Morphine sulphate injection	5 mg	iv/sc	10
Diamorphine injection	10 mg	iv/sc	30
Alfentanil injection	1 mg	sc	30
Oxycodone IR (oxynorm)	5 mg	po	10
Oxycodone MR (oxycontin)	5 mg	po	10
Oxycodone injection	2.5 mg	iv/sc	10
Tramadol	100 mg	po/im/iv	10
Codeine phosphate	60 mg	po	6
Dihydrocodeine	60 mg	po	6
Co-codamol 30/500	2 tabs	po	6

Example:

60-mg morphine sulphate IR po is equivalent to:	60-mg morphine sulphate MR po
	30-mg morphine sulphate injection
	20-mg diamorphine injection
	2-mg alfentanil injection
	30-mg oxycodone IR po
	15-mg oxycodone injection

Recommended conversion doses from morphine to a fentanyl patch:

Morphine dose in 24 hrs (mg)	4-hourly morphine dose (mg)	Fentanyl TTS (mcg/hr)
30–60	5–10	12
60–134	10–20	25
135–224	25–35	50
225–314	40–50	75
315–404	55–65	100
405–494	70–80	125
495–584	85–95	150
585–674	100–115	175
675–764	115–125	200
765–854	130–140	225
855–944	145–155	250
945–1034	160–170	275
1035–1124	175–190	300

Source: Adapted from The Royal Marsden Hospital Guidelines for Symptom Control.

The WHO Analgesic Ladder recommends the use of these drugs in combination with non-opioids and weak and strong opioids. Other interventions include nitrous oxide, local anaesthetics, and topical anaesthetics. Alongside these, non-pharmacological measures should be considered to help patients with pain management. Table 3 shows the options that can be considered.

NAUSEA AND VOMITING

Nausea and vomiting are common experiences of patients with advanced cancer, independent of exposure to chemotherapy (45). Approximately 60% of patients with advanced cancer report nausea and 30% report vomiting (46).

The most common causes of nausea and vomiting in advanced cancer are as follows:

- Gastric stasis
- Pharyngeal irritation such as candida and difficulty expectorating sputum
- Metabolic changes (hypercalcaemia and renal failure)
- Treatments
- Brain metastasis
- Pain
- Anxiety/fear
- Medication induced

Assessment is key in the management of nausea and vomiting and although there are no defined assessment tools for this symptom in palliative care there are key questions that can be asked and some of which are listed in Table 4. The choice of antiemetic will depend on the cause of the nausea and vomiting (47). The principles of treatment are based on knowledge regarding the emetic pathways (48).

TABLE 3 Non-Pharmacological Interventions

Gentle humour
Heat therapy
Cold therapy
Exercise
Rest
Relaxation
Education
Acupuncture
Psychological support
Trans cutaneous nerve stimulation (TENS)

TABLE 4 Questions to Consider in the Assessment of Nausea and Vomiting

When did the nausea/vomiting start?
Does anything make the nausea/vomiting better or worse?
Is there a pattern to the nausea and vomiting?
If vomiting is present is there any relief experienced afterwards?
Is undigested food present in the vomit?
What is the colour of the vomit?
Assess the current bowel pattern.
Differentiate between coughing that causes retching and the vomiting that occurs.

Watson et al. (49) suggest the following considerations in the management of nausea and vomiting:

- Give anti-emetics regularly
- Consider an alternative route of administration from the oral route if there is a concern over absorption, for example using a continuous sub cutaneous infusion
- Reverse any reversible causes such as hypercalcaemia
- Check urea and electrolytes and liver function

As with all symptom control, the key is reassessment and revaluation of response.

CONSTIPATION

Constipation can be referred to as "unduly, infrequent and difficult evacuation of the bowel" (50). Constipation does not just cause physical problems for the patient with advanced cancer (51). It has been recognised to cause psychological and social problems which can cause limitations in daily life for the patient. Undertaking a detailed history from the patient is pivotal in establishing the appropriate interventions for the patient. Adequate constipation assessment is the key prior to selection of the most appropriate treatment for the patient. Considerations in assessment of constipation will include these:

- The frequency of the stool being passed
- Consistency of the stool being passed
- The normal pattern of the patient's bowel prior to the illness
- Ease of defaecation
- Presence of nausea and/or vomiting

Causes of Constipation
- Drugs (e.g., 5HT3 receptor antagonists and opioids)
- Some chemotherapy agents
- Immobility
- Dehydration
- Bowel obstruction
- Low-fibre diet
- Hypercalcaemia
- Spinal cord compression
- Concurrent disease

Management of Constipation
The treatment of constipation is largely by the oral and rectal route. In the case of opioid-induced constipation, associated with vomiting or nausea that prevents the patient from tolerating oral laxatives, subcutaneous medication is available. Laxatives can be categorised as follows:

- Bulk forming
- Osmotic
- Stimulant
- Lubricating

Guidelines for the management of constipation are based mainly on practitioner preference and anecdotal evidence (51). See Table 5 for the classification of laxatives.

Constipation can be a significant problem for patients with advanced cancer. Each patient should be assessed on an individual basis taking into consideration the patient's pre-illness pattern. Following this, the correct laxative may be selected.

TABLE 5 Classification of Laxatives

Type of laxative	Notes	Preparation	Special instruction
Bulk-forming	These agents act by retaining water so the stool remains large and soft thus stimulating peristalsis	Ispaghula Husk (Fybogel)	Patients with strictures or partial obstruction must be cautious as intestinal obstruction could occur if insufficient quantities of fluid are taken
Stimulant	Cause water and electrolytes to accumulate in the intestines and stimulate motility through direct contact of the agent and the mucosa	Danthron[a*] (component of co-danthramer and co-danthrusate) Senna: tablets/liquid Bisacodyl: tablets/liquid Glycerinsuppository: rectal Phosphate enema: chronic constipation	This group should be avoided in bowel obstruction as they can exacerbate colic
Mixed stimulants and softeners	2 in 1 preparations	Co-danthramer:– liquid/capsules Danthron and poloxamer available in normal and strong strengths	Alert patients to orange/brown change in urine. Can cause perianal irritation and discolouration, avoid when patient has a catheter or is incontinent
		Docusate	Mild stimulant
Softeners	Attract/retain water in intestine	Milpar (liquid parafin and magnesium hydroxide)	Long-term use of softeners can cause gut granulomata and lipoid pneumonitis
		Docusate	
		Arachis oil enema	*Avoid if patient has nut allergy*
Osmotic	Agents act in the intestinal tract by increasing stimulation of fluid secretion and motility	Lactulose	Can cause bloating, flatulence, and abdominal discomfort. Not absorbed, used in the case of hepatic encephalopathy.
		Movicol Phosphate enema Microlax enema Magnesium sulphate mixture	For rapid bowel evacuation use with caution

[a]Licensed for constipation in terminally ill patients only; rodent studies indicate potential carcinogenic risk.
Source: Adapted from The Royal Marsden Hospital Guidelines for Symptom Control.

ASSESSMENT TOOLS IN PALLIATIVE CARE

Choosing the correct tool to measure symptoms must be guided by an understanding of the goals of assessment and the practicality, applicability, and acceptability of the tool (52). Careful consideration must be given to the potential burden placed upon patients in using such tools. There are several tools that are validated to be used to assess multiple symptoms, which are listed below. It is recognised that this list is not exhaustive but offers some of the recognised tools available.

- Memorial Symptom Assessment Scale: a validated patient-rated measure that provides multidimensional information about multiple symptoms (53)
- The Edmonton Assessment Scale: a validated tool that evaluates eight symptoms and has been used extensively in palliative care research
- The Rotterdam Symptom Checklist: a validated patient-rated measure that evaluates a spectrum of common symptoms in terms of patient-rated distress
- Symptom Distress Scale: a 13-item patient-rated scale that evaluates 11 symptoms. It is a valid and useful measure of global symptom distress (52).

There are more specific measures available for assessment of fatigue, pain, breathlessness, and impaired cognition

MANAGEMENT OF BREATHLESSNESS

Breathlessness, otherwise known as dyspnoea, is the subjective experience of breathing discomfort. It may arise as an interaction between physiological, psychological, social and environmental factors thus, as with other symptoms requires a holistic approach. Although objective measures may hint at an underlying pathology they do not reliably indicate the subjective experience. Breathlessness is a common complaint even when there appears to be no cardiac or lung involvement. One study revealed that 24% of cancer patients reported shortness of breath and did not have heart or lung involvement (54).

The primary focus of managing breathlessness should be on identifying the underlying cause and identifying reversible components. Palliation of breathlessness may occur during this stage of management but frequently is introduced once the symptom is deemed refractory to such interventions. Although the mechanism of action is not well understood, evidence supports the use of opioids as first-line therapy for the palliation of breathlessness (55). The benzodiazepine drugs are frequently employed for their hypnotic, sedative, anxiolytic, and muscle relaxant properties. There is a lack of evidence available to support their use as first-line therapy but since many patients with breathlessness feel anxious it appears rational and safe to support its use as second-line therapy. Bronchodilators, usually delivered by the nebulised route, may be employed where a degree of airway obstruction is suspected as may steroids if airway obstruction, stridor, superior vena cava obstruction, lymphangitis carcinomatosis, or radiation pneumonitis is present. Abernathy et al. (56) conducted an international, multicentre, double blind, randomised controlled trial to assess the symptomatic effectiveness of oxygen versus room air for patients with life limiting illness, who are breathless but do not meet the criteria for long-term oxygen therapy. The results demonstrated that oxygen therapy showed no significant benefit over room air for patients who met the inclusion criteria for the study. Since evidence to support the use of oxygen is lacking (and likewise to support not using it) good practice would be to assess response and have a low threshold to discontinuing it in the absence of symptomatic improvement. As previously mentioned, objective measures such as measuring the oxygen saturation does not always correlate with the subjective sensation of shortness of breath and thus the decision to continue with therapy should not be solely based on this reading. For a summary of interventions that might be employed for the management of breathlessness, see Table 6.

TABLE 6 Management of Breathlessness

Symptoms	Management options			
	Non-pharmacological	Comments	Pharmacological	Examples
Breathlessness	Breathing techniques Cognitive-behavioural techniques Electric fan Acupuncture	Non-pharmacological options are a very useful adjunct to pharmacological options, particularly in patients with less severe dyspnoea and/or "panic attacks". Electric fans can be helpful, although the flow of air needs to be directed towards the face of the patient	Systemic opioids	Morphine sulphate (immediate release) orally PRN/(maximum 1 hourly) and then consider 4 hourly
			Benzodiazepines	Lorazepam sublingually PRN (maximum 1 hourly) Diazepam orally tds or Midazolam 2.5-5 mg subcutaneously PRN (maximum one hourly)
			Bronchodilators	Salbutamol nebulised PRN (or regularly, qds)
			SteroidsOxygen therapy	Dexamethasone orally once daily (pragmatic approach to be reviewed at 5 days)

MANAGEMENT OF THE TERMINAL PHASE

Despite recent advances in the management of metastatic breast cancer with the introduction of new chemotherapeutic, biological, and hormonal agents, the disease remains incurable. At a variable point, the continuation of anticancer treatment will be deemed inappropriate by the MDT, or maybe limited by a lack of further treatment options available. At this point the focus of treatment shifts from attempting to control the disease to one of maximising symptom control and minimising unnecessary interventions. Recognition of this phase and open discussion with the patient is critical to optimising the management of the dying phase. The last 48 hours of life should ideally be met having established optimal symptom control with the patient's, and their carer's, wishes fulfilled.

In a large-scale survey conducted on behalf of the BBC, only 34% of the general population had reported their wishes for how they would like to die. In contrast, however, two-thirds had prepared a will (57). In 2008, the Department of Health (UK) developed the End-of-Life Care Strategy whose goal is to provide high-quality care for all patients at the end of life wherever the patient wishes to be. It emphasises a coordinated pathway approach [Fig. 3 (57)] with six steps recognising different elements necessary to deliver effective, high quality end-of-life care along an individual patient's journey. Throughout the pathway, attention must always be paid to the giving and sharing of information between health-care professionals, patients, and their carers. The strategy discusses the consequences of failure to discuss openly the preferences of patients and their carers for the dying phase (57):

- People may be unnecessarily frightened about the process of dying.
- Close relatives of people who are approaching the end of life may be unaware of their wishes and therefore do not know how best to help and support them. This is particularly important for those who may lose the capacity to make their own decisions.

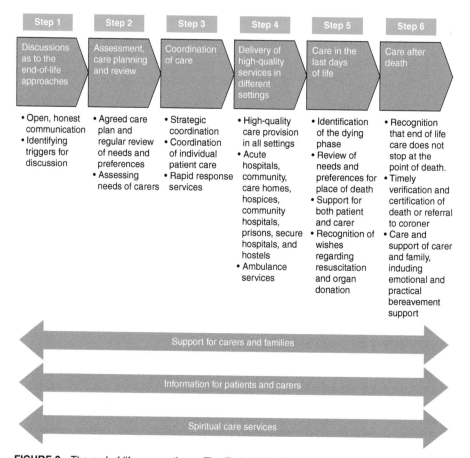

FIGURE 3   The end-of-life care pathway, The End-of-Life Care Strategy. *Source*: From Ref. (57).

- Inappropriate interventions may be tried if those caring for someone are not aware of the person's treatment preferences, including advance decisions to refuse treatment.
- People who would have wished their organs to be used for transplantation may not have discussed this with their relatives who have to make decisions after their death.
- People may not have discussed funeral wishes with their relatives.
- People may die without writing a will.
- Same sex partners may not have declared their status, with the consequence that professionals may exclude them from involvement in their partner's care.
- Fear of the unknown meaning that people sometimes tend to avoid those who are ill for fear of "upsetting them" or "making them worse".
- Lack of public and professional discussion about death and dying may be one of the reasons why this area has historically been given low priority by health and social-care services.
- People, including clinical staff, are ignorant of the possible options that could improve quality of life and restore independence.
- Lack of knowledge of the financial implications for the bereaved following a death and what needs to be put in place ahead of the event.
- Lack of public and professional discussion about grief and loss, which results in the isolation of the bereaved.

A qualitative systematic literature review published in 2000, which evaluated the views of both patients with advanced cancer and the general public concluded that the majority of people would prefer to die at home (58). However, data published by the Office of National Statistics (UK) from 2008 revealed that overall only around 18% people die at home, with 4% dying in hospices, and 58% in acute hospitals. For those with a diagnosis of cancer, the Figures remain similar with 25% dying at home, 16% in a hospice, and 52% in hospital (59). The ability to care for a patient at home in the dying phase and ultimately for a patient to die at home will depend upon local resources and the availability of professionals with the appropriate skills to manage a patient at this stage of the disease. These professionals will require the expertise to manage the challenges that being outside of the acute setting can bring which may be on a physical, psychological, social and/or, spiritual level. However, through coordinated care planning between professionals in the primary and secondary settings, this is often achievable, especially if early planning is made possible through early discussions with patients and those involved in their care. Nevertheless, the terminal phase remains a challenging period for all concerned.

SYMPTOM CONTROL IN THE LAST 48 HOURS

The symptom control issues encountered in patients with advanced metastatic breast cancer are essentially the same as those encountered in patients with other types of advanced cancer. As the patient proceeds to the later stages of the terminal phase, the professionals involved must continue to attend to pre-existing symptoms but be alert to those that more commonly present in the last 48 hours of life. These are primarily terminal agitation and the accumulation of respiratory secretions. The management of terminal agitation and respiratory secretions is briefly summarised in Table 7 When considering the management of these two symptoms it is assumed that reversible conditions have been excluded or are failing to respond to treatment. All efforts should be made to identify a tolerable therapy which does not compromise consciousness.

TABLE 7 Management of Common Symptoms in the Last 48 Hours

Symptoms	Management Options			
	Non-Pharmacological	Comments	Pharmacological	Comments
Terminal agitation	Environmental measures	Patients should be cared for in a quiet, well-illuminated room, which contains objects familiar to the patient (e.g., photographs), and objects that can help to orientate the patient (e.g., clock). In addition, patients are often reassured by the presence of non-professional carers although the emphasis should be on minimising external stimulation and the number of individuals involved	Common 1st-line agents include midazolam, levomepromazine, and haloperidol. If symptoms appear refractory to these agents, other agents such as phenobarbitone and propofol may be considered. Guidance for doses to use should be sought from the local palliative care team	Since the ability to tolerate the oral route is likely to be diminished (is likely to diminish further), these drugs are delivered via the parenteral, usually subcutaneous, route. In most circumstances assessment of response to an initial stat (immediate) dose is advised in order to calculate the 24-hr dose to be delivered by an infusional system
Excess respiratory secretions	Reassurance	Control of the 'death rattle' may only be effective in about a third to a half of patients (25). Efforts to control this symptom may not be necessary for patient comfort but may alleviate carer distress. Every effort should be made to explain this to carers	Hyoscine hydrobromide, hyoscine butylbromide, and glycopyrronium are common agents to use. Hyoscine hydrobromide crosses the blood–brain barrier and is thus more likely to cause confusion and agitation. Guidance for doses to use should be sought from the local palliative care team	The production of bronchial secretions is largely under parasympathetic control and thus anticholinergic drugs are the most effective although will have little effect on secretions that have already accumulated. It is wise, therefore, to act early to prevent the accumulation of secretions in the first instance
	Positioning	Promotion of drainage of secretions through repositioning to a lateral or more upright position, if possible, may be effective		
	Suctioning	This may cause significant distress and should be reserved for rare situation when secretions are visible and easily reachable		

FUTURE OF PALLIATIVE CARE

The presence of palliative medicine as a distinct speciality is variable. Its ongoing development and growth to parts of the world where it doesn't already exist is important for the development of evidence-based practice and not only for the ongoing education of health-care professionals involved in the care of patients in the terminal phase but also to support patients and their families at earlier stages of the disease process. With an ever-ageing population and advances in medicine which have changed the pattern of diseases, such as metastatic breast cancer, into chronic progressive types the demand for palliative care will only increase.

REFERENCES

1. World Health Organization. National Cancer Control Programmes. Policies and Managerial Guidelines, 2nd edn. Geneva: WHO, 2002.
2. Anonymous. Cancer care during the last phase of life. J Clin Oncol 1998; 16: 1986–96.
3. Department of Health. The NHS Cancer plan – A plan for investment. A plan for reform. London: Department of Health, 2000. [Available from: http://www.dh.gov.uk/prod_consum_dh/groups/dh_digitalassets/@dh/@en/documents/digitalasset/dh_4014513.pdf] (1st March 2010).
4. National Institute for Clinical Excellence. Improving Supportive and Palliative Care for Adults with Cancer. NICE: UK, 2004. [Available from: http://www.nice.org.uk/nicemedia/pdf/csgspmanual.pdf] (1st March 2010).
5. National Institute for Clinical Excellence. Advanced Breast Cancer: Diagnosis and Treatment. NICE: UK, 2009 (7th January 2011).
6. Portenoy RK, Thaler HT, Kornblith AB, et al. Symptom prevalence, characteristics and distress in a cancer population. Qual Life Res 1994; 3: 183–9.
7. IASP. Classification of chronic pain. Pain 1996; 3(Suppl): 51–226.
8. ANZCA and Faculty of Pain Medicine. Acute Pain Management. Melbourne: ANZCA and FPM, 2005: p9.
9. Foley K. Pain assessment and cancer pain syndromes, Oxford Textbook of Palliative Medicine. Oxford: Oxford University Press, 2005: 298–316.
10. Portenoy RK, Lesage P. Management of cancer pain. Lancet 1999; 353(9165): 1695–700.
11. Donnelly S, Walsh D. The symptoms of advanced cancer. Semin Oncol 1995; 22(Suppl 3): 67–72.
12. Twycross RG, Wilcock A. Symptom management in advanced cancer. Abingdon: Radcliffe Medical, 2001.
13. World Health Organization. Cancer Pain Relief, 2nd edn. With a Guide to Opioid Availability.
14. Hanks GW, Conno F, Cherny N, et al. Morphine and alternative opioids in cancer pain: the EAPC recommendations. Br J Cancer 2001; 84: 587–93.
15. Davis MP, Glare P, Hardy J. Opioids in cancer pain. Oxford: Oxford University Press, 2005.
16. Sindrup SH, Jensen TS. Efficacy of pharmacological treatments of neuropathic pain: an update and effect related to mechanism of drug action. Pain 1999; 83: 389–400.
17. McQuay H, Moore A, Justins D. Treating acute pain in hospital. BMJ 1997; 314: 1531–5.
18. Romsing J, Moiniche S, Dahl JB. Rectal and parenteral paracetamol, and paracetamol in combination with NSAIDs, for postoperative analgesia. Br J Anaesthesia 2002; 88: 215–26.
19. Reicin A, Brown J, Jove M, et al. Efficacy of single-dose and multidose rofecoxib in the treatment of post-orthopedic surgery pain. Am J Orthopedics 2001; 30: 40–8.
20. Rowbotham DJ. Non-steroidal anti-inflammatory drugs and paracetamol. Chronic Pain London: Martin Dunitz, 2000.
21. Macintyre PE, Jarvis DA. Age is the best predictor of postoperative morphine requirements. Pain 1996; 64: 357–64.
22. Quigley C. Opioid switching to improve pain relief and drug tolerability. Cochrane Database Syst Rev 2004: CD004847.
23. McQuay HJ, Moore RA. Oral tramadol versus placebo, codeine and combination analgesics. An Evidence-Based Resource for Pain Relief. Oxford: Oxford University Press, 1998.

24. Bamigbade TA, Langford RM. Tramadol hydrochloride: an overview of current use. Hosp Med 1998; 59: 373–6.
25. McQuay H, Edwards J. Meta-analysis of single dose oral tramadol plus acetaminophen in acute postoperative pain. Eur J Anaesthesiol 2003; 28(Suppl): 19–22.
26. Hardy J, Jackson K. Codeine. Opioids in cancer pain. Oxford: Oxford University Press, 2009.
27. Hanks GW, Conno F, Cherny N, et al. Morphine and alternative opioids in cancer pain: the EAPC recommendations. Br J Cancer 2001; 84: 587–93.
28. Hanks G, Cherny N, Fallon M. Opioid analgesic therapy. Oxford textbook of palliative medicine. Oxford: Oxford University Press, 2004.
29. Klepstad P, Kaasa S, Cherny N, et al. Pain and pain treatments in European palliative care units. A cross sectional survey from the European Association for Palliative Care Research Network. Palliat Med 2005; 19: 477–84.
30. McQuay H. Opioids in pain management. Lancet 1999; 353: 2229–32.
31. Riley J. An overview of opioids in palliative care. Eur J Palliat Care 2006; 13: 230–3.
32. Heiskanen T, Kalso E. Controlled-release oxycodone and morphine in cancer related pain. Pain 1997; 73: 37–45.
33. Mucci-LoRusso P, Berman BS, Silberstein PT, et al. Controlled-release oxycodone compared with controlled-release morphine in the treatment of cancer pain: a randomized, double-blind parallel-group study. Eur J Pain 1998; 2: 239–49.
34. Vondrackova D, Leyendecker P, Meissner W, et al. Analgesic efficacy and safety of oxycodone in combination with naloxone as prolonged release Tablets in patients with moderate to severe chronic pain. J Pain 2008; 9: 1144–54.
35. Ahmedzai S, Brooks D. Transdermal fentanyl versus sustained-release oral morphine in cancer pain: preference, efficacy, and quality of life. The TTS-Fentanyl Comparative Trial Group. J Pain Symptom Manage 1997; 13: 254–61.
36. BMA, Royal Pharmaceutical Society of Great Britain. Guidelines for prescribing of strong opioids. London: BMA, 2008.
37. Ling J. The use of transdermal fentanyl in palliative care. Int J Palliat Nurs 1997; 3: 22–5.
38. Zech D, Lehmann A, Ground S. A new treatment option for chronic cancer pain. Eur J Palliat Care 1994; 1: 26–30.
39. Dickman A, Littlewood C, Varga J. Drug information. The Syringe Driver: Continuous Subcutaneous Infusions in Palliative Care. Oxford: Oxford University Press, 2002.
40. Hays H, Hagen N, Thirlwell M, et al. Comparative clinical efficacy and safety of immediate release and controlled release hydromorphone for chronic severe cancer pain. Cancer 1994; 74: 1808–16.
41. Ellershaw J. Hydromorphone: a new alternative to morphine. Prescriber 1998; 9: 21–7.
42. Portenoy RK, Forbes K, Lussier D, Hanks G. Difficult pain problems: an integrated approach. Oxford textbook of palliative medicine. Oxford: Oxford University Press, 2004.
43. McMillan C. Breakthrough pain: assessment and management in cancer patients. Br J Nurs 2001; 10: 860–6.
44. Farrell A, Rich A. Analgesic use in patients with renal failure. Eur J Palliat Care 2000; 7: 201–5.
45. Glare P, Pereira G, Kristjanson LJ, et al. Systematic review of the efficacy of antiemetics in the treatment of nausea in patients with far advanced cancer. Support Care Cancer 2004; 12: 432–40.
46. Davis MP, Walsh D. Treatment of nausea and vomiting in advanced cancer. Support Care Cancer 2000; 8: 443–52.
47. Twycross R, Back I. Nausea and vomiting in advanced cancer. Eur J Palliat Care 1998; 5: 39–45.
48. Regnard C, Dean M. A guide to symptom relief in palliative care. Oxon: Radcliffe Publishing, 2010.
49. Watson M, Lucas C, Hoy A, et al. Oxford Handbook of Palliative Care. Oxford: Oxford University Press, 2009.
50. Miles C, Fellows D, Wilkinson S. Laxatives for the management of constipation in palliative care patients. Cochrane Database Syst Rev 2006: CD003448.
51. Stevens A, Droney J, Riley J. Managing and treating opioid induced constipation in patients with cancer. Gastrointestinal Nurs 2008; 6: 16–22.

52. Ingham JM, Portenoy RK. Patient evaluation and outcome measures. Oxford textbook of palliative medicine. Oxford: Oxford University Press, 2005.
53. Portenoy RK, Thaler HT, Kornblith AB, et al. Memorial Symptom Assessment Scale-An instrument for the evaluation of symptom prevalence, characteristics and distress. Eur J Cancer 1994; 9: 1326–36.
54. Reuben DJ, Mor V. Dyspnea in terminally ill cancer patients. Chest 1986; 89: 234–6.
55. Thomas JR, von Gunten CF. Textbook of palliative medicine. Edward Arnold (publishers) Ltd, 2006: 655–62.
56. Abernethy AP, McDonald CF, Frith PA, et al. Effect of palliative oxygen versus room air in relief of breathlessness in patients with refractory dyspnoea: a double blind, randomised controlled trial. Lancet 2010; 376: 784–93.
57. Department of Health. End of life care strategy - Promoting high quality care for all adults at the end of life. London: Department of Health, 2008. [Available from: http://www .dh.gov.uk/prod_consum_dh/groups/dh_digitalassets/@dh/@en/documents/digital-asset/dh_086345.pdf] (7th January 2011).
58. Higginson IJ, Sen-Gupta GJA. Place of care in advanced cancer: a qualitative systematic literature review of patient preferences. J Palliat Med 2000; 3: 287–300.
59. Office for National Statistics. Mortality rates. London, Office for National Statistics, 2008. [Available from: www.statistics.gov.uk].

Specialist support services and information needs for patients

Diane Mackie and Melissa Warren

INTRODUCTION

Among the large population of breast cancer survivors there is now another sizable, largely silent, and invisible population of patients living with metastatic breast cancer (MBC) (1).

The exact proportion of patients living with MBC in the United Kingdom is currently unknown as this data collection is variable (2,3). It has been estimated that over 100,000 patients are living with advanced/metastatic breast cancer at any one time in the United Kingdom (4).

In stark contrast to the primary breast cancer setting, the unique characteristics and needs of patients diagnosed with MBC often go unrecognised. Warren (5) describes how relatively little is known about patients' experiences of living with this condition in comparison with those diagnosed with primary breast cancer.

The National Institute of Health and Clinical Excellence (NICE) highlight that the welfare of all breast cancer patients is multidimensional and psychosocial support should be available at every stage of the disease pathway to help patients and their families cope with the effects of the disease (6).

Following the recommendations stated in the NHS Cancer Plan in 2000 (7), NICE Guidance on Improving Supportive and Palliative Care for Adults with Cancer in 2004 (8), the Cancer Reform Strategy in 2007 (9), and the National Cancer Survivorship Initiative Vision in 2010 (10) the provision of appropriate supportive care to cancer patients has become a national priority.

Separate guidelines were produced by NICE in 2009 (11) for advanced breast cancer as it was recognised by patients with MBC and professionals who care for these patients that despite the recommendations of 2002 (6), gaps in service remained for this patient group (11). A key priority recommended the assessment and discussion of patients' needs for physical, psychological, social, spiritual, and financial support and also to develop mechanisms to promote continuity of care which may include the nomination of a key worker (11).

Recognition of these unmet needs was also identified by the U.K. charity organisation, Breast Cancer Care (BCC) which established a task force in 2006 in direct response to people living with MBC who felt neglected as a patient group (2). Their remit was "to promote improvements in the treatment, support and care of people living with MBC by influencing national policy and guidelines, by raising awareness of the needs of MBC patients with health-care professionals and by disseminating best practice" (2).

As a result of the 2-year project carried out by the secondary breast cancer task force, several recommendations were made informing us what people with MBC would like and need. Key areas identified as priorities were access to better co-ordination of care, to nurse specialists with the skills and knowledge to manage MBC, to accurate information from the point of the MBC diagnosis for patients and their families, and psychosocial support (2).

SUPPORTIVE CARE

Although a relatively recent term, "supportive care" is now firmly established on the health-care agenda (7–10).

Supportive care needs have been defined "as requirements for care that arise during illness and treatment to manage symptoms and side effects, enable adaptation and coping, optimise understanding and informed decision making, and minimise decrements in functioning" (12). It has also been described as an umbrella term that covers a wide range of both generalist and specialist services, which aim to meet the informational, physical, psychosocial, spiritual, and practical needs of patients (8).

With improving outcomes for MBC due to more effective and better tolerated treatments arise more complex needs and problems among patients (13–15). Despite recent advances in the development of various systemic therapies MBC remains, at present, incurable (4). When patients have an incurable disease, optimising quality of life and meeting their psychosocial as well as information needs are central to excellent care (13). Quality of life has defied objective definition for centuries with authors seeking to either define or measure quality of life (16). It is a very individual concept for patients with MBC; each individual has a different priority about the aims of his or her care and how it will affect, improve, disrupt, or maintain his or her quality of life. Quality of life has been described by Bowling (17) as a multilevel concept reflecting a wide range of influences and concerns about individuals' experiences, circumstances, health, social well-being, values, perceptions, and psychology. Patient priorities will vary but may include alleviating suffering and distressing symptoms, maintaining independence and control, and for some, prolonging life.

Key to addressing the multidimensional needs of patients with MBC is to deliver patient-focused care adopting a multiprofessional approach (11). A multiprofessional approach is now well established in early-stage breast cancer. In MBC when the sole focus of the oncologist and the patient is on the evaluation of the disease and its response to treatment this approach can leave many aspects of patient care unaddressed (18). The National Cancer Survivorship Initiative (10) has identified the need to develop new models of care for patients with advanced disease, which will include the involvement of a multidisciplinary team. Clinical teams are responsible for all medical decisions and concurrent with anti-cancer treatment, nurse-led interventions addressing psychosocial issues, continuity of care, and care coordination can often achieve other needs being facilitated with beneficial outcomes (19).

Individualised assessment of needs and expectations is recommended as few characteristics of the patient predict his or her need for information and support (20).

It has been documented that patients do not always independently report their symptoms and concerns, and the responsibility of assessing the holistic needs rest with the health-care professional (21). Assessment at key points along the patient pathway is recommended, for example at the time of diagnosis, at each subsequent recurrence, and the terminal phase (8). However for patients with MBC, assessment should be an ongoing process. Like the disease, the needs of patients with MBC can be very variable and not necessarily related to the stage of disease, prognosis, or symptoms.

This chapter explores the main domains of specialist supportive care for patients and their families affected by MBC.

INFORMATION GIVING

For many patients the diagnosis of MBC is reported as more devastating than a primary diagnosis and gives rise to higher levels of psychological morbidity (13,14,22) Cella et al. (23) found that 78% (31/40) of patients reported that the recurrence was more upsetting than the initial diagnosis since they felt the threat of death to be stronger. In a prospective study carried out by Hall et al. (24) of 269 women diagnosed with early breast cancer, 61 developed a metastatic recurrence of their disease within the 3-year study period. Thirty-eight of these women were interviewed following recurrence and reported experiencing more distress than when initially diagnosed with their primary breast tumour (24). Similarly, in Davies and Sques' (25) study that comprised semi-structured interviews, 10 participants stated feeling more shocked and distressed when confronted with their disease recurrence since it had greater ramifications than their initial diagnosis.

The impact of recurrence upon hope compared with the time of the first primary diagnosis was vastly greater, with 98% of patients stating that they felt less hope after recurrence than they did after initial diagnosis (23). In Mahon and Casperson's (26) study, the meaning of their cancer recurrence was explored and patients spoke of their realisation that their disease would not go away. The realisation that it may considerably shorten their life expectancy also resulted in a loss of hope.

What is clear is that the effects of a diagnosis of MBC differ significantly from those after an initial diagnosis of primary breast cancer. The disease is no longer curable and how that news is communicated to the patient and family is paramount as it can affect their comprehension, adjustment, level of hopelessness, and satisfaction with care (27–29).

Communicating and imparting a diagnosis of MBC is a challenging area of practice. The most important aspect of breaking news is the way in which it is given, thus relying on the use of effective communication techniques of the person delivering the bad news (29).

The sensitivity of the clinician and how the information is conveyed in an honest, open, clear way, while maintaining hope were considered by patients and their families in studies by Wong et al. (30) and Kirk et al. (20) as most important at disclosure of the initial diagnosis. While patients recognise the incurable nature of their disease it was crucial that those clinicians and their teams were perceived to sustain hope and were not seen to be giving up (21,31) Patients often assumed that treatment was no longer a viable option, but hope was restored when told about treatment options aimed at controlling disease spread, optimising quality of life, and prolonging survival (25,31,32).

A continued interest, and demonstration of caring behaviours such as showing warmth, being present, taking the time to talk and answer questions and ensuring that everything would be done for the patient's well being by the specialist team raised and maintained hope for the patient (33).

At the time of a primary diagnosis it is standard practice to have a clinical nurse specialist (CNS)/breast care nurse (BCN) in attendance to offer support (6). Despite this a third (47/135) of BCNs in Reed et al.'s (34) study which surveyed the provision of breast care nursing for patients with MBC, stated it was not standard practice for a BCN to be present when patients had been given their diagnosis of MBC.

It is at this time when MBC patients are in most need of direction and support. It is vital a specialist nurse or an appointed key worker who has expert knowledge and skills in managing MBC is present to meet the patients' information needs, while helping to maintain emotional equilibrium (2,6,11).

More patients are living longer with MBC and subsequently require more comprehensive information to understand their illness, the increasing number of treatment options, and how to self-care/manage living with an incurable disease.

Assessment to ascertain what the individual patient's needs and preferences are is central to meeting the information needs and supporting patients with decision making (11). While some patients will want the maximal amount of information, other patients will want limited or staggered information. Patient factors such as cultural, educational, and social aspects also need to be considered as this can influence how patients seek and receive information and will guide healthcare professionals as to how best to communicate and provide individualised information (35).

Decisions about treatment can frequently be difficult as there may be several choices such as combined treatment approaches and clinical trials. This can be overwhelming, therefore, it is imperative that patients are given the time to understand their disease, thus empowering them to take control and participate together with their health-care professionals in making decisions about their management plan.

Evidence suggests that by fulfilling informational needs health-care professionals can improve psychological coping and quality of life for patients who are living with MBC and their families who are taking care of the patients (30,35,36).

PHYSICAL

An individual woman's perception of quality of life and the experience of physical symptoms appeared as a central theme in many studies assessing physical functioning and quality of life in women with MBC.

Women reported significantly more physical symptoms at the time of recurrence than they had at initial diagnosis (37). This was consistent with a study by Kenne-Sarenmalm et al. (38) where 56 consecutive women with MBC completed questionnaires measuring symptom occurrence, coping capacity, and coping effects. In their study women reported a wide variety of symptoms such as a lack of energy, difficulty sleeping, pain, sweats, problems with sexual interest, nausea, dizziness, cough, and lack of appetite; 65% of the women reported experiencing multiple concurrent symptoms.

These findings were consistent with other studies in which women with advanced breast cancer reported high multiple levels of physical symptoms, most commonly fatigue, weakness, insomnia, and pain (13,39–42).

As physical symptoms increased, the perceived quality of life appeared to decrease. The experience of physical symptoms was frequently associated with the site of metastasis (32,38,43). The sites of metastasis that frequently caused women the most physical symptoms were bone (65%), lung (25%), liver (25%), skin (20%), nodes (20%), and brain (8%) (32,43,44). This was supported by Hanson-Frost et al. (45), in their study that examined the differences in the physical and social well-being of 235 women during the various breast cancer states; in newly diagnosed, adjuvant therapy for stable disease and recurrent disease it was found that the recurrent group reported a greater impact on their physical function than any other group. The increased difficulties with physical functioning in the recurrent group were related to the sites of metastasis such as bone and lung, which resulted in more physical symptoms and physical limitations (45).

Despite symptom burden being high in this group of patients, treatable symptoms such as fatigue and pain, are not always appropriately assessed or managed (13,38,40). Patients frequently do not independently report their symptoms and there may be several reasons for this, such as not knowing who to turn to or not wanting to complain.

Luoma and Hakamies-Blomqvist (39) in their study, interviewed 25 women being treated for advanced breast cancer who were given the freedom to discuss the important issues in their own way. The findings showed that having limitations in physical functioning was a distressing experience and it impacted on the women's ability to perform usual activities of daily living, such as driving, walking, housework, family and leisure activities, and self-care. The over-riding impact of the physical limitations was the women's dependence on others and feelings of helplessness (39). Similarly, in a study of 105 women with MBC who completed a questionnaire about quality of life and supportive care needs, Aranda et al. (13) found that 80% of the women reported difficulty with their physical functioning and daily living, not being able to do the things they used to. Consistent with these findings was

DeSanto-Madeya et al.'s (42) study detailing the daily activities of 84 women with advanced breast cancer. The findings of the study reported that although women were living full and active lives they did experience numerous symptoms and reductions with physical functioning including engagement with work and leisure activities.

Invariably, physical functioning changed with the onset of MBC and treatment. In Luoma and Hakamies-Blomqvist's (39) study, a number of women felt their physical functioning would have been good without treatment and they suffered because of the treatment, which made them feel sick and tired. However in the same study, many women felt that the treatment had positive effects and women with treatment response experienced improvement in their physical function and quality of life. This was reflected in Karamouzis et al.'s (46) study, where patients reported chemotherapy treatment not only reducing their symptom burden such as fatigue and pain, but increasing their overall quality of life in terms of role, sexual, and emotional functioning. The woman's expectations of what she will gain from her treatment is crucial as it may not only be how the disease responds to treatment that is important to the woman, but also the improvement in quality of life and symptom management that makes having the treatment worthwhile (32).

Physical symptoms and altered physical functioning are significant but it is only a portion of the burden borne by patients with MBC. Even patients devoid of physical symptoms still need to be assessed as it may be the emotional aspects such as living with uncertainty, loss of hope and control, and so on that are impacting on the quality of life and need support to cope and adjust (5).

PSYCHOLOGICAL

Psychological problems can often be more traumatic and challenging to some patients with cancer than the physical aspects of the disease, thus contributing to significant overall suffering and reductions in quality of life (47).

Recognition of psychological and psychiatric disorders in cancer patients is generally poor. However in a study by MacMillan (48), which explored the emotional impact of cancer of 1751 people with and affected by cancer, more than 4 in 10 (45%) people with cancer said that the emotional aspects of cancer were most difficult to deal with, as compared with the practical and physical effects of the disease.

Research evidence has shown that psychiatric morbidity in patients with MBC is high, as patients perceive their situation as more hopeless and uncontrollable, resulting in a higher rate of psychological problems such as anxiety and depression (22,38,39,41,44,49–51).

Patients most at risk of developing psychological problems in response to MBC are those with a history of psychological illness, lack of social support, isolation, pre-existing relationship problems, and low expectations of the treatment working (15).

Common psychological problems experienced by patients with MBC include living with uncertainty, anxiety, depression, and emotional functioning.

Uncertainty is an over-riding theme of MBC and has many facets. In several studies women spoke about consciously suppressing thoughts related to their uncertain future in order to control the overwhelming range of emotions that uncertainty elicited (13–15,45,50). Living with a range of varying emotions was considered a powerful aspect of uncertainty in a number of studies. In Aranda et al.'s (13) study of 105 consecutive women with MBC, the highest unmet needs were in the psychological and health domains with uncertainty about the future and learning to feel to be in control being ranked highly. Uncertainty for the future was commonly associated with lack of control and was reported by one-third of 66 patients in Turner et al.'s (41) study as being one of the hardest things to come to terms with in MBC. Some patients likened the uncertainty to living with a "ticking bomb" in Davies and Sque's (25) study. Another factor contributing to women's lack of control is treatment. Women spoke frequently about their lives revolving around treatment plans and waiting for test results, while treatment effectiveness, whether positive or negative, influenced women's uncertainty and their ability to control their lives (41,50).

Simply by being able to talk about their uncertainty with another person helped women feel better even if it did not change the outcome (50). Thus, support from spouses, family members, friends, and health-care professionals resulted in women feeling more confident and hopeful for the future.

Anxiety and depression are frequently experienced by women with MBC (22,41); this was consistent with other studies. When determining the prevalence and persistence of affective disorders such as anxiety and depression in 222 patients with MBC, it was found that patients experienced high levels of psychological morbidity and exhibited high emotional distress (50). In Grabasch et al. (51) a study of 227 women to determine the frequency of psychiatric morbidity and assess the quality of life showed that 42% of the women had depression or anxiety, or both.

There was a general consensus from many of the women in the studies that their physical functioning and emotional functioning were intertwined (38,39,44,52). Women spoke about having good emotional functioning when they were without physical symptoms such as pain, fatigue, or insomnia, and decreased emotional functioning when physical symptoms were not controlled (39). Fulton (44) studied the physical and psychological sequelae of a MBC diagnosis and its treatment in 80 women, which also found that there was a strong association between physical function and mood, women reporting that their physical symptoms had an effect on their mood state. This was consistent with Kenne-Sarenmalm et al.'s (38) findings, where most of the 56 women completing questionnaires looking at physical symptoms, anxiety, and depression reported that the three were more likely to occur in tandem.

Psychological morbidity in patients with MBC is significant and if undetected can substantially affect quality of life attributes, such as adjustment, levels of hope, and coping and can also impact on their ability to make important treatment decisions.

There are a variety of psychological interventions available to patients with MBC and these will depend on the nature and severity of the patient's psychological problem. Critical to ensuring patients have their psychological needs met are assessments at regular intervals and appropriate psychological support (8,9). A four-level model of professional psychological assessment has been recommended by NICE (8) (Table 1).

TABLE 1   NICE Model of Psychological Assessment and Support (8)

Level 1	Effective information giving, communication, and general psychological care	Given by all members of the multidisciplinary team
Level 2	Psychological interventions such as crisis management—at key points in the patient pathway	Given by all members of the multidisciplinary team, but usually a designated health-care professional such as a nurse specialist
Level 3	Specific psychological interventions—counselling and specialist psychological support	Given by counsellors and psychological therapists
Level 4	Specialist psychological and psychiatric interventions	Given by a range of psychological therapists such as clinical psychologists, psychiatrists, and others

The multidisciplinary team has a vital role to play in meeting the psychological needs of the patients. Often the person best placed to support the patient will be the CNS in MBC. As the key worker, the CNS in MBC provides continuity, therefore is likely to detect any new signs and symptoms that may be impacting on the patient's psychological functioning. For patients having a key contactable health-care professional whose constant presence in their care pathway is important, as they feel better supported and are more likely to share their concerns and worries (53). When patients have moderate to severe psychological problems it is paramount that they are referred to the appropriate mental health-care specialists.

SOCIAL
Managing at Home and in the Community
Health-care restructuring (7) and the availability of more oral treatments for the management of MBC have resulted in an increase in patients being treated in the ambulatory setting with home based health-care services. Key to this model being a success is by the adoption of good working relationships between the hospital-based teams and the primary care teams involved in the patient care, with both teams having an understanding of the main areas of need for the patients and informal carers (54).

As the role of the family caregiver expands in our health-care system, it will be important to understand the factors that determine who becomes a caregiver, and if some of those factors indicate that a family requires additional resources, a formal social support should be implemented when needed (55).

Breast cancer is more prevalent with advanced age and half the patient population is over 65 at the time of the diagnosis (6). Many older women who go on to develop MBC live alone and may lack adequate support structures, both in the size of their support network and the quality of that support (56). As with any vulnerable group, help should be enlisted from statutory and voluntary organisations to minimise the risk of marginalisation (57).

The needs and concerns of the families and carers actively involved in the care of a patient with MBC should be continually assessed and addressed, it is important to be inclusive of all non-traditional structures (56), with support continuing into bereavement care (57).

Work and Finance
Mcllfatrick (55) highlights that for some patients concern about finances can potentially be one of the most worrying problems when they are ill.

MBC, its symptoms, and side effects from treatment can restrict someone's ability to work, whether in paid, unpaid, or voluntary work, or working as a carer. Loss of income from paid employment, plus the potential increased costs as a direct result of the cancer, can affect day-to-day financial managing, paying bills, meeting the cost of transport, etc. and in the long term affect the financial planning for the future (2,21). It is always difficult to alleviate the stressful financial implications associated with MBC; however, it is essential to assess whether or not this is a potential problem (27) and then initiate appropriate referrals to access expert financial and employment advice (2).

Family and Close Relationships
Relationships may or may not change with family members and significant others with a recurrence of breast cancer. Existing relationships may be strengthened or new problems may emerge (27). Mahon (27) notes that a variety of illnesses like MBC that are characterised by relapses or exacerbations require flexibility on the part of families and close relations.

Lewis and Deal's (58) study examined married couple's experience with breast cancer recurrence from each partner's own perspective. Their findings showed that couples actively worked at balancing their lives trying to keep the breast cancer a background, and not a foreground, issue. Results showed that for those consciously seeking to keep the cancer in the background exhibited a higher incidence of depression, mood disturbance, and marital problems. This finding was consistent with that of other studies (52,59).

Recommendations for health-care professionals suggested some couples may benefit from additional strategies, including help with working through and expressing sad thoughts or feelings instead of avoiding them and recognising and supporting each other's views (58,60). Support may be needed with how the illness is impacting on sexual relations, and issues of intimacy need to be sensitively dealt with (57).

Children of parents with MBC will require support practically, emotionally, and with answering questions, which is best managed through preparation and forward planning (61). Specialist palliative care teams and services should be used if needed for advice and support (57), and appropriate charities and voluntary organisations can also be utilised to help support children and families.

Social and Recreational

Luoma and Hakamies-Blomqvist's (39) study showed women's social functioning altered when they were treated for MBC. In their study, women reported missing mutual relationships even though they retreated from social relationships with friends, colleagues, and neighbours. This was consistent with the findings in Leadbeater and Larder's (62) study, which showed women's existing social networks dwindled as women backed away from others. Social isolation is used frequently by women as a way of controlling their illness experience and maintaining autonomy. What adds to the isolation is lack of understanding of what the diagnosis means. Because MBC can be variable during the disease trajectory with its different phases of active and stable disease, patients do not fit the true sick role or the true dying role (62,63).

Conversely, some of the literature suggest that the availability or an increase in social support during times of stress may ward off or lessen mood disturbances. This has been described as a "buffering hypothesis", surrounding oneself with close family and friends (64).

Keeping busy either through work or other activities can help distract the patient from thinking about what might happen in the future (51). However, the impact of the disease and its treatments can restrict or prohibit not only physical but also passive recreational activities. Support with trying to identify alternative interests may be needed.

Spiritual Well Being

The needs of patients for spiritual support are frequently not recognised by health-care professionals (8). This may be for varying reasons including the many definitions about what spirituality is, how it means different things to different people, and how in the past spirituality has been closely associated with religion (57,65). Buckley (57) states that it is generally agreed spirituality is much broader than religion and how we do more in our everyday caring approach of importance to an individual's spirituality than what we realise.

Watson et al. (66) identify some of the skills needed to provide spiritual care which are shown in Box 1.

BOX 1   Identified Skills Needed to Provide Spiritual Care (66)

- Giving good support and offering practical care
- Excellent communication skills
- Empathetic and active listening
- Detachment from our own orthodoxies
- Helping patients deal with past, present, and future issues
- Ability to foster hope and provide strategies to support or restore hope in some way
- A broad perspective

With a diagnosis of MBC spiritual issues such as "making sense of it all, fostering hope, conserving one's dignity, feeling connected to one's self, one's family, one's God" (67), all become more important as the individuals contemplate their own mortality. Telling someone that his or her illness can no longer be cured has the ability to impinge on all aspects of his or her life: personhood, physical, emotional, intellectual, social, and spiritual (57). This may include feelings of pain, hopelessness, grief, loss of control, and loss of identity.

The provision of spiritual care is the response to the specific and unique spiritual needs expressed by the patient (65).

Spiritual care can be provided by all disciplines, for example clinicians, nurses, and occupational therapists (8) and there may be times when the expertise of people with more advanced skills is necessary to help with spiritual pain, for example mental health practitioners, chaplains, and those with advanced communication training skills (57). NICE (8) recommends that patients, carers, and staff should all have access to spiritual caregivers to act as a resource with staff being aware of the availability of local community spiritual support services.

CHANGES IN PRACTICE/MODEL OF CARE

In recent years, practice has changed as a result of natural evolution and identified initiatives (68) (Box 2).

Mackie and Doyle (68) describe an example of effective multiprofessional approach working at the MBC clinic at The Royal Marsden NHS Foundation Trust.

Communication strategies for patients with MBC at the Royal Marsden Hospital are aimed at meeting supportive care needs, based on the individual and not the stage of the disease. These strategies have developed since the establishment of a highly specialised, multiprofessional service which is provided in designated clinics for patients with MBC and led by a consultant medical oncologist who specialises in the treatment of MBC.

Before each clinic session, a multiprofessional meeting is held to help streamline the service provided, to identify and prioritise each patient's clinical and supportive care needs and to ensure these will be met. The range of health-care professionals who attend the clinic is shown in Box 3 along with the list of other professionals that the team has access to for further advice and information as shown in Box 4.

A recent addition to the multiprofessional MBC team in some hospital trusts in the United Kingdom has been the clinical nurse specialist (CNS) in MBC. The role of CNS in MBC has evolved as this patient group has become a distinct entity (11). While medical staff make decisions, advice, and offer treatments to people it was recognised that the patients' emotional and psychological needs were often overlooked and how having a specialist nurse to provide that information, advice, and support to patients was important (11).

BOX 2   Factors Contributing to Changes in Practice

- Move to patient-centred, rather than disease centred, clinical practice (11)
- Multiprofessional team approach (6,8,10,11)
- Appointment of key workers such as clinical nurse specialists in MBC (2,11)
- Availability of courses in advanced communication skills
- Increased patient awareness
- Improved communication links between services
- Establishment of the U.K. Secondary Breast Cancer Task Force (2)
- NICE guidelines for advanced breast cancer (11)
- NCSI—recognition of advanced disease as potential long-term illness (10)

BOX 3   Health-Care Professionals Who Attend Routinely (68)

- Medical oncologists with an interest in metastatic breast cancer (MBC)
- Clinical oncologists
- Clinical nurse specialist—MBC
- Specialist palliative care team
- Specialist breast pharmacist
- Clinic nurses—oncology trained
- Research nurses

BOX 4   Other Professionals and Services Available (68)

- Medical specialists e.g., Orthopaedic, Cardiac, Chest, Neurology
- Appliance officers
- Chaplains
- Complementary therapies
- Complex discharge coordinators
- Dieticians
- Lymphoedema team
- Menopausal clinic
- Occupational therapists
- Physiotherapists
- Psychological care
- Clinical psychologist—family support
- Psycho-sexual practitioner
- Support groups—outside agencies including charities
- Tissue viability nurse
- Welfare benefits advisors

CONCLUSION

The common goal identified by policy makers, clinicians, nurses, and all other health-care professionals involved in the care of patients with MBC is to optimise the patient's quality of life with appropriate treatment and specialist supportive care (8,11,13,37,51,56,69). It is well recognised how variable the disease, its pathway, and current treatment options are (4). The supportive care needs, including the meaning of quality of life, are also very individual and variable within this patient group.

The aim of a health-care professional, be an oncologist or a CNS, is to establish an understanding of the individual patient's perceptions and expectations of how he or she wants his or her care managed now the disease is no longer curable. Individual patient's choice about treatment, information, and support available, and even treatment cessation must be valued and respected.

The domains of supportive care that have been discussed in this chapter may or may not be relevant to each individual patient but in order to deliver quality care, each of the separate domains needs to be assessed to establish the supportive care input required to achieve an optimal quality of life for patients and their families.

REFERENCES

1. Mayer M, Grober SE. Silent Voices. Woman with advanced (metastatic) breast cancer share their needs and preferences for information, support and practical services. [Available from: http://www.lbbc.org/data/news/LBBCsilentvoices.pdf(March2010)]
2. Breast Cancer Care. Improving the care of people with metastatic breast cancer. Final report; 2008.
3. Remak E, Brazil L. Cost of managing women presenting with stage IV breast cancer in the United Kingdom. Br J Cancer 2004; 91: 77–83.
4. Johnston SR, Swanton C. Handbook of Metastatic Cancer. London: Informa Healthcare, 2006.
5. Warren M. Uncertainty, lack of control and emotional functioning in women with metastatic breast cancer: a review and secondary analysis of the literature using the critical appraisal technique. Eur J Cancer Care 2010; 19: 564–74.
6. National Institute for Health and Clinical Excellence. Improving outcomes in breast cancer: NICE, London, UK, 2002.
7. Department of Health. The NHS Cancer Plan. A plan for investment. A plan for reform. HMSO, London, 2000.
8. National Institute for Health and Clinical Excellence. Improving supportive and palliative care for adults with cancer: NICE, London, UK, 2004.
9. Department of Health Cancer Reform Strategy. HMSO, London, 2007.
10. Department of Health. National Cancer Survivorship Initiative Vision. HMSO, London, 2010.
11. National Institute for Health and Clinical Excellence. Advanced breast cancer. Diagnosis and treatment: NICE, London, UK, 2009.
12. Ream E, Quennell A, Fincham L, et al. Supportive care needs of men living with prostate cancer in England: A national survey Br J Cancer 2008; 98: 1903–9.
13. Aranda S, Schofiled P, Weih L, et al. Mapping the quality of life and unmet needs of urban women with metastatic breast cancer. Eur J Cancer Care 2005; 14: 211–22.
14. Vilhauer RP. A qualitative study of the experiences of women with metastatic breast cancer. Palliat Support Care 2008; 6: 249-258
15. Svensson H, Brandberg Y, Einbergi Z, et al. Psychological reactions to progression of metastatic breast cancer-an interview study. Cancer Nurs 2009; 32: 55–63.
16. Leary A. Quality of life in advanced cancer. In: Leary A, ed. Lung Cancer a Multidisciplinary Approach. Oxford: Wiley-Blackwell, 2010; In press.
17. Bowling A. Current state of art in quality of life measurement. In: Carr A, Higginson I, Robinson PG, eds. Quality of Life. London: BMJ, 2003: 1–18.
18. Miles D. The management of metastatic breast cancer. Breast Cancer Forum. [Available from: www.breastcancer.org.uk] 2010; 45: 1–6.
19. Bakitas M, Lyons K, Hegel M, et al. Effects of a palliative care intervention on clinical outcomes in patients with advanced cancer. JAMA 2009; 302: 741–9.
20. Kirk P, Kirk I, Kristjnason L. What do patients receiving palliative care for cancer and their families want to be told? A Canadian and Australian qualitative study. BMJ 2004; doi:10.1136/38103.423576.55
21. Richardson A, Tebbit P, Brown V, et al.; On behalf of the Cancer Action Team. Assessment of Supportive and Palliative Care Needs for Adults with Cancer. London: King's College London, 2006.
22. Kissane DW, Grabsch B, Love A, et al. Psychiatric disorder in women with early-stage and advanced breast cancer: a comparative analysis Aust NZ J Psychiatry 2004; 38: 320–6.

23. Cella D, Mahon S, Donovan M. Cancer recurrence as a traumatic event Behav Med 1990; 16: 15–22.
24. Hall A, Fallowfield L, A'Hern R. When breast cancer recurs: A 3 year prospective study of psychological morbidity. Breast J 1996; 2: 197–203.
25. Davies M, Sque M. Living on the outside in: A theory of living with advanced breast caner. Int J Palliative Nurs 2002; 18: 583–90.
26. Mahon S, Casperson D. Exploring the psychological meaning of recurrent cancer: A descriptive study. Cancer Nurs 1997; 20: 178–86.
27. Mahon S. Managing the psychosocial consequences of cancer recurrence: implications for nurses. Oncol Nurs Forum 1991; 18: 577–83.
28. Fallowfield L, Lipkin M, Hall A. Teaching senior oncologists communication skills: results from phase 1 of a comprehensive longitudinal program in the UK J Clin Oncol 1998; 16: 1961–8.
29. Baile W, Buckman R, Lenzi R, et al. SPIKES- A six-step protocol for delivering bad news: Application to the patient with cancer. Oncologist 2000; 5: 302–11.
30. Wong R, Franssen E, Szumacher E, et al. What do patients living with advanced cancer and their cares want to know? – A needs assessment. Support Care Cancer 2002; 10: 408–15.
31. Dixon R, Lee-Jones C, Humphris G. Psychological reactions to cancer recurrence. Int J Palliative Nurs 1996; 2: 19–21.
32. Burnet K. An overview of the management of recurrent breast cancer. Int J Palliative Nurs 2000; 6: 318–30.
33. Chi GC. The role of hope in patients with cancer. Oncol Nurs Forum 2007; 34: 415–24.
34. Reed E, Scanlon K, Fenlon D. A survey of provision of breast care nursing for patients with metastatic breast cancer: implications for the role. Eur J Cancer Care 2010; 19: 575–80.
35. Zarbock S. Meeting the information needs of patients with metastatic breast cancer. Home Care Provider 2001; 37–40.
36. Gray R, Greenberg M, Fitch M, et al. Information needs of women with metastatic breast cancer. Cancer Prev Control 1998; 2: 57–62.
37. Bull A, Meyerowitz B, Hart S, et al. Quality of life in women with recurrent cancer. Breast Cancer Res Treat 1999; 54: 47–57.
38. Kenne-Sarenmalm E, Ohlen J, Jonsson T, et al. Coping with recurrent breast cancer: predictors of distressing symptoms and health-related quality of life. J Pain Symptom Manage 2007; 34: 24–39.
39. Luoma M, Hakamies-Blomqvist L. The meaning of quality of life in patients being treated for advanced breast cancer: a qualitative study. Psycho-oncology 2004; 13: 729–36.
40. Thornton A, Madlensky L, Flatt S, et al. The impact of a second breast cancer diagnosis on health related quality of life. Breast Cancer Res Treat 2005; 92: 25–33.
41. Turner J, Kelly B, Swanson C, et al. Psychosocial impact of newly diagnosed advanced breast cancer. Psycho-oncology 2005; 14: 396–407.
42. DeSanto-Madeya S, Bauer-Wu S, Gross A. Activities of daily living in women with advanced breast cancer. Oncol Nurs Forum 2007; 34: 841–6.
43. McEvoy M, McCorkle R. Quality of life issues in patients with disseminated breast cancer. Cancer 1990; 66: 1416–21.
44. Fulton C. Patients with metastatic breast cancer: their physical and psychological rehabilitation needs. Int J Rehabil Res 1999; 22: 291–301.
45. Hanson-Frost M, Suman V, Rummans T, et al. Physical, psychological and social well-being of women with breast cancer: the influence of disease phase Psycho-oncology 2000; 9: 221–31.
46. Karamouzis MV, Ioannidis G, Rigatos G. Quality of life in metastatic breast cancer patients under chemotherapy or supportive care: a single-institution comparative study. Eur J Cancer Care 2007; 16: 433–8.
47. Fawzy FI, Fawzy NW, Armdt LA, et al. Critical review of psychosocial interventions in care. Arch Gen Psychiatry 1995; 52: 100–13.
48. MacMillan Report: Worried Sick: The Emotional Impact of Cancer Opinion Leader Research, 2006
49. Hopwood P, Howell A, Maguire P. Psychiatric morbidity in patients with advanced cancer of the breast: prevalence measured by two self-rating questionnaires. Br J Cancer 1991; 64: 349–52.

50. Nelson J. Struggling to gain meaning: living with the uncertainty of breast cancer. Adv Nurs Sci 1996; 18: 59–76.
51. Grabasch B, Clarke D, Love A, et al. Psychological morbidity and quality of life in women with advanced breast cancer: a cross-sectional survey. Palliat Support Care 2006; 4: 47–56.
52. Kershaw T, Northouse L, Kritprachia C, et al. Coping strategies and quality of life in women with advanced breast cancer and their family caregivers. Psychol Health 2004; 19: 139–55.
53. Fincham L, Copp G, Caldwell K, et al. Supportive care: experience of cancer patients. Eur J Oncol Nurs 2005; 9: 258–68.
54. Coristine M, Crooks D, Grunfeld E, et al. Caregiving for women with advanced breast cancer. Psycho-oncology 2003; 12: 709–19.
55. McIlfatrick S. Assessing palliative care needs: views of patients, informal carers and healthcare professionals. J Adv Nurs 2007; 57: 77–86.
56. Booth S. Palliative care consultations in advanced breast cancer. Oxford: Oxford University Press, 2006.
57. Buckley J. Palliative care an integrated approach. Oxford: Wiley-Blackwell, 2008.
58. Lewis F, Deal L. Balancing our lives: a study of the married couple's experience with breast cancer recurrence. Oncol Nurs Forum 1995; 22: 943–53.
59. Badr H, Carmack CL, Kashy DA, et al. Dyadic coping in metastatic breast cancer Health Psychol 2010; 29: 169–80.
60. Northhouse L, Dorris G, Charron-Moore C. Factors affecting couple's adjustment to recurrent cancer. Soc Sci Med 1995; 41: 69–76.
61. Rauch PK, Muriel AC, Cassem NH. Parents with cancer: Who's looking after the children. JCO 2003; 21: 117s–21s.
62. Leadbeater M, Larder M. Living with secondary breast cancer. Cancer Nurs Pract 2008; 7: 29–34.
63. Burnet K, Robinson L. Psychosocial impact of recurrent cancer. Eur J Oncol Nurs 2000; 4: 29–38.
64. Koopman C, Hermanson K, Diamond S, et al. Social support, life stress, pain and emotional adjustment to advanced breast cancer. Psycho-oncology 1998; 7: 101–11.
65. Stirling I. The provision of spiritual care in a hospice. moving towards a multi-disciplinary perspective. Scott J Healthcare Chaplain 2007; 10: 21–7.
66. Watson M, Lucas C, Hoy A, et al. Oxford Handbook of Palliative Care Oxford. Oxford University Press, 2005.
67. Keubler K, Davis M, Moore C. Palliative practices : an interdisciplinary approach. Missouri: Elsevier Mosby St Louis, 2005.
68. Mackie D, Doyle N. The management of metastatic breast cancer. Breast Cancer Forum. [Available from: www.breastcancer.org.uk] 2010; 45: 1–6.
69. Carlson RW. Quality of life issues in the treatment of metastatic breast cancer. Oncology 1998; 12: 27–31.

Index